Phlebotomy Handbook
Third Edition

Diana Garza, EdD, MT(ASCP), CLS
Associate Professor and Coordinator
Department of Health Care Administration
College of Health Sciences
Texas Woman's University—Houston Center

Clinical Associate Professor Program in Medical Technology/Cytogenics
School of Allied Health Sciences
University of Texas Health Science Center

Adjunct Associate Professor
Division of Laboratory Medicine
University of Texas MD Anderson Cancer Center
Texas Medical Center
Houston, Texas

Kathleen Becan-McBride, EdD, MT(ASCP), CLS(NCA)
Professor, Department of Clinical Laboratory Sciences
Programs in Medical Technology and Clinical Cytogenics
School of Allied Health Sciences

Associate Professor
Department of Pathology and Laboratory Medicine
Medical School

UTHHSC Texas-Mexico Border Coordinator for Health Services Projects
UTHHSC Coordinator for Primary Health Care Education
The University of Texas Health Science Center (UTHHSC)
Texas Medical Center
Houston, Texas

APPLETON & LANGE
Norwalk, Connecticut

0-8385-7900-0

Copyright © 1993 by Appleton & Lange
Simon & Schuster Business and Professional Group
Copyright © 1989 by Appleton & Lange
Copyright © 1984 by Appleton-Century-Crofts

94 95 96 97 / 10 9 8 7 6 5 4 3

Prentice Hall International (UK) Limited, *London*
Prentice Hall of Australia Pty. Limited, *Sydney*
Prentice Hall Canada, Inc., *Toronto*
Prentice Hall Hispanoamericana, S.A., *Mexico*
Prentice Hall of India Private Limited, *New Delhi*
Prentice Hall of Japan, Inc., *Tokyo*
Simon & Schuster Asia Pte. Ltd., *Singapore*
Editora Prentice Hall do Brasil Ltda., *Rio de Janeiro*
Prentice Hall, *Englewood Cliffs, New Jersey*

Library of Congress Cataloging-in-Publication Data

Garza, Diana.
    Phlebotomy handbook / Diana Garza, Kathleen Becan-McBride. — 3rd
ed.
        p.   cm.
    Includes bibliographical references and index.
    ISBN 0-8385-7900-0
    1. Phlebotomy—Handbooks, manuals, etc. I. Title.
    [DNLM: 1. Blood Specimen Collection—handbooks. 2. Bloodletting—
handbooks.   QY 39 G245p]
    RB45.15.G37   1992
    616.07'561—dc20
    DNLC/DLC   92-49812
    for Library of Congress   CIP

Acquisitions Editor: Cheryl L. Mehalik
Production Editor: Elizabeth Ryan
Designer: Michael J. Kelly

PRINTED IN THE UNITED STATES OF AMERICA

To my husband Peter McLaughlin, daughters Lauren and Kaitlin, and my parents for their affection and constant support.

Diana Garza

*To my husband Mark, sons Patrick and Jonathan,
parents, sister, and parents-in-law
for their support and devotion.*

Kathleen Becan-McBride

Contents

Preface

We have put forth major time and effort in this third edition to encompass the constantly changing, dynamic area of blood collection. Since it is imperative to remain current in phlebotomy, the aim of this edition is to reflect the most up-to-date information on specimen collection. It features the latest safety blood collection equipment and techniques with many photographs of phlebotomy safety apparatus. The *Phlebotomy Handbook*, third edition, has been enhanced and revised with:

- The Recent OSHA requirements as related to specimen collection
- Two additional chapters on Total Quality Management (TQM) and quality assurance/quality control with their impact on phlebotomy
- Expanded sections on bedside glucose testing and problems to avoid
- Updates on legal aspects and professional liability as they directly relate to blood collection
- Increased communicative terms in several foreign languages (Spanish, French, German, Russian, and Japanese) to assist the blood collector in his or her responsibilities
- Latest updates on AIDS-related issues including needlesticks
- Expanded information on interpersonal communication skills, management techniques, and educational methodologies with specific emphasis on specimen collection
- Information on drug interference and factors that may interfere in blood test results

The third edition continues as a practical instruction manual, but also a comprehensive textbook, reference book, and review book. Key terms and chapter outlines are major new features to enhance the reader's time and efficiency as he or she pursues the presented information. The *Phlebotomy Handbook*, third edition, has the companion review book, *Phlebotomy Exam*

Review, to prepare the reader for national certification examinations and includes review for required continuing education.

The overall goal of the third edition is to link the health professional performing blood collection to the latest safety phlebotomy techniques, skills, and equipment for the improvement of laboratory testing and, ultimately, for the provision of superior patient care services.

Acknowledgments

We were indebted to many individuals for assistance in preparing the first and second editions of this textbook. We would like to express appreciation to Bill Fetter, David Payne, Barbara Nemitz, Debra Hines, Jim Hixton with Becton-Dickinson Vacutainer Systems, Bob McEwen with Ulster Scientific, Inc., Tuyet-Van Phung, Lydia Morris, Inga Danville, Peggy McCall, Helen Harrell, Ann Cork, Pam Chamallas from Beckman Instruments, Martin Valaske, and Gordon Briggs, the College of American Pathology, and Coulter Electronics.

In addition, we acknowledge the contributing authors of the first edition who provided a frame of reference for the second edition. These individuals are Karen Hlavaty, Carrie Ventura, Pam Bollinger, Dr. Annot Littlepage, and Amelia Carr. Special thanks are given to Dr. Doris Ross for her contributions to the first edition and continued support for the second edition.

For the third edition, we particularly wish to thank Dr. Jose Trujillo, Sandra Murdock, Judy Hays, Estella Woodard, Mimi Gugsden, and all the phlebotomists at University of Texas MD Anderson Cancer Center and Margaret Gordon at Hermann Hospital.

Appreciation is also due to Texas Woman's University, the University of Texas School of Allied Health Sciences, the University of Texas MD Anderson Cancer Center, and Hermann Hospital. In addition, appreciation is due to Martha Garza for her assistance in manuscript preparation of the third edition. We gratefully acknowledge the efforts of the translators: Mr. and Mrs. S. A. Garza, Ann Blume, Dr. Kenji Nishioka, Lee Vining, and Tatiana Morozov. We also wish to thank the photographer, Donald Kelley, and artist, Martha Burton. These individuals worked diligently under short time constraints.

We are indebted to our families for tolerating the many hours we spent writing the three editions of this textbook.

1 Phlebotomy and the Health Care Setting

CHAPTER OUTLINE

INTRODUCTION TO PHLEBOTOMY

The development of new diagnostic techniques, clinical laboratory technology, and automated instruments has greatly increased the volume of laboratory testing. As a result, a member of the clinical laboratory team, the *phlebotomist,* has emerged with a greater role in facilitating the specimen collection process.

The main function for this vital laboratory member is to obtain patients' blood specimens by venipuncture and microcollection techniques and to facilitate collection and transportation of other clinical laboratory specimens.

In the past, phlebotomists were trained on a one-to-one basis as part of on-the-job training. Due to the increase in laboratory assays and need for quality assurance in laboratory test results, however, many colleges, universities, and hospitals have implemented phlebotomy curricula to prepare individuals to assume the responsibilities and tasks of phlebotomists. Consequently, the field of phlebotomy has expanded, and the phlebotomist now is an integral member of the health care team.

THE HEALTH CARE TEAM IN HOSPITALS AND CLINICS

Clinical laboratories are located in various types of settings and institutions having different levels of care. The levels are usually referred to as primary, secondary, and tertiary care.

Primary care is care given to maintain and monitor normal health and to prevent diseases through immunizations. Examples of this level of care include treatment of minor injuries, diagnosis and treatment of minor disorders such as a "cold" or "sore throat," regular checkups for babies, immunizations, prenatal care in a normal pregnancy, and treatment of chronic illnesses and diseases such as diabetes mellitus.

A primary care physician is usually called a family practitioner or a general internist. A major task of the primary care physician is to refer patients to the correct specialist if the patient needs a higher level of care.

Secondary care is specialized care involving a physician who is an expert in one particular group of diseases, group of organ systems, or organ. For example, a specialist may exclusively diagnose and treat eye disorders and is referred to as an ophthalmologist.

Tertiary care is highly specialized and oriented toward unusual and complex problems. Sophisticated instrumentation such as CAT scanners are used in the treatment and diagnosis of patients in this setting.

Clinical laboratories with a high level of technologic and organizational complexity are frequently in secondary and tertiary care hospitals; and, consequently, that is where many phlebotomists work. Hospitals are classified in many different ways. For example, one type of classification referred to as "clinical" is based on the type of patients treated. Clinical hospitals include general types that serve patients with various illnesses, and special-care hospitals are those that treat only a few types of illnesses. Included in special-care classification are pediatrics, cancer, maternity, and psychiatric hospitals.

Another type of classification for hospitals pertains to the type of ownership or control (government or nongovernment). Within the governmental classification are federal hospitals such as the Veterans Administration hospitals, military hospitals, and the United States Public Health Service hospitals.

Other types of governmental hospitals include state, county, and city facilities. Governmental hospitals have a public tax base for support of health care facilities.

State hospitals usually provide long-term psychiatric and chronic care. Also, some state hospitals are affiliated with state medical universities and, thus, serve as a teaching facility that provides short-term general acute care.

Teaching hospitals usually provide highly specialized services (tertiary services) such as organ transplantations and cardiac bypasses.[1] These hospitals are generally committed to the threefold mission of education, research, and patient care. In addition, teaching hospitals provide a disproportionate number of charity patient services.

Nongovernmental hospitals differ in ownership and, thus, control. For example, the largest group of nongovernmental hospitals are referred to as community hospitals because they are owned by the community. The governing board has representatives from the community and relates the needs of the community to the hospital. Other types of nongovernmental hospitals include church hospitals and privately owned hospitals.

Hospital size is commonly designated by the number of inpatients and outpatients seen per day. Another measurement is the number of beds the hospital contains. This bed number may be recorded as adult beds, pediatric beds, or both.

Other examples of health care facilities and services in which phlebotomists may be employed include ambulatory care facilities, *Health Maintenance Organizations (HMOs),* multiphasic screening centers, community health centers, home health care services, and medical group practices.

Ambulatory care is personal health care provided to an individual who is not a bed patient in a health care institution. It includes all health services, other than community or public health services, provided to noninstitutionalized patients.

Most hospitals provide two levels of ambulatory care: emergency services and outpatient clinic care. Freestanding ambulatory care facilities providing emergency services and urgent care for noninstitutionalized patients now operate throughout the United States. Some, such as the emergicenter, have the same 24-hours, 7-days-a-week access that hospital emergency services provide. Urgicenters provide less comprehensive emergency services and are commonly open 12 hours a day, 7 days a week.

An HMO is a comprehensive group practice center financed by prepayment or regular monthly accounts. Facilities are usually integrated with the hospital, screening center, clinic, and physicians' offices located in one central area. Multiphasic screening centers have laboratory, radiologic, and electrocardiographic screening examinations for preventive medicine and early detection of disease. Community health centers (CHCs) offer services to the community and are supported to a great extent by federal money. Most of these centers are primary care centers that are located in low-income areas and treat and diagnose members of the community on an ambulatory basis.[2]

Home health care services are medical services that are provided in a patient's home under a physician's direction. These services are becoming more popular since it is less costly for a patient to be home rather than in a hospital when recovering from a disease, illness, or injury. Phlebotomists are now being employed by companies and hospitals having home health care services. The phlebotomist travels to homes throughout the community collecting blood from these patients and then transports the blood to the clinical laboratory for testing.

Medical group practices usually consist of physicians, nurses, and other health professionals offering medical care to individuals in need of diagnosis and treatment. The services may be general or specific, depending upon the practice group. The number of medical group and physician's office laboratories is increasing because (1) new developments in laboratory technology have produced complex laboratory analyzers that are now simple to operate and relatively inexpensive, (2) the laboratory results can be obtained while the patient is in the office, and (3) the amount of money generated by these laboratories is providing an additional incentive for physicians.

Phlebotomists are employed in all these health care facilities. Because each institution or facility has its own philosophy, rules, and regulations, the phlebotomist must become familiar with them in order to perform in the manner expected.

DEPARTMENTS WITHIN THE HEALTH CARE SETTING

The rapid scientific advances in diagnostic and treatment instrumentation within health care settings has led to numerous departments with which the phlebotomist must interact. The larger the health care setting and the more specialized the medical services, the greater the number of separate medical departments. Departments in health care facilities can be listed according to medical specialties, as shown in Table 1–1. More subspecialized medical departments are usually organized around organ and organ systems, as shown in Table 1–2. Also, they may be categorized according to therapy or services provided to the patient (i.e., occupational therapy, pharmacy, physical therapy). Within the hospital setting, the phlebotomist should become familiar with radiology, nuclear medicine, radiation therapy, occupational therapy, physical therapy, electrocardiography, encephalography, pharmacy, and of course, the clinical laboratory.

Radiology/Medical Imaging

The radiology department uses ionizing radiation for treating disease, fluoroscopic and radiographic x-ray instrumentation and imaging methods for diagnosing, and radioactive isotopes for both diagnosing and treating (Fig. 1–1). These procedures involve fluoroscopy, tomography, and radiographic analysis

TABLE 1-1. DEPARTMENTS FOUND IN MOST LARGE HEALTH CARE FACILITIES

Department	Brief Description
Internal medicine	General diagnosis and treatment of patients for problems of one or more internal organs
Pediatrics	General diagnosis and therapy for children
Surgery	Diagnosis and treatment in which the physician physically alters a part of the patient's body
Anesthesiology	Preparing the patient for specialized treatment and/or surgery
Pathology and laboratory medicine	Diagnosis, both before and after treatment using anatomic and/or clinical laboratory test results
Obstetrics/gynecology	Diagnosis and treatment relating to the sexual reproductive system of females, using both surgical and nonsurgical procedures
Psychiatry/neurology	Diagnosis and treatment for people of all ages with mental, emotional, and nervous system problems, using primarily nonsurgical procedures
Radiology/medical imaging	Diagnosis and treatment, primarily through the use of x-ray, ultrasonography, and other internal imaging procedures
Allergy	Diagnosis and treatment of persons who have allergies or "reactions" to irritating agents
Geriatrics	Diagnosis and treatment of the elderly population
Oncology	Diagnosis and treatment of malignant (life-threatening) tumors
Proctology	Diagnosis and treatment of diseases of the anus and rectum
Rheumatology	Diagnosis and treatment of joint and tissue diseases, including arthritis
Family medicine/general practice	Cares for the medical problems of all members of a family, so it is not necessary to have a different physician for each family member by age-level or sex
Neonatal perinatal	Study, support, and treatment of newborn and prematurely born babies and their mothers
Physical medicine	Diagnosis and treatment of disorders and disabilities of the neuromuscular system
Plastic surgery	Concerned with correction of the loss or deformity of tissues, including skin

of the chest, abdomen, heart, bones, and other parts of the body using manual, automated, stationary, or mobile equipment.

Almost every patient admitted to a hospital (inpatient or outpatient) or to another health care facility becomes a patient in the department of radiology at some time during his or her stay. In radiology, patients and employees must be protected against unnecessary irradiation from radiologic instrumentation. On occasion, the phlebotomist may have to go to the radiology department in order to collect laboratory specimens from the patient. Thus, the phlebotomist should become acquainted with the location and safety requirements of this department.

Radiology studies sometimes require that the patient be injected with dye. If the phlebotomist finds that the patient has received radiology dyes prior to

TABLE 1–2. MEDICAL DEPARTMENTS LISTED BY ORGAN AND ORGAN SYSTEMS

Department	Organ and Organ Systems Diagnosed and Treated
Orthopedics	Bones and joints
Ophthalmology	Eye
Otolaryngology	Ear, nose, and throat
Urology	Male sexual and reproductive system and renal system for both females and males
Cardiology	Heart
Dermatology	Skin
Neurology	Nervous system
Hematology	Blood system
Immunology	Immune system
Gastroenterology	Esophagus, stomach, and intestines
Nephrology	Kidney
Endocrinology	Organs and tissues that produce hormones (e.g., estrogens, testosterone, cortisol)
Cardiovascular	Heart and blood circulation
Pulmonary	Lungs

blood collection, he or she should communicate the patient's name and possible dye interference to the clinical laboratory supervisor in charge of specimen control. The supervisor then can communicate with the laboratory director, clinical pathologist, and attending physician to determine if the dye will interfere in the requested laboratory assays.

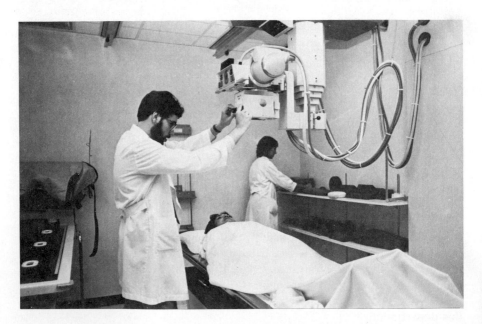

Figure 1–1. X-ray equipment.

Nuclear Medicine

The nuclear medicine department uses radioactive materials in the diagnosis and treatment of patients and in the study of the disease process. This department is used primarily in diagnosis, and in procedures requiring introduction of a radiotracer into the patient, usually by intravenous injection. The resulting emitted rays are detected by sensitive crystals on the complex instrumentation, which provide sequential imaging and graphic representation of radioactivity. The nuclear medicine procedures differ from radiology predominantly in that the latter use rays transmitted through the patient whereas the former use radiation emitted from the patient, resulting in images that provide more anatomic than functional information. As in radiology, phlebotomists should acquaint themselves with the location and safety requirements of the nuclear medicine department.

The radioisotopes, which are introduced into a patient for nuclear medicine studies, may interfere in laboratory assays. Thus, the phlebotomist who finds that the patient from whom he or she must collect blood is not in the hospital room but rather in the nuclear medicine department should ask employees in nuclear medicine if the patient has already had a radioisotopic injection. If so, the phlebotomist should report this information to the specimen control supervisor, who will then follow up to determine if the injection will interfere with laboratory assays.

Radiation Therapy

The department of radiation therapy applies high-energy x-rays, cobalt, elution, and other types of radiation in the treatment of disease—especially cancer (Fig. 1–2). The instrumentation used in radiation therapy presents a problem of irradiation greater than that of the radiology department. Thus, safety precautions against unnecessary irradiation are extremely important for patients and employees.

Occupational Therapy

The department of occupational therapy helps the patient to become as independently active as feasible within the limitations of his or her mental or physical problem. The occupational therapist collaborates with other health professionals (i.e., social workers, nursing staff, attending physician, physical therapist) to plan a therapeutic program of rehabilitating activities for the patient.

Since the patient may spend a considerable amount of time in the occupational therapy department, phlebotomists should become aware of this department's location if they must collect blood from patients who have been taken to this department to undergo therapy.

Physical Therapy

The role of the physical therapy department is to eliminate the patient's disability or to restore as completely as possible his or her mental or physical

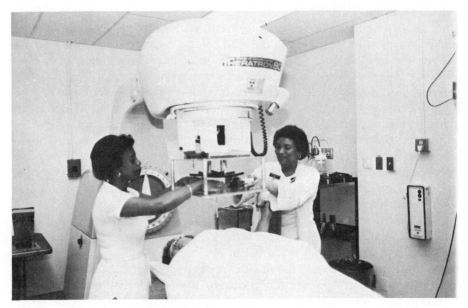

Figure 1–2. Radiation therapy equipment.

abilities that have been impaired by illness or injury (Fig. 1–3). Rehabilitation within this department requires the use of heat, cold, water exercise, ultrasound or electricity, and other physical techniques to restore useful activity. Because the rehabilitative service to the patient is usually quite extensive and time consuming, the phlebotomist may, on occasion, need to collect specimens in the physical therapy department.

Encephalography and Electrocardiography

Another department that the phlebotomist should become aware of is the encephalography department. The electroencephalograph (EEG) is an instrument that records brain waves. It is a sensitive instrument, and therefore the patient must be taken to a special shielded area that is protected against outside electrical or static interference.

The department of electrocardiography is used as a diagnostic service for the patient. The electrocardiograph (ECG or EKG) records the electric current produced by the contractions of the heart muscle and is used to assist in the diagnosis of heart disease or indicate progress in recovery from heart disease.

Pharmacy

Almost everyone knows that the pharmacist dispenses medications ordered by a physician. In addition, however, the pharmacist is involved with members of the health care team as a primary consultant on drug therapy. On many occasions, the pharmacist must communicate with clinical laboratory personnel

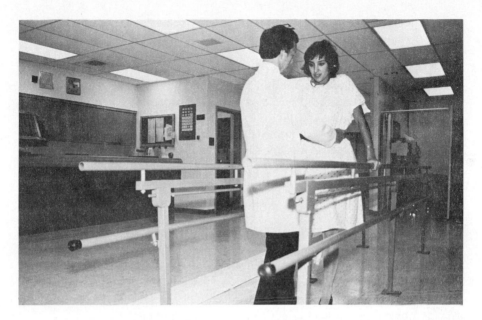

Figure 1–3. Physical therapist and patient.

concerning a patient's blood level of a certain drug when the patient is on drug therapy. In order to monitor therapeutic drug levels, the blood specimens must be drawn at certain time intervals. The phlebotomist may have the responsibility to collect the blood specimens for therapeutic drug monitoring and may need to communicate with the pharmacy department regarding time intervals of the blood collections.

Support Services
In addition to the forementioned departments, most hospitals and many other types of health care facilities have *support service departments*. These support services include the following: dietary, housekeeping, physical plant, grounds, security, medical records, purchasing, personnel, and laundry. These service departments are indirectly involved with patient care, and, thus, the phlebotomist will usually not be involved directly with activities of these departments. However, as a health care provider in the health care environment, the phlebotomist should be knowledgeable of departments in his or her work setting.

Quality Management Department
Health care institutions must have some means to identify if quality health care is being provided to the patients. The *Quality Management Department* in a health care facility usually has a quality assurance model composed of the following four basic components: (1) Quality Assurance, (2) Risk Management, (3) Utilization Management, and (4) Infection Control.[3] The fundamen-

tal goal of Quality Assurance is to identify and take advantage of opportunities for improvement in care. Risk Management's primary goal is to protect the financial assets of the health care organization and to prevent unforeseen events. The Utilization Management area is concerned with appropriate use of the health care facility's resources. Last, Infection Control is an area focusing on prevention, identification, and resolution of problems related to infections occurring in the health care environment.

Laboratorians and phlebotomists are directly affected by these four components. Thus, the phlebotomist needs to become knowledgeable of the Quality Management Department and its overall responsibilities and tasks. These areas will be discussed in greater depth in other chapters of the book.

DEPARTMENT OF CLINICAL LABORATORY MEDICINE

The rapid advances in clinical laboratory automation and procedures are reflected in the fact that the clinical laboratory has grown faster in past years than has hospital growth in general. Sophisticated technology and automation have provided new dimensions in the diagnosis and treatment of disease.

The clinical laboratory department is composed of two major areas. In the clinical pathology area, blood and other types of body fluids and tissues [such as urine, cerebrospinal fluid (CSF), biopsy specimens, and gastric secretions] are analyzed (Fig. 1–4). The area of anatomic pathology is involved in the performance of autopsies, cytology, and surgical pathology procedures. The clinical laboratory is primarily interested in patient services, but is also usually involved in research and development and teaching in order to ensure high quality of laboratory service.

Clinical Laboratory Personnel

Laboratory Directors. The laboratory personnel are frequently directed by a pathologist or clinical laboratory scientist with a doctorate degree, as shown in the organizational structure of Figure 1–5. The organizational structure of the clinical laboratory is constantly being revised as shown in Figure 1–6; with this structure the personnel are directed by a complementary relationship between the pathologist and administrative technologist.

The pathologist is a physician who usually has extensive education in pathology (the study and diagnosis of diseases through the use of laboratory test results). He or she directs the physician–patient services of the clinical laboratory and has the following responsibilities[4]: assists in the establishment of policies and test protocols; provides consultation services concerning laboratory results to medical–dental staff; teaches continuing education programs for laboratory personnel; and provides consultation and interpretation on surgical and autopsy tissues, cytological specimens, and bone marrows.

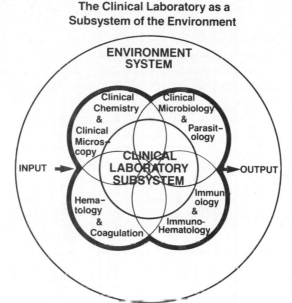

Figure 1–4. Clinical laboratory areas.

The administrative technologist is a medical technologist who has had additional education in management and administration. He or she is the director of administrative and technical services and has the following responsibilities[4]: sets up laboratory procedures and policies; employs laboratory personnel; performs budgetary functions of the laboratory; and provides for orientation and training of new personnel, continuing education of technical and supervisory staff, and assignment of duties to personnel commensurate with their qualifications.

Technical Supervisors of Clinical Laboratory Sections.   The technical supervisor in each of the clinical laboratory sections is a medical technologist with additional experience and education in his or her section, such as specimen control, hematology, microbiology, or clinical chemistry. He or she assumes the following responsibilities[4]: prepares daily work schedules to provide adequate coverage and effective use of personnel; maintains levels of supplies and reagents commensurate with workload; ensures that policies and procedures are followed by clinical laboratory personnel; provides technical instructions and training of personnel in his section; provides direct supervision of personnel in his section; maintains a current procedural manual; assists the administrative technologist in budget preparation; and recommends to the administrative technologist the selection, transfer, discipline, and discharge of personnel.

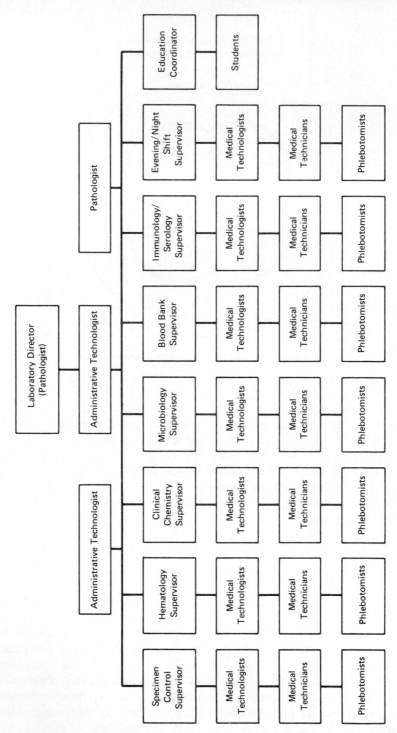

Figure 1–5. Organizational structure of a typical clinical laboratory.

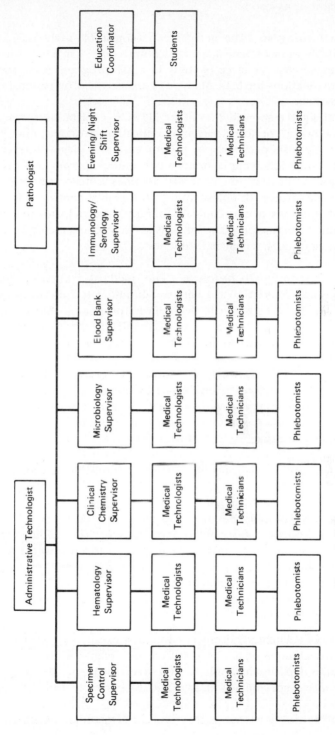

Figure 1–6. Organizational structure becoming increasingly common in clinical laboratories.

Medical Technologist.   The medical technologist (MT), who is also referred to as clinical laboratory scientist, has a bachelor's degree in a biologic science, which includes a year or more of study in a MT program. Some states have licensing examinations for MTs. Many MTs are certified by national certification examinations.

The duties and responsibilities of the MT (clinical laboratory scientist) include the following[5]: performs various chemical, microscopic, microbiologic, or immunologic tests pertaining to patient care and diagnosis, records and reports test results following laboratory procedures; participates in research and development of new test methods; assumes a major responsibility for preventive maintenance, troubleshooting, and quality control of instruments and safety conditions in the clinical laboratory; participates in continuing education and in-service programs; and assists in teaching medical technology and medical laboratory technician students.

Medical Laboratory Technician.   The medical laboratory technician (MLT), who is also referred to as a clinical laboratory technician, is a graduate of a 2-year certificate or associate degree MLT program. Some states require licensing for the MLT and have a licensing examination for this category. Many medical laboratory technicians are certified by MLT or CLT national certification examinations.

Under supervision by a MT or technical supervisor, the MLT performs routine tests and procedures in any assigned laboratory department. He or she records and reports results following laboratory procedures and reports abnormal results to the supervisor. Other duties and responsibilities include: prepares specimens for reference laboratories; prepares reagents as needed; draws blood as required; observes safety procedures and maintains laboratory area and equipment; and participates in continuing education and in-service programs.[5]

Phlebotomist.   The phlebotomist is usually required to be a high school graduate or equivalent to enter phlebotomy training. The training varies from one health care center to another and may take from a few weeks to months, depending on the institution. The phlebotomist may become certified by passing a national certification examination.

Under supervision of the specimen control technical supervisor, the phlebotomist has the following typical duties and responsibilities[6]:

1. Collects adequate and correct blood specimens by venipuncture or microtechnique on adults, children, and infants
2. Follows departmental policies to correctly identify the patient before any blood specimen is drawn and to correctly label all specimens drawn
3. At all times shows concern for and understanding of the patient and

promotes the comfort and well-being of the patient as much as possible while performing collecting duties. Patience and persistence are needed when dealing with patients from whom blood specimens are difficult to obtain

4. Starts glucose tolerance procedures and collects remaining specimens at required times; draws other timed specimens as indicated
5. Picks up and delivers to the laboratory a variety of clinical specimens other than blood
6. Sorts and processes specimens received in central specimen receipt area of department. Maintains orderly and timely flow of specimens to the technical areas
7. Maintains accurate and orderly log records and worksheets where required according to established departmental and hospital protocol
8. Projects an image of professionalism in appearance and conduct at all times

Clinical Laboratory Sections

Clinical Chemistry. The clinical chemistry section is one of the largest areas in the clinical laboratory. Here, the laboratory procedures that are run (Table 1–3) include the quantitative measurement of serum proteins, blood glucose, serum lipids (triglycerides, cholesterol), serum iron and iron binding levels, serum electrolytes (sodium, potassium, bicarbonate, and chloride), blood gases (PO_2, PCO_2, pH), serum creatinine, blood urea nitrogen (BUN), vitamins (i.e., ascorbic acid, vitamin B_{12}, folic acid), enzymes (i.e., lactate dehydrogenase, alanine aminotransferase, creatine phosphokinase). Also, the clinical chemistry section usually has a toxicology area for drug analysis and an area for the analysis of hormones. Other procedures generally included in clinical chemistry are bilirubin and liver function analysis and CSF and gastric fluid analysis.

The clinical chemistry section has become highly automated, and, thus, most of the chemical procedures use less patient's blood for each analysis than in the past. Automation has greatly increased the efficiency and quality assurance within the clinical chemistry section (Fig. 1–7).

Hematology. The hematology section is concerned with laboratory assays used to identify diseases of blood-forming tissues. In addition, other processes can be evaluated through changes in the blood. Coagulation, clinical microscopy, and urinalysis are frequently housed in the hematology section. Hematologic results are extremely valuable diagnostic tools and are an integral part of a patient's examination. Most health care facilities require that the hematologic assay referred to as the complete blood count (CBC) be run on every individual admitted as a patient to the health care facility. The five components of the CBC are:

1. Red blood cell count (RBC)
2. White blood cell count (WBC)
3. Hemoglobin (Hgb or Hb)
4. Hematocrit (Hct or Crit)
5. Differential white count (Diff)

Other assays evaluated in the hematology section include: reticulocyte count, erythrocyte sedimentation rate (ESR), and erythrocyte indices [mean corpuscular volume (MCV), mean corpuscular hemoglobin (MCH), and mean corpuscular hemoglobin concentration (MCHC)]. Many of these assays are automated and can simultaneously test a blood specimen for various hematologic parameters (Fig. 1–8). Also, these hematologic instruments can electronically compute results for these assays.

Coagulation tests, usually performed in the hematology section, are run to determine the clotting ability of the blood. The two most common coagulation assays are prothrombin time (PT) and partial thromboplastin time (PTT). Screening tests and confirmatory assays for classical hemophilia are performed in the coagulation area. Also, other procedures, such as platelet counts and fibrinogen assays, help to detect coagulation problems such as disseminated intravascular coagulation disease (DIC).

The clinical microscopy and urinalysis area uses microscopic and chemical procedures to screen urine specimens for abnormalities. Generally, each patient admitted to a health care facility must have a urinalysis performed on his or her random sample (see Chapter 3 for urine collection information). Assays performed on a urine specimen include the determination of pH, specific gravity, protein, sugar, ketones, bilirubin, nitrates, urobilinogen, ascorbic acid, and occult blood. Also, a microscopic examination may be performed to identify the presence or absence of crystals, casts, white blood cells, and red blood cells.

Clinical Microbiology.   The section of clinical microbiology has the principal tasks of culturing and identifying bacterial pathogens and their toxins. In addition, this section evaluates bacterial sensitivity to a particular antibiotic. Thus, when a microbiological specimen is collected, the physician usually requests a culture and sensitivity test (C and S). Sensitivity refers to the inhibition of bacterial growth by an antibiotic.

The bacterial pathogens are classified according to (1) how they appear after Gram staining; (2) shape of the microorganisms—rod-shaped (bacilli), circular-shaped (cocci), or spiral-shaped (spirochetes); and (3) the microorganism requirements for oxygen (aerobic) or lack of oxygen (anaerobic).

Major methods for analysis in this section include: (1) how these microorganisms grow in culture, (2) their biochemical properties, and (3) sensitivity of the microorganisms to antibiotics. In addition to analysis of bacterial pathogens, this section identifies pathogenic parasites, fungi, and viruses.

TABLE 1–3. A SUMMARY OF MAJOR TESTS PERFORMED IN THE CLINICAL LABORATORY SECTIONS

Clinical Chemistry Procedures

Total proteins
Serum protein electrophoresis
Glucose and glucose tolerance
Glycated hemoglobin
Triglycerides
Cholesterol
Iron
Total iron binding capacity (IBC or TIBC)
Electrolytes [sodium (Na^+), potassium (K^+), chloride (Cl^-), bicarbonate (HCO^{-3})]
Magnesium
Blood gases [pH, partial pressure of carbon dioxide (Pco_2), partial pressure of oxygen (Po_2)]
Creatinine
Uric acid
Blood urea nitrogen (BUN)
Enzymes (e.g., lactate dehydrogenase (LH), alanine aminotransferase (ALT), creatine phosphokinase (CK)]
Drug analysis (e.g., gentamicin, tobramycin, primidone, phenytoin, digoxin, quinidine, salicylates, blood alcohol, barbiturate)
Bilirubin
Hormones [e.g., thyroxine (T_4), insulin, testosterone, renin activity, luteinizing hormone, parathyroid hormone, prolactin, cortisol]

Clinical Microbiology Procedures

Acid-fast bacilli (AFB) smear	Fungus direct smear	Ova and parasites
Anaerobic culture	GC culture	Pinworm preparation
Culture and sensitivity	Gram stain	Stool culture
AFB culture	Occult blood	Strep screen
Fungus culture	Nose/throat culture	Urine culture
Blood culture		

Hematology and Coagulation Procedures

CSF cell count	Hemoglobin	RBC
Differential	Hemoprofile	Reticulocyte count
Eosinophil count	LE cell preparation	Sedimentation rate
Fecal leukocyte	Nasal eosinophil	Sickle cell preparation
Hematocrit	Platelet count	WBC
CBC	Partial thromboplastin time	Thrombin time
Fibrin split product	Prothrombin time	
Fibrinogen		

Clinical Microscopy and Urinalysis Procedures

	Routine UA		
Hemosiderin			Synovial fluid analysis
Pregnancy test			Seminal fluid analysis
	pH	Bilirubin	
	Specific gravity	Nitrates	
	Protein	Urobilinogen	
	Sugar	Ascorbic acid	
	Ketones	Occult blood	

(*continued*)

TABLE 1–3. (*Continued*)

Immunohematology Procedures (Transfusion Medicine)		
ABO and Rh_0 (D) Type	Antibody SCR indirect	Rh phenotype and
ABO group	Coombs' test	genotype
Antibody identification	Antibody titer	Rh_0 (D) type
Hepatitis B core antigen and antibody	Direct Coombs' test	
Hepatitis B surface antigen and antibody		
HIV-1 testing		

Clinical Immunology/Serology Procedures		
Amebiasis screen	Cold agglutinins	Rheumatoid factor
Antinuclear antibody (ANA)	CSF/VDRL	RPR
ASO screen	Syphilis antibody (FTA-ABS)	RPR quantitative
ASO titer	Infectious mononucleosis	Salmonella agglutinins
Brucella antibody	MHA-TP	Q Fever
C-reactive protein	Proteus OX antibodies	
Borrelia Burgdorferi (Lyme Disease) antibody	Rubella HIA	
Francisella tularensis antibody		
Legionnaires' disease antibody		

Abbreviations: GC, gonococcus; HIA, hemagglutination-inhibition antibody; LE, lupus erythematosus; MHA-TP, microhemagglutination–*Treponema pallidum*; UA, urinalysis.

The occult (hidden) blood test (Guaiac test) is frequently performed in the clinical microbiology section. This procedure tests for blood in feces (stool), urine, and other patient secretions.

The specimens for microbiologic analysis may be highly infectious and, thus, are considered biohazardous. Extreme caution and care must be taken in collecting and processing them.

Clinical Immunology–Serology. The serology section has the major tasks of running procedures to determine antigen–antibody reactions and identifying diseases having antigen–antibody pathogenesis. Common serologic tests run in the serology–clinical immunology section include: Venereal Disease Research Laboratory (VDRL), rapid plasma reagin (RPR), fluorescent treponemal antibody absorption (test) (FTA-ABS), cold agglutinins, febrile agglutinins, rubella, ASO titer, anti-DNase B, fungus antibody tests, and Monospot. As an example of diseases that are identified in this section, the VDRL and RPR tests are used to test for syphilis. Fluorescent treponemal antibody absorption test

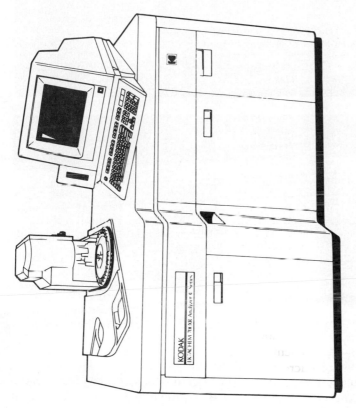

Figure 1–7. Kodak Ektachem 700XR Analyzer. (*Courtesy of Eastman Kodak Co., Rochester, N.Y.*)

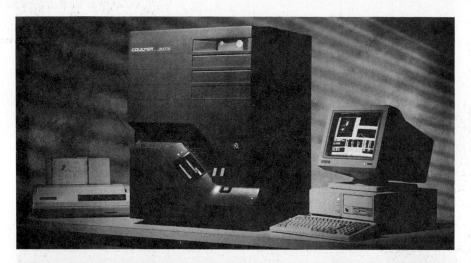

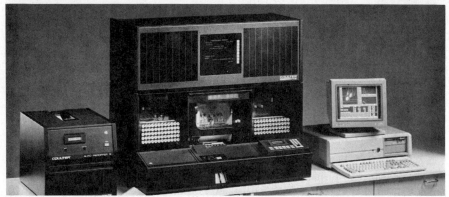

Figure 1–8. Coulter Counter Systems. (*Courtesy of Coulter Electronics, Inc., Hialeah, Fla.*)

(FTA-ABS) is a procedure used to confirm a syphilitic infection with the spiral-shaped bacteria. The cold agglutinins test is primarily for primary atypical pneumonia. Febrile agglutinins is a procedure used to test for typhoid fever, paratyphoid, brucellosis, and tularemia. The ASO titer is used to test for a streptococci infection and Monospot (Ortho Diagnostics) tests for infectious mononucleosis.

Blood Banking (Immunohematology)—Transfusion Medicine. The blood bank, sometimes referred to as immunohematology or transfusion medicine, has the major tasks of providing blood products to patients. These products, collected from volunteer donors and given to the patients (recipients), include whole blood, packed red blood cells, platelets, and fresh frozen plasma.

In order to give blood to patients, the donor and recipient must have their blood grouped and typed. In addition, other procedures run in the blood bank include: antibody screening test, Rh antibody titer test, direct antiglobulin (Coombs') test, and hepatitis B surface antigen (HB$_s$Ag).

Cytology.   The cytology section of the laboratory processes body fluids and other tissue specimens for detection and diagnostic interpretation of cell changes that might indicate cancer. Cytology is usually known as the section that screens "Pap" smears for early diagnosis of malignant diseases of the female genital tract.

Histology.   The preparation and processing of tissue samples removed during surgery, autopsy, or other medical procedures are the primary tasks of the histology section. Following preparation of the tissue, the anatomic pathologist microscopically examines and evaluates the patient's tissue sample.

Cytogenetics.   The section of cytogenetics is relatively new in the clinical laboratory. Within this section, cytogenetic techniques provide detailed study of individual chromosomes (Fig. 1–9) that detect relationships to clinical disease, both congenital and acquired. The cytogenetic tasks require competence in preparing specimens of peripheral blood, bone marrow, solid tissue, and amniotic fluid through cell cultures and chromosomal analysis. The phlebotomist, on occasion, may draw blood specimens for chromosomal analysis.

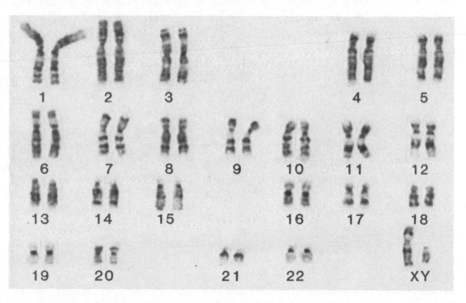

Figure 1–9. Photograph of karyotype. (*Courtesy of University of Texas M. D. Anderson Hospital, Division of Laboratory Medicine.*)

DNA Probe Analysis. The DNA probe analysis section is a fairly new section in the clinical laboratory. Dependent upon the type of health care facility, this section may test for genetic disorders, malignant disorders, infectious pathogens, or DNA fingerprinting in forensic medicine. The genetic disorders that have been diagnosed with DNA probes include sickle-cell anemia, Duchenne muscular dystrophy, and cystic fibrosis.[7] Some leukemias and lymphomas can be identified and classified with the use of DNA probes; human immunodeficiency virus (HIV) is an example of an infectious pathogen that can be detected with this analysis technique. Since the DNA probe technology is expected to grow rapidly in the next few years, it is very likely that the phlebotomist will be collecting many blood specimens for this section of the clinical laboratory.

Education and Research. The large clinical laboratory usually has ongoing research in the development of new procedures recently described in the medical literature, as well as basic research contributing to the clinical laboratory sciences. This work is performed by the pathologists, other doctorate staff, and the medical technologists.

In addition to research, the large clinical laboratory department generally provides or is affiliated with a university for teaching programs. The educational programs include (1) a pathology residency program to teach physicians the subspecialty of pathology; (2) a medical technology program to teach qualified college seniors or graduates the concepts, theories, and techniques in clinical laboratory sciences; (3) a medical laboratory technician program to train college freshmen and sophomores the basic techniques and concepts in clinical laboratory sciences; and (4) a phlebotomy program to train individuals on how to collect blood.

INTERDEPARTMENTAL RELATIONSHIPS

Clinical laboratory test results provide important data to the physician in diagnosing and monitoring patients and depend on smooth interrelationships with all other hospital departments. For example, a physician requests laboratory tests to be performed on a patient. The laboratory tests are performed on admission of the patient to the hospital. When the patient's specimens and the requisition slips specifying the clinical laboratory procedures to be performed arrive at the clinical laboratory, they are sent to the appropriate section(s) for analysis. The test results are recorded in the clinical laboratory and returned to the patient's medical chart to be reviewed by the attending physician. This information must be as timely as possible, and coordination between the clinical laboratory and nursing staff is important. The appropriate charges for the laboratory tests are directed to the patient's account at the business office.

Information resulting from the laboratory test requires that clinical laboratories coordinate activities with other hospital departments such as nursing, pharmacy, and dietary. Because the effects of diet and medication(s) on laboratory test results have been well-documented, coordination and cooperation between the laboratory, medical staff, nursing staff, dietary department, and the pharmacy are required to prevent false test results. This team of health care providers must be aware of the total patient care plan in relation to the clinical laboratory collection and test procedures so that laboratory test results can be efficiently used for the best possible patient care.

THE LABORATORY IN THE PHYSICIAN'S OFFICE

As described earlier, physician's office and medical group laboratories are increasing in numbers throughout the nation. Each group practice of physicians has unique office laboratory needs owing to their subspecialty. For example, a medical group of internists specializing in medical care of the diabetic patient needs laboratory tests for glucose monitoring, whereas obstetric group practices need laboratory assays related to pregnancy testing. In addition, since the laboratory services are provided only for the office patients, the office laboratories are usually small and have all the clinical laboratory areas (e.g., clinical chemistry, hematology, clinical microbiology) located in one room.

The phlebotomist working in a medical group or physician's office laboratory will quite frequently need to acquire multidisciplinary laboratory skills to assist in all phases and areas of laboratory testing.

KEY TERMS

ambulatory care	medical group	physical therapy
clinical laboratory	practices	primary care
medicine	medical laboratory	quality management
community health	technician	department
centers	medical specialties	radiation therapy
electrocardiography	medical technologist	radiology/medical
encephalography	multiphasic screening	imaging
Health Maintenance	centers	secondary care
Organizations	nuclear medicine	support service
(HMOs)	occupational therapy	departments
home health care	pharmacy	tertiary care
services	phlebotomist	

STUDY QUESTIONS

1. Which of the following hospital departments uses ionizing radiation for treating diseases and fluoroscopic and radiographic x-ray instrumentation for the diagnosis of diseases?

a. radiology   **c.** nuclear medicine
b. radiation therapy   **d.** occupational therapy

2. The electroencephalograph (EEG) is an instrument that records

   a. the electric current produced by the contraction of the heart muscle
   b. brain waves
   c. signals from the skeletal muscles

3. Which of the following clinical laboratory sections performs the VDRL?

   a. clinical chemistry   **c.** clinical immunology
   b. hematology   **d.** clinical microbiology

4. Blood glucose determinations are usually performed in which of the following laboratory sections?

   a. clinical chemistry   **c.** clinical immunology
   b. hematology   **d.** clinical microbiology

5. From the following personnel, which individual is sometimes referred to as clinical laboratory scientist?

   a. medical laboratory technician
   b. medical technologist
   c. phlebotomist

REFERENCES

1. Kovner A: *Health Care Delivery in the United States.* New York, Springer, 1990.
2. Himmelstein DU, Woolhander S: A national health program for the United States. *N Engl J Med* 320:102, 1989.
3. Graham NO (ed): *Quality Assurance in Hospitals: Strategies for Assessment and Implementation.* Rockville, MD, Aspen Pub, 1990.
4. Price G: American Society for Medical Technology's alternative proposal (ASMT's comments on the notice of proposed regulations on clinical laboratory personnel standards). *Am J Med Technol* 46:2, 1980.
5. Becan-McBride K: *Textbook of Clinical Laboratory Supervision.* New York, Appleton-Century-Crofts, 1982.
6. Hermann Hospital, Department of Pathology and Laboratory Medicine Personnel Policies. Houston, 1982.
7. Dawson B: DNA diagnostic uses grow. *Clin Chem News,* p 12, Sept 1989.

Basic Anatomy and Physiology of Body Systems

2

CHAPTER OUTLINE

ANATOMIC REGIONS

The design of the human body is very elaborate and sophisticated. Billions of cells make up each individual. Similar groups of cells are combined into tissues such as muscle or nerve tissue; and tissues are combined into systems such as the circulatory or reproductive systems. These organ systems work simultaneously to serve the needs of the body. No system works independently of the others.

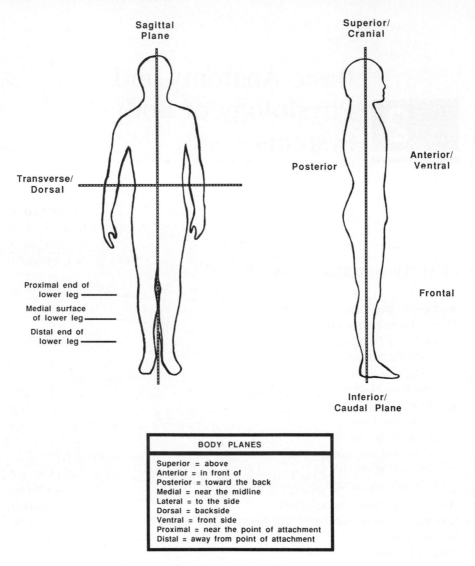

Figure 2–1. Body planes.

The human body has distinctive characteristics, that is, a backbone, bisymmetry, body cavities, and nine major organ systems: skeletal, muscular, nervous, respiratory, digestive, urinary, reproductive, endocrine, and circulatory. This chapter highlights each system and emphasizes the role of the circulatory system.

Body regions can be categorized in various ways. One way is to begin at the top and work down. In this manner the body can be described with the following regions[1]:

- Head and neck
- Upper torso
- Lower torso (female and male)
- Back
- Arms
- Legs
- Hands and feet

The body can also be described by surface regions and body cavities. The front, anterior, or ventral surface of the body is separated into thoracic, abdominal, and pelvic cavities. The back, posterior, or dorsal surface is divided into cranial and spinal cavities. Each of these cavities houses one or more organs. Areas of the body can be described by their distance from or proximity to one of the *body planes* (Fig. 2–1). The sagittal plane runs lengthwise from front to back, dividing the body into right and left halves. The frontal plane runs lengthwise from side to side, dividing the body into anterior and posterior sections. The transverse plane runs crosswise or horizontally, dividing the body into upper and lower sections. Normal anatomic position refers to an erect standing position with arms at rest and palms forward.[1,2]

MAJOR BODY FUNCTIONS

Before progressing to the major body systems and their functions, it is important to have a basic understanding of the human cell. Figures 2–2 and 2–3 illustrate a basic cell and its structures and some examples of specific cell morphologies.

Every body contains trillions of cells, and their size and shape depend on their function. Some cells fight disease-causing viruses and bacteria, some transport gases such as oxygen and carbon dioxide, some produce movement, store nutrients, or manufacture proteins, chemicals, or liquids, others such as the egg and sperm cells can create a new life. Yet other cells can contribute to thoughts and emotions. Even with such complexity, there are basic structural elements common to all.

The cell membrane encloses the contents of the cell. It serves as a protective barrier that selectively allows certain substances to move in or out. Nutrients and oxygen are taken in through the membrane only when needed, and wastes are eliminated as they build up.

Most cells have a *nucleus,* which is enclosed inside a nuclear membrane. The nucleus (or "nuclei" for 2 or more) is commonly thought of as the control mechanism of the cell that governs the functions of the individual cell (i.e., growth, repair, reproduction, and metabolism). Inside the nucleus is a *nucleolus* and threadlike chromatin. The nucleus contains a blueprint of itself in the genetic material so that it can reproduce itself when necessary. If the nucleus of a cell is damaged or destroyed, most cell types will usually die.

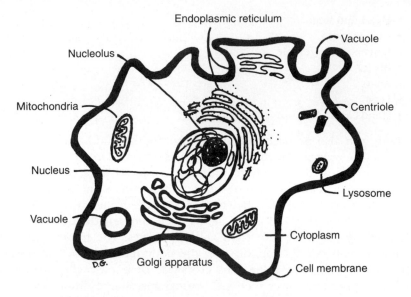

Figure 2–2. Basic cellular structure and components.

However, red blood cells lose their nuclei when they mature, but the cells continue to live and function to carry oxygen for several months.

The *cytoplasm* of the cell contains mostly water with dissolved nutrients and fills up the rest of the cell membrane. Within the cytoplasm are smaller structures called organelles. The names and functions are as follows:

Mitochondria. Energy production for the cell

Ribosomes. Assemble amino acids into proteins

Endoplasmic reticulum. Transport channels between the cell membrane and the nuclear membrane

Lysosomes. Release digestive enzymes into vacuoles or small pouches for digestion of food particles

Golgi apparatus. Storage of proteins

Cells communicate with each other in sophisticated reactions using electrical impulses (such as from one nerve cell to another) or chemical reactions that result in the release of hormones or other enzymes and proteins to stimulate a particular function.

The study of cellular structures and processes have captivated clinical laboratory scientists for years. With technologies such as flow cytometry, amplification of genetic material, and specific probing, there continue to be new and additional ways of seeking answers to cellular functions.

One of the most progressive areas of study is the study of *deoxyribonucleic acid,* or *DNA*. DNA is a long molecule commonly described as a "double helix" or "twisted ladder." The molecule contains thousands of *genes,* which carry the code for an individual's genetic makeup, such as color of eyes, gender, and height. The DNA of an individual contains the "DNA-coded blueprint," which was inherited from the parents. Genes also instruct the body to make the necessary proteins needed to sustain life. While each nucleus has a complete set of genes (except the egg and sperm, which contain half a set), only certain ones are used in each cell to do its own specific functions. DNA also functions to duplicate exact copies of itself. An individual's DNA directs the development, growth, and functioning of all body systems. It makes each individual's body different and unique, except in the case of identical twins.

Survival is the primary function of the human body and many complex processes work independently and together to achieve this function. In human physiology, the body strives for a steady state or homeostasis. Literally, *homeostasis* means remaining the same. It is a condition in which a healthy body, although constantly changing and functioning, remains in a normal healthy condition. Homeostasis, or a *steady-state* condition, allows the normal body to keep in balance by compensating with changes. For example, if the body is taking in too much water, it responds to this imbalance by excreting water from the kidneys (urine), skin (perspiration), intestines (feces), and lungs (water in expiration) (Fig. 2–4). A healthy body maintains constancy of its chemical components and processes in order to survive. All organ systems and body structures play a part in maintaining homeostasis.

Another important function of the human body is metabolism. This is the

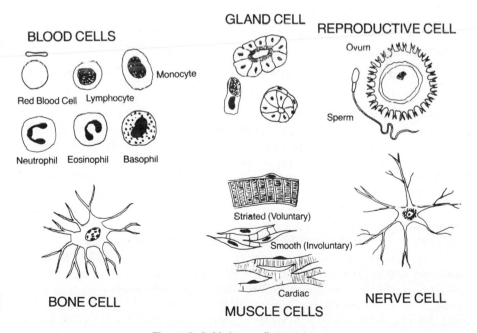

Figure 2–3. Various cell structures.

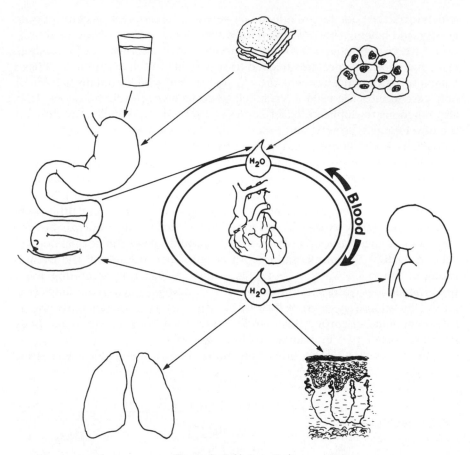

Figure 2–4. Homeostasis.

process of making necessary substances or breaking down chemical substances in order to use energy. Catabolism is a series of chemical reactions produced in cells to change complex substances into simpler ones while simultaneously releasing energy. It provides energy for all functions of the body, whether by moving a chair or allowing a heart to beat. Anabolism is a process by which cells use energy to make complex compounds from simpler ones. It allows for the synthesis of body fluids such as sweat, tears, saliva, or chemical constituents (enzymes, hormones, and antibodies). Both phases are required to maintain metabolic functions in a healthy individual.

A normal healthy body integrates both structural and functional aspects of anatomy and physiology. Organization of all the body structures such as cells, tissues, organs, and systems, together with proper functioning such as digestion, respiration, circulation, nerve sensitivity, movement, and secretion provide for a healthy individual. Systems working together can keep a body metabolizing properly and in homeostasis, which is the basis of survival.

Laboratory testing can provide a wealth of information about the individual organ systems and the integrated processes. Specimens, such as blood, bone marrow, urine, cerebrospinal fluid, pleural fluid, biopsy tissue, seminal fluid, and others, can be microscopically analyzed, assayed, and cultured to determine pathogenesis.[1,2]

MAJOR BODY SYSTEMS

This section summarizes the functions of the organ systems, with particular emphasis on cellular components and on the circulatory system. Refer to Table 2–1 for a brief summary of body systems.

Skeletal System

The *skeletal system* refers to all bones and joints of the body. This system is comprised primarily of two types of tissue: bone and cartilage. Bone is composed of cells surrounded by calcified intercellular substances that allow for a rigid structure. *Cartilage* is composed of similar cells, but these are surrounded by a gelatinous material instead of calcified substances, thus allowing for more flexibility. The skeletal system serves the body in five major ways: support, protection for softer tissues (brain or lungs), movement and leverage, *hematopoiesis* (blood cell formation) in the bone marrow, and calcium storage.

There are over 200 bones in the human body, classified into four groups based on their shapes. Long bones include leg bones, for example, femur, tibia, fibula; and arm and hand bones, for example, humerus, radius, ulna, and phalanges. Short bones include carpals and tarsals or wrist and ankle bones, respectively. Flat bones include several cranial bones, ribs, and scapulae or shoulder blades. And irregular bones include cranial bones, for example, sphenoid, and ethnoid; and bones of the vertebral column, for example, vertebrae, sacrum, and coccyx (Fig. 2–5).

Bones are connected to each other by a variety of joints that permit

TABLE 2–1. BODY SYSTEMS

Function	Systems
Systems for standing and moving	Skeletal
	Muscular
Systems for energy and waste disposal	Circulatory
	Digestive
	Respiratory
	Urinary
Systems for coordination and control	Nervous
	Sensory
	Endocrine
System for producing new life	Reproductive

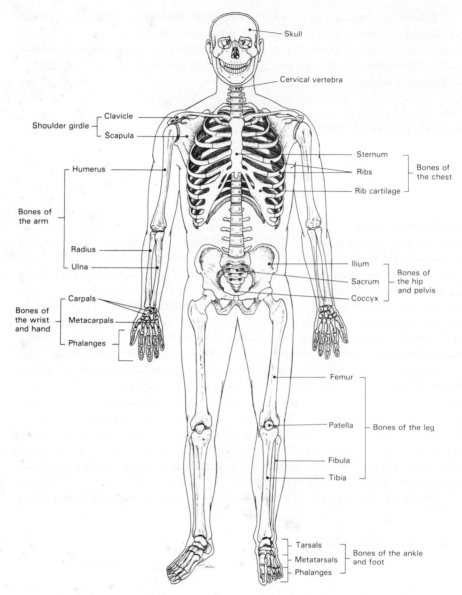

Figure 2–5. The skeletal system. *(Adapted from Evans WF: Anatomy and Physiology, 3rd ed. Englewood Cliffs, N.J., Prentice-Hall, 1983, with permission.)*

flexion, extension, abduction (away from median), adduction (toward median), rotation, and combinations of these. Bone structure differs between male and female skeletons. Aside from being somewhat larger and heavier, men have a pelvis that is deeper with a narrow pubic arch. The female pelvis is shallow, broad and with a wider pubic arch, to facilitate childbirth.

Bones, in general, consist of several layers covered by a membrane, the periosteum. The periosteum contains blood vessels that bring blood from inside to the outer layer. The outer layer, compact bone, is more rigid and heavier than the inner layer, which is like a honeycomb. It is called spongy bone but is just as strong as compact bone. In the center of bones is the marrow, which produces most blood cells. Approximately 5 billion red cells are produced daily by about half a pound (227 g) of bone marrow. It is located in all bones of an infant, but in adults it is in the skull, sternum or breastbone, vertebrae, hipbones, and ends of the long bones.[1]

Minerals that are stored in bones include calcium and phosphorus. When these minerals are needed in other parts of the body, they are released from bone through the bloodstream.

Laboratory assessment of the skeletal system can include serum calcium and phosphate levels, serum alkaline phosphatase (ALP) levels, microscopic analysis, and microbial culture of the bone marrow and synovial fluid (fluid between joints and bones).

Muscular System

The muscular system refers to all muscles of the body, including those attached to bones and those along walls of internal structures such as the heart. Based on location, microscopic structure, and nervous control, muscles are classified as follows: (1) *skeletal* or *striated voluntary*—attached to bones; (2) *visceral* or *nonstriated* (smooth) *involuntary*—line the walls of internal structures such as veins and arteries; (3) *cardiac* or *striated involuntary*—make up the wall of the heart (see Fig. 2–3). Muscles provide movement, maintain posture, and produce heat. Movement takes place not only during locomotion but also during body movements, changes in size of openings, and propulsion of substances, for example, blood through veins or passage of food through intestines. Posture is maintained during sitting and standing by continued partial contraction of specific muscles. Muscle cells that provide mechanical energy for movement also release energy in the form of heat. All three types of muscles work by extending, contracting, conducting, and being easily stimulated.

Skeletal muscles (over 400 in humans) comprise approximately 40 percent of a man's body. In contrast, women have a lower amount of muscle and the proportion of fat is greater than in men. Muscles are strongest at about age 25, but through proper nutrition and exercise, they can remain strong throughout life. Without sufficient exercise they become smaller and weaker. Glycogen is the form of stored glucose in muscles. Exercise increases the amount of glycogen available for muscles, which, in turn, makes it easier for them to function. Without stores of glycogen, muscles must wait for glucose, which is transported through the bloodstream.[1]

Laboratory testing of the muscular system often involves clinical assays of specific muscle enzymes, such as creatine kinase (CK), microscopic examination, or culturing of biopsy tissue.

Nervous System

The nervous system provides communication in the body, sensations, thoughts, emotions, and memories. Nerve impulses and chemical substances serve to regulate, control, integrate, and organize body functions. The nervous system is composed of specialized nerve cells (*neurons*), brain, spinal cord, brain and cord coverings, fluid, and the nerve impulse itself. It is estimated that there are over 10 billion neurons (nerve cells) in the human body, most of which are in the brain. Sensory neurons transmit nerve impulses to the spinal cord or brain from muscle tissues. Motor neurons transmit impulses to muscles from the spinal cord or brain. Both the brain and spinal cord are covered by protective membranes (*meninges*). Between these protective membrane layers are spaces filled with cerebrospinal fluid that provide a cushion for the brain and spinal cord. The brain has many vitally important areas. In conjunction with the cranial nerves, its functions include all mental processes and many essential motor, sensory, and visceral responses. The spinal cord and spinal nerves control sensory (touch), motor (voluntary movement), and reflex (kneejerk) functions. Reflexes are responses to stimuli that do not require communication with the brain. A simple reflex, such as moving a finger from something hot, occurs even before the brain realizes the pain. Specific cranial and spinal nerves exist to control all complex or simple action processes in the body.

Laboratory diagnosis of nervous disorders is not very specific. Chemical assays can reveal drug interactions, as well as hormonal, protein, and enzyme alterations. Meningitis can be detected by bacterial, viral, or fungal culture or by detection of specific antibodies in the cerebrospinal fluid (CSF).

Respiratory System

Respiration allows for the exchange of gases between blood and air. Once gases enter the blood, the circulatory system transports them between lungs and tissues. Together, the respiratory and circulatory systems get oxygen (O_2) to the cells and remove carbon dioxide (CO_2) from tissue cells.

O_2 allows the body to burn its fuel from the nutrients eaten. O_2 makes up about a fifth of the air around us. The average person inhales and exhales about 15 times per minute, or approximately 20,000 times per day.[1] As a person breathes in, the O_2 travels through air passages to the lungs. Here the exchange of gases takes place. O_2 is exchanged for CO_2, which is then breathed out as the person exhales. The main components of the respiratory system are in the head, neck, and thoracic cavity and include the nose, pharynx, larynx, trachea, bronchi, and lungs.

Receptors in the nose provide the sense of smell and allow for changes in voice. The nose also functions as the primary filter for air entering the body. It catches impurities and chemical substances that may be irritating to the respiratory system. In the nose, throat, and bronchial tree, mucus is continuously produced to trap unwanted particles and prevent them from entering the lungs. Tiny hairlike cilia line the passageways and function to sweep the mucous to the nose and mouth so it can be coughed, sneezed, or swallowed.[1] The pharynx is a tubelike structure that allows for both food and air to pass before reaching the appropriate pathway. Along with the larynx (voice box), it determines the quality of voice. The trachea and bronchial passages provide openings for outside air to reach the lungs. Within the bronchi are grapelike alveolar sacs that are enveloped by capillaries and allow for diffusion between air and blood. The lungs are structured into millions of branches of alveoli with surrounding capillaries. They can quickly take in large amounts of O_2 and release amounts of CO_2 if they are functioning properly.

Lungs are soft and spongy and reach from just above the collarbone down to the diaphragm. Lungs have no muscles; so the diaphragm and other surrounding muscles help enlarge and contract the chest cavity as respiration occurs. Humans have 2 lungs, the right one with 3 lobes and the left one with 2 lobes. The left side allows room for the heart. An adult's lungs hold 3 to 4 qt (approximately 3 to 4 L) of air depending on how vigorously one is moving or exercising.[1] In patients with pneumonia, the alveolar sacs become inflamed and fluid or waste products block the minute air spaces, thus making normal O_2 and CO_2 exchange very difficult.

Blood transports O_2 and CO_2 as part of molecules of certain chemical compounds such as hemoglobin. When O_2 and CO_2 are exposed to blood, they rapidly combine with hemoglobin to form oxyhemoglobin and carbaminohemoglobin, respectively (Fig. 2–6).

Association and dissociation with hemoglobin depends on the gaseous pressure. In lung capillaries, O_2 pressure [partial pressure of oxygen (Po_2)] increases and CO_2 pressure [partial pressure of carbon dioxide (Pco_2)] decreases, allowing O_2 to rapidly associate, or combine chemically, with hemoglobin and CO_2 to dissociate, or be released, from carbaminohemoglobin. In tissue capillaries, the opposite occurs: O_2 pressure is decreased and CO_2 pres-

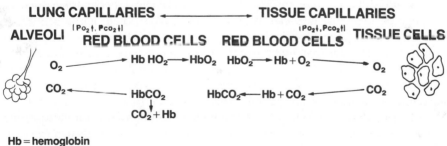

Hb = hemoglobin
PO_2 = pressure of O_2
PCO_2 = pressure of CO_2

Figure 2–6. O_2 and CO_2 transport via hemoglobin.

sure increased; therefore allowing O_2 to dissociate from oxyhemoglobin and CO_2 to combine with hemoglobin.

Gas pressure can be measured in the clinical laboratory from appropriate blood samples (see Chapter 5). In addition, other tests for chemical constituents (sodium, chloride, bicarbonate, and potassium) in the blood often indicate respiratory abnormalities. Lung biopsies, throat swabs, sputum, and bronchial washings can be examined microscopically or cultured for pathogenic microorganisms such as fungi, bacteria such as acid-fast bacilli, and parasites. Pathogenic microorganisms can cause respiratory infections such as the common cold, sore throats, coughs, sneezes, runny noses, bronchitis, and more serious diseases such as tuberculosis, pneumocystis pneumonia, Legionnaires' disease, and other types of pneumonia. Tuberculosis is caused by acid-fast bacilli that destroy lung tissue. In pneumonia, the air sacs in the lungs fill with fluid and gaseous exchanges cannot occur. Pneumocystis infections are considered opportunistic infections, e.g., they become pathogenic when the patient is immunosuppressed and are associated with acquired immunodeficiency syndrome (AIDS).

Digestive System

The digestive system functions, first, to break down food chemically and physically into nutrients that can be absorbed and used by body cells, and second, to eliminate the waste products of digestion. The gastrointestinal (GI) tract is made up of the following components: mouth, pharynx, esophagus, stomach, intestines, and some vital accessory organs such as salivary glands, teeth, liver, gallbladder, pancreas, and appendix. Many proteins, enzymes, and juices are released by these components to facilitate digestion, absorption, and movement through the GI tract. The passageway of the GI tract where food passes is known as the alimentary canal. It begins at the mouth and ends at the anus. In an adult, the average length of the alimentary canal is 27 feet. Circular muscles that surround the intestines contract to assist the movement of food through the body. These wavelike contractions are called *peristalsis*. One meal can take 15 hours to 2 days to pass through the alimentary canal. Peristalsis is such an effective process that one can even swallow upside down. If the process is reversed, vomiting enables the body to reject food.[1] Saliva moistens food and contains an enzyme that helps begin the breakdown of carbohydrates into simple sugars such as glucose. (If one chews a salt cracker a long time, it may begin to taste sweet).[1] Also, the liver secretes bile, which aids in fat digestion and absorption. In addition, it is involved in carbohydrate metabolism, protein and fat catabolism, and synthesis of many vital blood proteins for clotting and regulating functions. Each component functions either mechanically or chemically to keep the body in homeostasis. The digestive system helps regulate the intake and output of essential proteins, carbohydrates, fats, minerals, vitamins, and water. The body can then use these substances by catabolizing them for stored energy, or anabolizing them to build other complex compounds such as hormones, other tissue proteins, and enzymes. Levels of these constituents can be clinically measured in the laboratory from blood specimens and other body fluids. Materials that are not digested in the alimentary canal are eliminated from the body as waste.

Urinary System

The urinary system serves primarily to produce and eliminate urine. It consists of two kidneys and ureters, one bladder, and one urethra.

The kidney's main function is to regulate the amount of water, electrolytes (sodium, potassium, chloride), and nitrogenous waste products (urea) from protein metabolism. The proper concentration of these blood constituents is vital to life. As blood passes through the specialized kidney cells called glomeruli, water and solutes are filtered out. Only the necessary amounts of these substances are reabsorbed into the blood. The rest are excreted as waste products in the urine. Ureters collect urine as it is formed and transport it to the bladder. The bladder serves as a reservoir until it can be voided. The urethra is the terminal component of the urinary system. In women, it is merely a passageway from the bladder. In men, it eliminates both urine and semen from the body.

Two thirds of human body weight is water. About 60 percent of the body's water is inside cells and the rest is in the bloodstream or tissue fluids.[1] The salt content of the body's water is extremely important for survival. When excess salt is in the tissues, the kidneys eliminate salt; if there is excess water, kidneys will eliminate that. If the kidneys are not functioning properly, a mechanical filtering process (dialysis) must be used or a kidney must be transplanted.

Laboratory assessment of urinary function includes detection of chemical constituents, blood, microorganisms, and cells in the urine, as well as chemical analysis of the blood. A variety of urine collection techniques and preservatives are available.

Reproductive System

Male reproductive structures include testes, seminal vesicles, prostate, epididymis, seminal ducts, urethra, scrotum, penis, and spermatic cords. Primary functions of this system are spermatogenesis (sperm production), storage, maintenance and excretion of seminal fluid, and secretion of hormones (the most important of which is testosterone). Female reproductive structures include ovaries, fallopian tubes, uterus, vagina, and vulva. These structures play a role in ovulation, fertilization, menstruation, pregnancy, labor, and secretion of hormones (estrogens and progesterone).

A sperm is one of the smallest cells in the body. In contrast, the mature egg is the largest.[1] Each of these cells contains a nucleus with 23 chromosomes. Since the mother's egg and father's sperm contain different sets of DNA, a variety of genetic characteristics are paired with each other. One of the pairs of chromosomes determines gender of the baby. The egg contains only an X chromosome; however, the sperm may contain an X or Y chromosome. If an X sperm fertilizes the egg, an XX pair of chromosomes will form and the baby will be a girl. If a Y sperm fertilizes the egg, an XY pair will form and the baby will be a boy. The 46 combined chromosomes will contain the DNA-coded blueprint for the new baby. The DNA controls not only gender but all characteristics such as height, eye, hair, and skin color, immunity to diseases, allergies, and many other factors.

Laboratory tests of these reproductive functions might include semen, hormonal and cytogenetic analysis, as well as microbiologic cultures of infected areas.

Endocrine System

The human body has two types of glands. Exocrine glands secrete fluids such as sweat, saliva, mucus, and digestive juices, which are transported via channels or ducts. Endocrine glands, or ductless glands, release their secretions (hormones) directly into the bloodstream. This glandular system has the same functions as the nervous system, that is, communication, control, and integration. *Hormones* play an important role in metabolic regulation that influences growth and development, in fluid and electrolyte balance, energy balance, and acid-base balance. Hormonal imbalances can lead to severe disorders such as dwarfism, giantism, and sterility. Endocrine glands include pituitary, thyroid, parathyroid, thymus, adrenal, ovaries, and testes. The *pituitary gland,* or "master gland" as it is sometimes called, stimulates the other glands to produce hormones as needed. It controls and regulates hormone production through chemical feedback. The pituitary hormones also regulate retention of water by the kidneys, cause uterine contractions during childbirth, stimulate breast milk production, and produce growth hormone. This hormone controls growth by regulating the nutrients that are taken into cells. It also works with insulin to control blood sugar levels. If blood sugar is not controlled, diabetes mellitus can result. It is the most common disorder of the endocrine system. The thyroid gland produces a hormone that affects cell metabolism and growth rate. Parathyroid glands regulate calcium and phosphorus in the blood and bones. The thymus gland affects the lymphoid system. The *adrenals* (2 glands) produce hormones as a result of emotions like fright or anger. This causes an increase in blood pressure, widened pupils, and heart stimulation. The adrenals also produce hormones that regulate carbohydrate metabolism and electrolyte balance.[1] Ovaries and testes, as mentioned earlier, produce estrogens and progesterone, and testosterone, respectively.

Because hormones are transported via the bloodstream, it is easy to detect abnormalities by analyzing blood samples. Chemical assays are available for all types of hormones and provide very specific and sensitive patient results.

Circulatory System

The circulatory system transports water, electrolytes, hormones, enzymes, antibodies, cells, gases, and nutrients to all cells. In addition, it contributes to body defenses and the coagulation process and controls body temperature. This discussion centers on the processes by which these functions occur, composition of blood, and formation of blood.

The lymphatic system is also considered to be part of the circulatory system. Its main purpose is to circulate lymph fluid to and from the tissues and to produce blood cells. Lymph tissue is found in nodes, thymus, spleen, intestine, bone marrow, liver, and tonsils.

Blood.   Blood is composed of water, solutes, and cells. Normally, humans have approximately 5 qt (4.75 L) of blood. It is composed of approximately 3 qt of plasma and 2 qt of cells. Plasma contains water and solutes. Circulating blood cells are classified as *red blood cells* (RBCs or *erythrocytes*), *white blood cells* (WBCs or leukocytes), and *platelets* (*thrombocytes*). White blood cells are divided further into granulocytes (*basophils, neutrophils, eosinophils*), *lymphocytes,* and *monocytes* (Figs. 2–7 and 2–8). All these blood cells develop from undifferentiated stem cells in the *hematopoietic* (blood forming) tissues, such as the bone marrow. Stem cells are considered immature cells because they have not developed into their functional state. As the stem cells mature, they differentiate into the different cell lines mentioned. (Figure 2–9

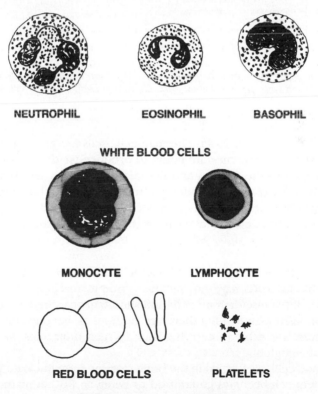

Figure 2–7. Human blood cells.

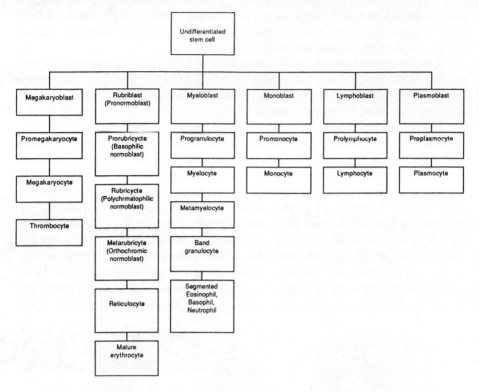

Figure 2–8. Blood cell formation. *(From Diggs LW, Sturm D, Bell A: The Morphology of Human Blood Cells, 5th ed. Abbott Park, Ill., Abbott Laboratories, 1985, with permission.)*

and Tables 2–2, 2–3, and 2–4). The maturing cells are given specific names based on which cell type they are going to produce. As they mature the cells undergo changes in the nucleus and cytoplasm so that when they reach the circulating blood, they become fully mature and functional (see Figure 2–7). These changes are clearly visible using staining techniques and light microscopy or can be distinguished by some of the more sophisticated hematology instruments.

Erythrocytes.   RBCs measure about 7 μm in diameter. Normally, when in the circulating blood, RBCs have no nucleus. Prior to reaching maturity in the bone marrow, RBCs lose their nucleus and simultaneously become biconcaved disks. Within each mature RBC there are millions of hemoglobin molecules; each molecule is capable of carrying four oxygen molecules. As previously mentioned, hemoglobin can also carry CO_2.

Red blood cells are formed in the bone marrow from nucleated stem cells. Once the stem cell becomes committed to being an RBC, it matures through several stages, all of which are morphologically different. The process takes several days and the stages are called rubriblast, prorubricyte, rubricyte, meta-rubricyte, reticulocyte, and mature RBC. Nomenclature differs among laboratories. The terms pronormoblast, basophilic normoblast, polychromatophilic normoblast, orthochromic normoblast are also used as indicated in Figure 2–8. The life span of RBCs is approximately 120 days in the circulating bloodstream. After this time, they begin to fragment and rupture. Cells in the liver, spleen, and bone marrow phagocytize the destroyed RBCs and begin to break down hemoglobin into iron-containing pigments (hemosiderin) and bile pigments (bilirubin and biliverdin). The bone marrow reuses the iron for new RBCs and the liver excretes bile pigments into the intestines.

Millions of RBCs are continually being formed and destroyed daily. The bone marrow must have an adequate supply of several substances to maintain a normal blood supply. These substances include amino acids, vitamin B complexes, and minerals such as iron. Deficiencies of any of these substances or failure of the bone marrow to function properly may result in anemia.

The surface membranes of RBCs contain antigens that designate the individual's blood type. RBCs with A antigen are type A; those cells with "B" antigen are type B; RBCs containing both A and B antigens are type AB; and RBCs with neither A or B antigens are type O. These antigens constitute the *ABO* blood group system. Another commonly recognized blood group system contains the Rh factor. If the RBCs contain the antigen for Rh factor, the individual is considered Rh positive. Rh-negative people do not have the Rh factor antigen on their RBCs. Many other blood group systems exist as well.

It is vitally important that blood transfused into a patient never contain *antibodies* to the patient's blood group *antigens* on the red cells. Antibodies can react with specific RBC antigens and destroy the red cells. This happens when a patient is transfused with blood that has been accidentally mistyped or confused with another patient's. It can be rapidly fatal to the inappropriately

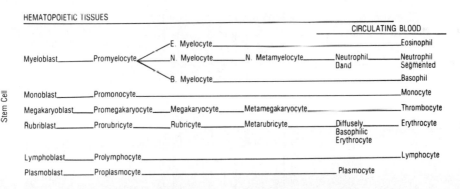

Figure 2–9. Blood cell development. *(From Diggs LW, Sturm D, Bell A: The Morphology of Human Blood Cells, 5th ed. Abbott Park, Ill., Abbott Laboratories, 1985, with permission.)*

TABLE 2–2. NOMENCLATURE

Prefix	Suffix	Myelocytic Series	Monocytic Series	Megakaryocytic Series	Erythrocytic (Rubricytic) Series	Lymphocytic Series	Plasmocytic Series
	___blast	myeloblast	monoblast	megakaryoblast	rubriblast	lymphoblast	plasmoblast
pro___	___cyte	promyelocyte	promonocyte	promegakaryocyte	prorubricyte	prolymphocyte	proplasmocyte
	___cyte	myelocyte	monocyte	megakaryocyte	rubricyte	lymphocyte	plasmocyte
meta___	___cyte	metamyelocyte		metamegakaryocyte	metarubricyte		

From Diggs LW, Sturm D, Bell A: *The Morphology of Human Blood Cells*, 5th ed. Abbott Park, Ill., Abbott Laboratories, 1985, with permission.

TABLE 2–3. PERIPHERAL BLOOD CELLS: NORMAL ADULT VALUES

	Percent	Per mm^3
N. Band	1–5	50–500
N. Segmented	50–70	2,500–7,000
Eosinophil	1–3	50–300
Basophil	0–1	0–100
Lymphocyte	20–40	1,000–4,000
Monocyte	1–6	50–600

From Diggs LW, Sturm D, Bell A: *The Morphology of Human Blood Cells,* 5th ed. Abbott Park, Ill., Abbott Laboratories, 1985, with permission.

transfused patient. (See Table 2–5 for antibodies present in various blood types.)

Type O RBCs can be transfused into any ABO type because the RBCs do not contain A or B antigen to react with either antibodies to A or B (anti-A, anti-B) present in type A or B patients.

Leukocytes.   WBC types differ in color, size, shape, and nuclear formation. Neutrophils, eosinophils, and basophils contain cytoplasmic granules, hence they are called granulocytes. Neutrophilic granules stain bluish with neutral dyes. Their nuclei generally have two or more lobes and are often referred to as polymorphonuclear (PMN) leukocytes. Eosinophilic granules stain orange-red with acidic dyes. Their nuclei normally have two lobes. Basophilic granules stain dark purple or black with basic dyes and their nuclei are often S-shaped. Lymphocytes and monocytes are nongranular and have relatively large nuclei (see Figs. 2–7 and 2–8).

Leukocytes function primarily as part of the body's defense mechanism. The cells phagocytize or ingest pathogenic microorganisms. Lymphocytes play a role in immunity and in production of antibodies (Table 2–3).

WBCs are formed in bone marrow and lymphatic tissues. The exact life span varies with cell type from days up to several years. Normally, blood contains 5000 to 9000 leukocytes/mm^3 with designated percentages for each cell line (Table 2–4).

The morphology of leukocytes and erythrocytes is routinely analyzed by using special staining techniques and visualizing the cells under the microscope. Categorization of cells and abnormalities are noted on the test report called a *differential.* More recently, hematology instruments have become very refined and many are now able to produce automated differentials at a higher speed and in a more cost-effective manner.

Leukocytes also contain specific cell surface antigens that can be characterized with sophisticated techniques, such as flow cytometry and monoclonal antibodies, in the clinical laboratory. Specific antigens are expressed at certain times during the development of the various WBC types. Using these labora-

TABLE 2–4. SUMMARY OF BLOOD CELLS

Cells	Number/Size	Function	Formation	Destruction
Erythrocytes (RBC)	4.5–5.5 million/mm³; size 6–7 μm	Transport O_2 and CO_2	Bone marrow	Fragmentation and removal in spleen, liver, and bone marrow; life span $\cong$ 120 days
Leukocytes (WBC)	5000–9000 per cu mm; size 9–16 μm	Defense	Granulocytes in bone marrow; nongranular WBCs in all lymphatic tissue	Removed in spleen, liver, bone marrow; life span 24 hr to years
Thrombocytes (platelets)	250,000–450,000/mm³; size 1–4 μm	Clotting	Bone marrow	Removed in spleen; life span 9 to 12 days

Abbreviations: RBC, red blood cells; WBC, white blood cells.

TABLE 2–5. ABO BLOOD TYPES

Blood Type	Antigens on RBC	Antibodies in Serum/Plasma
A	A	Anti-B
B	B	Anti-A
AB	AB	Neither anti-A or anti-B
O	None	Anti-A, anti-B

tory techniques, clinicians can tell more precisely how mature or immature the WBCs are in the bone marrow, peripheral blood, or both.

Thrombocytes.   Platelets are much smaller than other blood cells. They are fragments of megakaryocytes (located in the bone) and help initiate the clotting sequence. Normally there are 250,000 to 450,000 platelets/mm³ (see Table 2–3).

Plasma.   The liquid portion of the blood, without cells, is called *plasma*. If a chemical agent or anticoagulant is added to prevent clotting, a blood sample can be separated by centrifugation into the cells and plasma (Fig. 2–10). Chapter three contains additional information on anticoagulants.

Plasma is composed of 90 percent water and 10 percent solutes, which include nutrients such as glucose, amino acids, fats, metabolic wastes (urea, uric acid, creatinine, and lactic acid), respiratory gases (O_2 and CO_2), regulatory substances (hormones, enzymes, and mineral salts), and protective substances (antibodies).

Serum.   If a blood specimen is allowed to clot, the result is *serum* plus blood cells meshed in a fibrin clot. Serum contains essentially the same chemical constituents as plasma except that clotting factors and blood cells are contained within the fibrin clot.

Heart.   The human heart is a muscular organ about the size of a man's closed fist (Fig. 2–11). It contains four chambers and is located slightly left of the midline. The heart's function is to pump sufficient amounts of blood to all cells of the body by contraction (systole) and relaxation (diastole).

The average heart beats 60 to 80 times per minute. Children have faster heart rates than adults; and athletes have slower rates because more blood can be pumped with each beat. During exercise the heart beats faster to supply muscles with more blood; during and after meals it also beats faster to pump blood to the digestive system; and during fever, the heart pumps more blood to the skin surface to release heat. Heart rate is measured by feeling the pulse. One way to do this is to place 2 fingertips on the radial artery of the wrist (at the base of the thumb) and count the pulses for 60 seconds.[1]

The heart has 2 collection chambers (atria) that allow entry of blood from

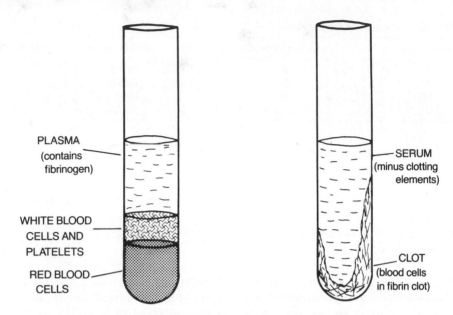

Figure 2–10. Blood specimens with and without anticoagulant. The blood specimen on the left is prevented from clotting by the addition of an anticoagulant and shows settling or centrifugation. Plasma is approximately 90 percent H_2O. The remaining constituents are proteins (coagulation factors, etc.), inorganic substances (sodium, chloride, potassium, etc.), organic substances (urea, creatinine, sugars, fats, cholesterol, etc.), and dissolved gases (O_2, CO_2, etc.). RBCs are heavier than WBCs or platelets so they sink to the bottom. The layer of WBCs is often referred to as the *buffy coat.* The blood specimen on the right will clot without anticoagulants. Serum is normally a clear, straw-colored fluid that contains everything that plasma contains except the coagulation factors. A fibrin clot forms that traps RBCs, WBCs, and platelets.

the pulmonary veins (bringing O_2-rich blood) and from the vena cava (bringing O_2-poor blood). Below the atria are the pumping chambers (ventricles), which have valves to control the flow. If a valve malfunctions, blood flows backwards causing a "heart murmur." The right side of the heart pumps O_2-poor blood to the lungs to pick up more O_2; the left side pumps O_2-rich blood toward legs, head, and organs.[1]

Blood Vessels.   There are three kinds of blood vessels: arteries, veins, and capillaries. The largest artery (aorta) and veins (vena cavas) are approximately 1 in. wide. Normally, blood vessels have smooth, flexible walls. However, with age, the walls of arteries may harden ("hardening of the arteries," also called arteriosclerosis). The inner walls of the vessels become rough because of cholesterol or calcium deposits. As the deposits worsen, blood clots may form that clog up the artery further, and the blood supply to tissues is reduced. In serious cases this can result in a stroke (if this happens in the brain) or a heart attack (if it happens in the coronary or heart vessels).

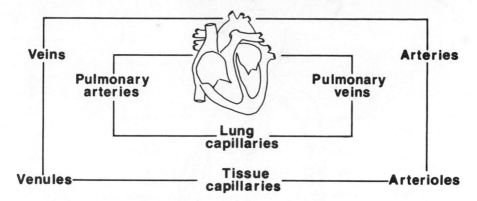

Figure 2–11. Schematic representation of blood pathway. O_2 and CO_2 exchange occurs in both the pulmonary and tissue capillaries.

Blood pressure is measured by an instrument called a sphygmomanometer. Values on the instrument relate to millimeters of mercury in a tube at certain points. Systolic pressure, the highest, is measured when the artery receives blood. Diastolic pressure, the lowest, is measured when the heart's ventricles relax. Therefore blood pressure is reported with 2 numbers, the systolic and then the diastolic pressure, for example 120/80. The systolic pressure measures 120 mm of mercury and the diastolic pressure measures 80 mm of mercury. High blood pressure can also cause a stroke when a body vessel ruptures in the brain. Slightly low blood pressure is generally considered to be a healthier state than having high blood pressure; however, if a person's pressure is too low, blood will not flow to the head and a faint feeling may result. In these cases it is best to lower the head to restore and increase blood flow to the head.

Arteries.   Vessels that carry blood away from the heart are highly oxygenated. *Arteries* branch into smaller vessels called arterioles. Principal arteries of the body are indicated in Figure 2–12.

Veins.   Blood is carried toward the heart by the smaller venules and *veins.* Since the blood flow in veins is against gravity in many areas of the body, they have one-way valves and rely on weak muscular action to move blood cells. The one-way valves prevent backflow of blood. All veins except the pulmonary veins contain deoxygenated blood. Principal veins of the body are indicated in Figure 2–13. Phlebotomists should be familiar with the principal veins of the arms and legs (Figs. 2–14 and 2–15).

Capillaries.   Microscopic vessels that carry blood and link arterioles to venules are called *capillaries.* Capillaries may be so small in diameter as to allow only one blood cell to pass through at any given time.

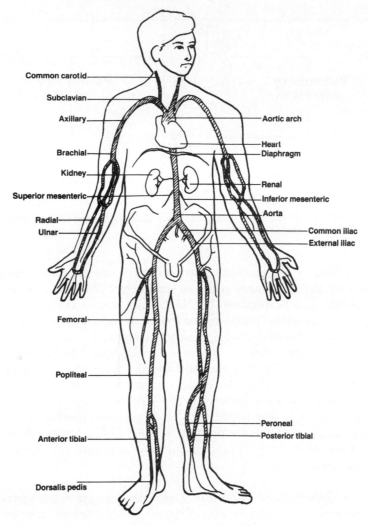

Figure 2–12. Principal arteries. *(From Anderson PD: Clinical Anatomy and Physiology for the Allied Health Sciences. Philadelphia, WB Saunders, 1976, with permission.)*

HEMOSTASIS AND COAGULATION

Hemostasis (not to be confused with homeostasis) is the maintenance of circulating blood in the liquid state and helps retain blood in the vascular system. When there is injury to a small blood vessel, the hemostatic process serves to repair the break and arrest the hemorrhage. The first step in this process is vasoconstriction, which decreases the blood flow to the injured vessel and the surrounding vascular bed. Platelets then degranulate, clump together, and adhere to the injured vessel in order to form a plug and inhibit bleeding. Many specific coagulation factors are released and interact to eventually form a fibrin meshwork or clot. Once bleeding has stopped, final repair and regeneration of the injured vessel takes place, and the clot slowly begins to degenerate.

The coagulation process is due to numerous coagulation factors. For purpose of simplicity, it is divided into two systems, intrinsic and extrinsic. All coagulation factors required for the intrinsic system are contained in the blood. The extrinsic factors are stimulated when tissue damage occurs. Blood

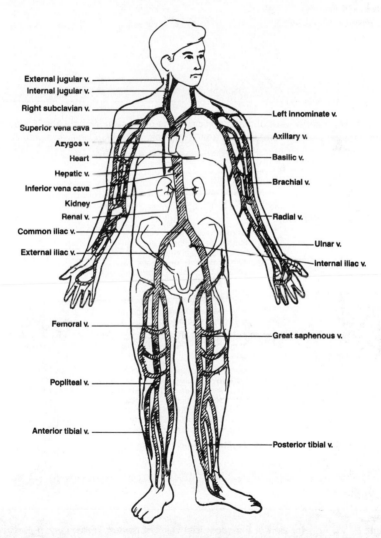

Figure 2–13. Principal veins. *(From Anderson PD: Clinical Anatomy and Physiology for the Allied Health Sciences. Philadelphia, WB Saunders, 1976, with permission.)*

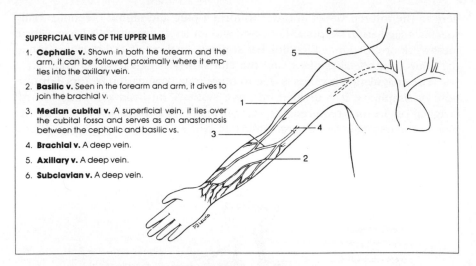

SUPERFICIAL VEINS OF THE UPPER LIMB

1. **Cephalic v.** Shown in both the forearm and the arm, it can be followed proximally where it empties into the axillary vein.

2. **Basilic v.** Seen in the forearm and arm, it dives to join the brachial v.

3. **Median cubital v.** A superficial vein, it lies over the cubital fossa and serves as an anastomosis between the cephalic and basilic vs.

4. **Brachial v.** A deep vein.

5. **Axillary v.** A deep vein.

6. **Subclavian v.** A deep vein.

Figure 2–14. Anterior view of the superficial veins of the arm. *(From Guy JF:* Learning Human Anatomy—A Laboratory Text and Workbook. *Norwalk, Conn, Appleton & Lange, 1992.)*

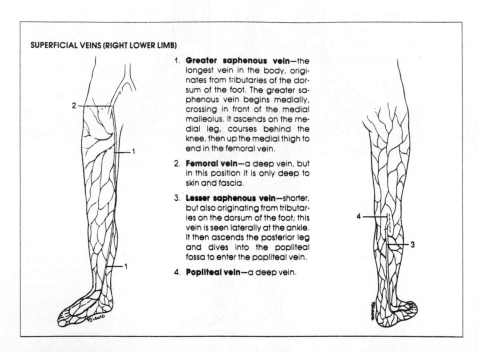

SUPERFICIAL VEINS (RIGHT LOWER LIMB)

1. **Greater saphenous vein**—the longest vein in the body, originates from tributaries of the dorsum of the foot. The greater saphenous vein begins medially, crossing in front of the medial malleolus. It ascends on the medial leg, courses behind the knee, then up the medial thigh to end in the femoral vein.

2. **Femoral vein**—a deep vein, but in this position it is only deep to skin and fascia.

3. **Lesser saphenous vein**—shorter, but also originating from tributaries on the dorsum of the foot; this vein is seen laterally at the ankle. It then ascends the posterior leg and dives into the popliteal fossa to enter the popliteal vein.

4. **Popliteal vein**—a deep vein.

Figure 2–15. Anterior view of the superficial veins of the leg. *(From Guy JF:* Learning Human Anatomy—A Laboratory Text and Workbook. *Norwalk, Conn, Appleton & Lange, 1992.)*

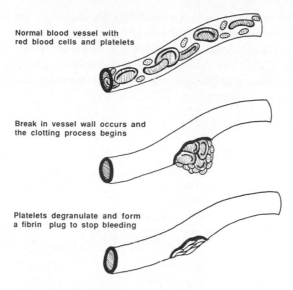

Normal blood vessel with
red blood cells and platelets

Break in vessel wall occurs and
the clotting process begins

Platelets degranulate and form
a fibrin plug to stop bleeding

Figure 2–16. Sequence of hemostatic plug formation.

vessels are lined with a single layer of flat endothelial cells and are supported by subendothelial cells and collagen fibers. Normally, endothelial cells do not react or attract platelets; however, they do produce and store some clotting factors. When the clotting sequence is initiated by vessel injury, they react with degranulated platelets in forming the fibrin plug (Fig. 2–16).

Large- or medium-sized veins and arteries require rapid surgical intervention to prevent bleeding. However, small arteries and veins are able to control bleeding by means of the platelet/fibrin plug and simultaneous vasoconstriction.

LABORATORY ASSESSMENT OF THE CIRCULATORY SYSTEM

The number of RBCs, their morphology, and hemoglobin content can be measured from an anticoagulated blood specimen in the clinical hematology laboratory. Platelets and WBCs can be assessed on the basis of number and morphology. The results of a laboratory procedure known as a WBC differential count enumerate specific cell lines in percentages. Platelet function, as well as each coagulation factor, can be measured from anticoagulated blood specimens in the coagulation section of the clinical hematology laboratory. Bone marrow can also be assessed in the hematology laboratory. It is removed by a physician from the iliac crest of the hip, stained, and studied microscopically for the detection of abnormal numbers and morphology of blood cells.

Tests for blood types and cross-matches for donor blood are done in an immunohematology, transfusion, or blood banking laboratory.

Serum and plasma constituents including nutrients, metabolic wastes, respiratory gases, regulatory substances, and protective substances can all be evaluated in the clinical chemistry laboratory. For further information on laboratory testing, see Chapter 3.

KEY TERMS

ABO	eosinophils	plasma
adrenals	genes	platelets
arteries	hematopoietic	(thrombocytes)
basophils	hemopoiesis	red blood cells
blood pressure	homeostasis (steady	(erythrocytes)
body planes	state)	reproductive system
buffy coat	hormones	respiratory system
capillaries	lymphocyte	serum
cardiac (striated	meninges	skeletal (striated
involuntary) muscle	monocyte	voluntary) muscle
cartilage	muscular system	skeletal system
circulatory system	nervous system	urinary system
cytoplasm	neurons	veins
deoxyribonucleic acid	neutrophils	visceral (nonstriated
(DNA)	nucleolus	involuntary) muscle
differential	nucleus	white blood cells
digestive system	peristalsis	(leukocytes)
endocrine system	pituitary gland	

STUDY QUESTIONS

1. Name the source(s) of water entry into the bloodstream.

    a. tissue metabolism   c. kidneys
    b. food   d. skin

2. Laboratory assessment of the endocrine system routinely includes which of the following?

    a. blood cell analysis   c. lymph tissue analysis
    b. biopsy   d. hormonal analysis

3. Normal lung capillaries have which of the following conditions?

a. increased P_{O_2}

c. increased P_{CO_2}

b. decreased P_{O_2}

d. decreased P_{CO_2}

4. Leukocytes are formed primarily in which organs?

a. central nervous system

c. heart

b. lymphatic tissue

d. bone marrow

5. What is the liquid portion of an anticoagulated blood specimen from veni-puncture called?

a. serum

c. plasma

b. capillary blood

d. arterial blood

REFERENCES

1. Bruun RD, Bruun B: *The Human Body.* New York, Random House, 1982.
2. Anthony CP, Thibodeau GA: *Textbook of Anatomy and Physiology,* 11th ed. St Louis, CV Mosby, 1983.
3. Anderson PD: *Laboratory Manual and Study Guide for Clinical Anatomy and Physiology for Allied Health Sciences.* Philadelphia, WB Saunders, 1976.
4. Diggs LW, Sturm D, Bell A. *The Morphology of Human Blood Cells,* 5th ed. Abbott Park, Ill., Abbott Laboratories, 1985.

Collection Reagents, Supplies, and Interfering Chemical Substances

3

TYPES OF CLINICAL LABORATORY SPECIMENS

As described in Chapter 2, blood is composed of plasma and cells (erythrocytes, leukocytes, and thrombocytes). Almost all of the cells in the blood are erythrocytes. Plasma may be separated from blood cells by centrifugation. As shown in Figure 3–1, plasma is differentiated from serum in that *plasma* retains the protein clotting component, fibrinogen, which is removed from serum during the clotting process. Plasma can be obtained from whole blood that has been mixed with a chemical, an anticoagulant, to prevent clotting in the collection tube. This centrifuged blood yields plasma, which contains fibrinogen in addition to the major proteins, albumin and globulin. *Serum* is obtained from *whole blood* that is not mixed with any anticoagulant. This centrifuged blood yields serum, which contains albumin and globulin, but no fibrinogen.

Most clinical laboratories use serum, plasma, or whole blood to perform various assays. More recently, heparinized whole blood has become the specimen of choice for the latest clinical laboratory instruments used in STAT situations. Using whole blood as a specimen decreases the time involved in acquiring the patient's result since centrifugation is not required prior to laboratory testing. Each assay may require a different type of anticoagulant. (A discussion of these anticoagulants is included in a following section of this chapter.)

For all types of blood specimens, the phlebotomist must label the speci-

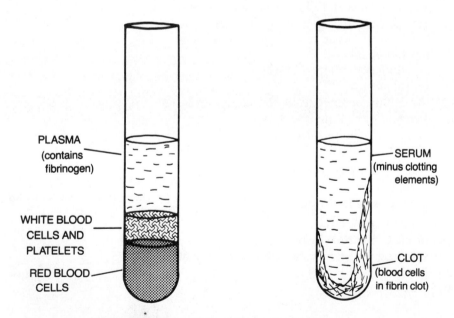

Figure 3–1. Differentiation between plasma and serum.

men with the following information: patient's name, patient's admission number, room number (applies to hospital patient, not outpatient), date, time, and initials of phlebotomist. The properly labeled specimens should be transported to the specimen collection area in the clinical laboratory accompanied by the laboratory request slip.

Other Body Fluids

In addition to blood specimens, other types of body fluids are analyzed in the clinical laboratory for their various constituents. These body fluids include: (1) *gastric secretions* obtained by gastric intubation, (2) *cerebrospinal fluid* (CSF) obtained through a spinal tap or lumbar puncture, (3) *synovial fluid* extracted aseptically from joint cavities, (4) fluid aspirated from body cavities (e.g., *pleural fluid* obtained from the lung cavity; *pericardial fluid* from the heart cavity, *peritoneal fluid* from the abdominal cavity), (5) fluid that bathes the fetus within the amniotic sac, called *amniotic fluid,* and (6) *seminal fluid,* which is composed of products formed in various male reproductive organs. Phlebotomists are usually not involved in the collection of these body fluids. However, they are sometimes involved in transporting these types of specimens to the laboratory for the necessary analyses. Chemical examination, cell count, microscopic examination, and microbiologic analysis are some of the body fluid tests usually requested. When transporting amniotic fluid to the laboratory, the specimen must be protected from light and transported immediately. Since metabolism in these collected fluids may affect the laboratory test results, it is very important to transport any body fluid specimens to the laboratory as quickly as possible.

The phlebotomist should be careful in the transportation of body fluids because they are difficult to obtain and may be biohazardous. Just as for blood specimens, a laboratory request slip must accompany the body fluid specimen and the body fluid must be properly labeled (patient's name, patient's admission number, date, and time specimen collected, type of specimen, attending physician).

Urine Collections

Because a basic urinalysis is almost always included in the routine hospital admission of a patient, the phlebotomist should be aware of the protocol for collecting the urine specimen in order to explain to the patient the proper collection technique, if such an occurrence arises. First, it is essential that the urine collection containers be clean and dry prior to the collection process. Appropriate containers include plastic, disposable cups, jars, and bags with a capacity of 50 to 100 mL for routine urinalysis procedures. They are available from various manufacturers in several sizes.

Midstream specimens are commonly used for routine admission urinalysis. The patient is instructed to void approximately one-half of the urine into the toilet, a portion is collected in a readily available container, and the rest is allowed to pass into the toilet.[1]

If asked, "What is a *clean-catch urine specimen?*" the phlebotomist may describe the procedure and mention that this type of specimen is used to detect the presence or absence of infecting organisms as well as routine urinalysis. The specimen must be free of contaminating matter that may be present on the external genital areas. Thus, the following steps should be explained to a female patient who is to obtain a clean-catch urine specimen:

1. The woman should separate the skin folds around the urinary opening and clean this area with a mild antiseptic soap and water.
2. Holding the skin folds apart with one hand and after urinating into the toilet, the patient should urinate into a sterile container. The container should not touch the genital area.
3. The patient should label the container with her name and time of collection and deliver to the requested place.
4. The urine specimen should be refrigerated immediately by hospital personnel.

For a male patient, the following procedure should be adhered to for obtaining a clean-catch urine specimen:

1. The man should wash the end of his penis with soapy water and then let dry.
2. After allowing some urine to pass into the toilet, the urine should be collected in the sterile container without touching the penis; and steps 3 and 4 are the same as for a woman.[2]

For some laboratory assays, it is necessary to analyze a *24-hour urine specimen*. Incorrect collection and preservation of this type of specimen are two very frequent errors in laboratory medicine. As part of the laboratory team, the phlebotomist should be aware of the protocol for a 24-hour urine collection in order to assist other health professionals and the patient in avoiding collection errors. The following steps should be followed for a 24-hour urine collection:

1. The patient should be given a chemically clean wide-mouthed, properly labeled large container for a 24-hour urine specimen. The laboratory personnel add required preservatives to the container prior to submitting it to the patient. Patients should NOT be allowed to submit urine specimens in their own jars because they may not be chemically clean and do not contain the required preservatives.
2. The patient should be instructed verbally that the collection of the 24-hour urine begins with emptying the bladder and discarding the first urine passed. This first step in the collection process should start between 6 and 8 AM with the exact time written on the container label.

3. Except for the first urine discarded, all urine should be collected during the next 24-hour period. The patient should be reminded to urinate at the end of the collection period and include this urine in the 24-hour collection.
4. Because urine is an ideal culture medium for microorganisms that decompose chemical constituents, the entire specimen should be refrigerated during collection with each specimen added during the 24-hour collection period. The patient should be told to urinate before having a bowel movement because fecal material in the urine specimen will make the specimen unacceptable for collection.
5. Some preservatives for 24-hour urine collection are very corrosive if accidentally spilled or contact is made during collection. Thus, the patient should be warned of any preservatives in the container.
6. The patient should be informed not to add anything except urine to the container and not to discard any urine during this collection period.
7. A normal intake of fluids during the collection period is desirable unless otherwise indicated by the physician.
8. Some laboratory assays require special diet restrictions, and thus, these instructions should be given to the patient.
9. If possible, medications should be discontinued for 48 to 72 hours preceding the urine collection as a precaution against interference in the laboratory assays.
10. The 24-hour urine specimen should be transported to the clinical laboratory as soon as possible. The specimen should be placed in an insulated bag or portable cooler to maintain the cool temperature.
11. Following all verbal instructions for the 24-hour urine collection, the patient should be provided with written instructions as a reminder.[3]

Culture Specimens

Other specimens that the phlebotomist may be requested to transport to the clinical laboratory include sputum (fluid from the lungs containing pus), throat and sinus drainage cultures, wound cultures, ear or eye cultures, skin cultures, and feces. The phlebotomist should be extremely careful in the transportation of each type of specimen because they can be easily contaminated and may be biohazardous. For safety, the phlebotomist needs to wear *gloves* when handling and transporting these specimens in their containers.

INTERFERENCE OF DRUGS AND OTHER SUBSTANCES IN BLOOD

Many prescribed drugs can interfere with clinical laboratory determinations or physiologically alter the levels of blood constituents measured in the clinical laboratory. Interference of drugs and other substances is so complicated and

dependent upon the chemical procedures used that only general recommendations are described here.

The direct analytical interference of drugs is decreasing with the advent of
more specific and sensitive chemical procedures. However, the physiologically
induced abnormalities from various types of drugs are the major causes of
interference from medications. Drugs administered to alleviate an illness can
induce physiologic abnormalities in one or more of the following systems:
hepatic, hematologic, hemostatic, muscular, pancreatic, and renal, with the
resultant obscuration of the clinical diagnosis.

Prior to the laboratory measurement of chemical constituents, the attending physician should take the necessary precautions in prescribing drugs to the
patient. If the patient must be maintained on medication that may cause interferences in laboratory assays, the medication should be written on the laboratory request form. Unless interference of medications can be avoided by ordering different laboratory assays, medications should be discontinued if at all
possible, and assays repeated when false laboratory values are suspected.

Direct analytical interference in laboratory determinations is least likely
to occur in blood assays because drug concentrations are usually very low.
However, some drugs or drug metabolites in blood can directly cause falsely
decreased or falsely elevated values in laboratory methodology.[4]

Drug interferences leading to falsely decreased results in blood specimens
may be caused by inhibition of the chromogenic or fluorescent reaction. Examples of such drugs are indicated in Table 3–1. A more complete list of such
drugs can be found in Hansten's *Drug Interactions.*[12] These drugs can

1. diminish fluorescence of the blood analyte by quenching the fluorescent energy, and thus falsely decrease the analyte's concentration.
2. compete with the blood analyte for a chromogenic reagent, and thus
   falsely decrease the resultant color and concentration of the analyte.
3. compete with the chromogenic reagent for peroxide in a peroxide-
   generating reaction, and thus falsely decrease the chromogen oxida-
   tion and concentration of the blood analyte.

The falsely decreased values of the blood analyte can be mistakenly interpreted as normal or subnormal if the blood analyte was truly in an elevated
range or normal range, respectively.

Drug interferences leading to falsely elevated results of blood analytes
may be caused by increasing the color or fluorescence produced in the laboratory methodology, altering the binding characteristics in radioimmunoassays
and enzyme immunoassays, or both. Examples of such drugs are shown in
Table 3–2.

Interference from medications usually causes falsely elevated values
rather than falsely decreased values. Some drugs, such as acetaminophen and
erythromycin, can increase serum aspartate aminotransferase and bilirubin
and, thus, falsely create a clinical interpretation of hepatic dysfunction without

TABLE 3–1. DRUG INTERFERENCES LEADING TO FALSELY DECREASED RESULTS IN BLOOD SPECIMENS

Analyte	Method	Drug Interference
Albumin	Colorimetric	Aspirin[5]
Bilirubin	Colorimetric (Diazo reaction)	Ascorbic acid[26] (vitamin C)
Cholesterol	Colorimetric	Thiouracil[7]
Glucose	Colorimetric	Ascorbic acid[8]
	Chromogenic oxidation (hexokinase reaction)	L-dopa[9] Ascorbic acid[3]
	Chromogenic oxidation (oxidase reaction)	Tetracycline[10]
Phosphate	Colorimetric	Phenothiazine[11]
Protein	Colorimetric	Cytarabine[7]
Uric acid	Colorimetric (phosphotungstate)	Salicylates[24] Lithium[7]
	Enzymatic	Ascorbic acid[27]

the true presence of hepatic abnormality.[6,8] Drug-induced elevations of blood constituents can be mistakenly interpreted as falsely increased or normal whereas the true values are in the normal range or subnormal range, respectively.

In addition to prescribed oral medications, interference in laboratory test results can occur after intravenous injections of medications and dyes. For example, the results of laboratory tests performed after fluorescein angiography may be erroneous owing to interference by the intravenous fluorescein.[29] The results for blood creatinine, cortisol, and digoxin are altered by this dye. If the phlebotomist collects blood in a cardiology section or specialized health care institution for heart patients, he or she needs to be alert of this potential hazard for laboratory test interference. If he or she is aware of collecting blood from a patient who has just had a dye injection, this information needs to be communicated promptly to the specimen collection supervisor.

Physiologically, drugs can alter blood analytes through various metabolic reactions; the production of blood cells and platelets and their survival times can be changed. Chemotherapeutic drugs can lead to a decrease in all forms of blood cellular elements and, thus, their metabolic and immunologic processes.

A variety of medications (Table 3–3) are toxic to the liver and thus can lead to acute hepatic necrosis.[16] The hepatic dysfunction, in turn, leads to an increase in blood liver enzymes such as alanine aminotransferase, alkaline phosphatase, and lactate dehydrogenase. Also, the production of globulins and clotting factors are decreased in drug-induced hepatotoxicity.

Patients receiving medications that may result in renal impairment should be monitored for possible electrolyte imbalance and elevation of blood urea

TABLE 3–2. DRUG INTERFERENCES LEADING TO FALSELY ELEVATED RESULTS
IN BLOOD SPECIMENS

Analyte	Method	Drug Interference
Alanine aminotransferase	Colorimetric	Erythromycin[13]
Catecholamines	Fluorescent	Ampicillin[10]
		Ascorbic acid[10]
		Methyldopa[14]
Cholesterol	Colorimetric	Corticosteroids[7]
		Salicylates[7]
Creatine kinase	Colorimetric	D-Penicillamine[15]
Creatinine	Colorimetric	Dexamethasone[15]
Iron	Colorimetric	Dextran
Protein	Colorimetric	Sulfobromophthalein[7]
		Phenazopyridine[7]
		Tetracycline[7]
Thyroxine	Radioimmunoassay	Oral contraceptives[3]
Total leukocytes count	Automated counting system	Azathioprine[15]
Triglyceride	Enzymatic with color development	Aspirin[28]
Uric acid	Colorimetric (phosphotungstate)	Ascorbic acid[7]
		Caffeine[7]

nitrogen. Antihypertensive agents given over a long period of time can lead to kidney damage if not monitored closely.

Pancreatitis can be caused by corticosteroids, estrogens, and diuretics[17] and causes elevations of serum amylase and lipase values. Aspirin causes hypobilirubinemia (decrease in bilirubin) by expelling bilirubin from the plasma to the surrounding tissue cells.[25]

Because many metabolic activities can be altered by medications as described in the examples above, the attending physician must note on the laboratory request form the presence of medications being taken by the patient. As a general rule, the College of American Pathologists (CAP)[18] recommends that medications that might interfere in laboratory assays be avoided for

TABLE 3–3. DRUGS TOXIC TO THE LIVER

Salicylates	Penicillin	Acetaminophen
Mitomycin	Isoniazid	Chlorpromazine
Actinomycin	Halothane	Methyldopa
Thiazides	Chloramphenicol	Acetohexamide
Trifluoperazine	Sulfamethoxazole	Chlorpropamide
Sulfachlorpyridazine	Tetracycline	Paramethadione
Phenytoin		

Adapted from Sher PP: Drug interferences with clinical laboratory tests, *Drugs* 24:24, 1982; and Sherlock S: Progress report: Hepatic reaction to drugs. *Gut* 20:634, 1979, at least 4 to 24 hours prior to blood studies and 48 to 72 hours prior to urine studies. This recommendation should be followed only if no risk or serious discomfort will result in the patient.

The phlebotomist is the link between the clinical laboratory and the patient. Laboratory tests are often ordered without knowledge of the drugs taken by a person. Yet these drugs, as discussed above, will lead to falsely elevated or decreased values. Sometimes during blood collection, a patient will mention that he or she has taken over-the-counter drugs such as Tylenol (acetaminophen). It is important for the phlebotomist to communicate the patient's name and possible drug interference to the clinical laboratory supervisor in charge of specimen collection. The supervisor can then communicate with the attending physician to determine if the medication(s) will or will not interfere in the laboratory assays. The follow-up communication by the phlebotomist and clinical laboratory supervisor can lead to better patient care by avoiding interfering substances in laboratory determinations.

SELECTION AND USE OF EQUIPMENT

Blood is the most frequent specimen analyzed in the clinical laboratory. Venipuncture with a *vacuum tube (Vacutainer),* as shown in Figure 3–2, is the most direct and efficient method to obtain a blood specimen. Vacuum tubes may contain silicon to decrease the possibility of hemolysis and prevent the clot from adhering to the wall of the tube. This convenient system eliminates the need for syringes and uses disposable needles and tubes. The tubes are available in different sizes. The external tube diameter and length plus the maximum amount of specimen to be drawn into the vacuum tube are the two criteria to describe vacuum tube size (see Table 3–4). The smaller sizes (e.g., 2 mL) are useful for pediatric and geriatric collections and can be purchased

TABLE 3–4. TYPICAL SIZES OF BLOOD COLLECTION VACUUM TUBES

External Diameter × Length (mm)	Draw Volumes (mL)
13 × 75	2.0
13 × 75	4.0
13 × 75	5.0
13 × 100	4.2
13 × 100	6.0
13 × 100	7.0
13 × 100	15.0
16 × 75	7.0
16 × 100	10.0

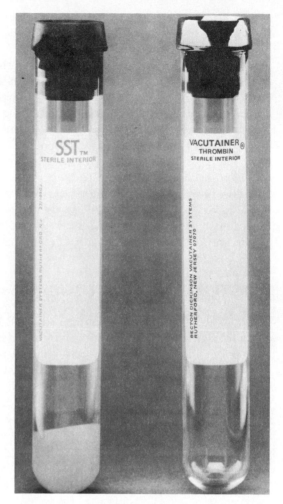

Figure 3–2. Vacuum tube (Vacutainer). *(Courtesy of Becton-Dickinson and Company, Rutherford, N.J.)*

with different types of anticoagulants as well as chemically clean or sterile glassware. The tubes are used in conjunction with a holder–needle combination as shown in Figure 3–3. Because these items are disposable, it eliminates the hazard of transmitting hepatitis, AIDS, or other infectious agents. Each vacuum tube is color-coded according to the anticoagulant contained within the tube (Table 3–5).

Anticoagulants and Blood Collection Tubes

Many coagulation factors are involved in blood clotting, and coagulation can be prevented by the addition of different types of anticoagulants. These *anticoagulants* often contain preservatives that can extend the metabolism and life span of the red blood cells (RBCs) after blood collection. Anticoagulants

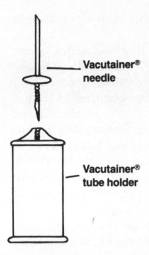

Vacutainer® needle

Vacutainer® tube holder

Figure 3–3. Holder-needle combination.

and preservatives are used extensively in blood donations to ensure the biochemical balance of certain components of RBCs such as hemoglobin, pH, adenosine triphosphate (ATP), and glucose. Once transferred, anticoagulants such as *citrate phosphate dextrose* (CPD) and *acid citrate dextrose* (ACD) ensure that the RBCs provide the recipient with the means of delivering oxygen to the tissues.

Another major use of anticoagulants and preservatives is in the collection of plasma for laboratory analysis. Specific anticoagulants or preservatives must

TABLE 3–5. SPECIMEN TYPE AND COLLECTION VACUUM TUBES

Specimen Type	Collection Tubes (Stopper Color/Type)	Additive
Blood/serum	Gray and red	Inert polymer barrier
	Yellow and red	Inert polymer barrier
	Red	None
Blood/plasma	Green and gray	Inert polymer barrier and lithium heparin
	Green and red	Inert polymer barrier and lithium heparin
	Blue	Trisodium citrate
	Lavender	EDTA(K_3) or EDTA(K_2) or EDTA (Na_2)
	Gray	Sodium fluoride and potassium oxalate
	Green	Lithium heparin
	Green	Sodium heparin
Blood/serum	Royal blue	No additive; but sterile tube for trace elements
	Brown	No additive; but lead-free glass and sterile for lead determinations
Whole blood	Lavender	EDTA(K_3) or EDTA(K_2) or EDTA (Na_2)
	Green	Lithium heparin or sodium heparin
	Yellow	Sodium polyanethole sulfonate (SPS)

be used depending on the test procedure ordered. Anticoagulants cannot be substituted one for another.

Coagulation of blood can be prevented by the addition of oxalates, citrate, *ethylenediaminetetraacetate (EDTA)*, or *heparin*. *Oxalates, citrates,* and EDTA prevent the coagulation of blood by removing calcium and forming insoluble calcium salts. These three anticoagulants cannot be used in calcium determinations; however, citrates are frequently used in coagulation blood studies. EDTA prevents platelet aggregation and is therefore used for platelet counts and platelet function tests. Fresh EDTA-anticoagulated blood allows for the preparation of blood films with minimal distortion of white blood cells (WBCs). Heparin prevents blood clotting by the inactivation of the blood clotting chemicals—thrombin and thromboplastin. Heparin is a mucopolysaccharide used in assays such as ammonia and plasma hemoglobin.

In addition to using the correct anticoagulant for a specific laboratory assay, the correct amount or dilution of anticoagulant in the blood specimen is important. An incorrect amount of anticoagulant may lead to latent fibrin formation in the serum.

Gray-stoppered Vacutainer tubes usually contain: (1) potassium oxalate and sodium fluoride or (2) *sodium fluoride and thymol*. This type of collection tube is used primarily for glycolytic inhibition tests. Since fluoride destroys many enzymes, this additive should not be used to collect blood for enzyme (e.g., CK, ALT, AST, and ALP) determinations. Oxalate distorts cellular morphology. Thus, gray-stoppered tubes should not be used for hematology studies.

The anticoagulants sodium heparin and lithium heparin are found in green-stoppered vacuum tubes. These tubes are used in various laboratory assays requiring plasma or whole blood. For potassium measurement, heparinized plasma or whole blood rather than serum is preferred since sporatic increased potassium results can occur in serum due to potassium released from platelets during blood clotting.[34] Lithium heparin tubes may be used for glucose, BUN, creatinine, and electrolytes; however, this anticoagulant is not suitable for the measurement of ionized calcium or lithium. Sodium heparin tubes should not be used for measurement of sodium.

The green-stoppered vacuum tube should not be used in preparation of blood smears to be stained with Wright's stain. The heparin causes the Wright's stain to have a blue background. Some procedures require sodium heparin without lithium or vice versa. When used for cytogenetic studies, it is important for these tubes to be sterile.

The purple-stoppered vacuum tubes (containing EDTA) are used for most hematology procedures. Many coagulation procedures are done on blood collected in blue-stoppered vacuum tubes, which contain sodium citrate at a concentration of 3.8 percent.

Dependent upon the needs of the laboratory procedure, the tubes may be ordered with or without sterilization. Sterile vacuum collecting tubes are fre-

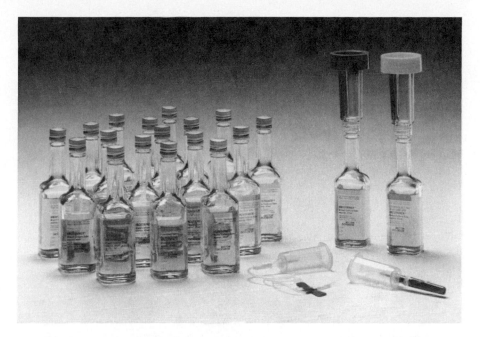

Figure 3-4. Vacutainer Microbiology Specimen Collection Units. *(Courtesy of Becton-Dickinson and Company, Rutherford, N.J.)*

quently used in the following procedures: prothrombin time, sedimentation rate, trace element studies, and activated clotting time. Sterile blood specimens are also ordered for blood cultures when the patient is suspected of having septicemia (symptoms of sepsis). A major problem with collecting blood for culture is that the patient's sample can become contaminated with microorganisms from the skin. Thus, the blood must be collected in a sterile container (vacuum tube or syringe) under aseptic conditions.

As shown in Figure 3-4, blood can be collected directly into vacuum tubes that contain culture media. This type of collection minimizes the risk of specimen contamination. The vacuum tubes can be purchased with (1) different types of culture media, (2) an unplugged venting unit for aerobic incubation, or (3) a plugged venting unit for anaerobic incubation.

Blood collecting vacuum tubes can be ordered in different sizes to allow for the different amounts of blood needed for various types of clinical laboratory assays. Table 3-6 lists the laboratory assays with the types of anticoagulants required and the approximate milliliters of blood needed to be drawn.

Becton-Dickinson and Company has developed a new safety vacuum tube called the B-D Vacutainer Brand Tube with Hemaseal. The Becton-Dickinson's glass-in-plastic tube construction is designed to (1) resist breakage, (2) reduce

TABLE 3–6. LABORATORY ASSAYS AND THE REQUIRED TYPES OF ANTICOAGULANTS

Test Name	Specimen Type/ Stopper Color	Whole Blood Minimum Volume (mL)
ABO group and type	Whole blood (purple)	3
Acetaminophen	Serum (red)	2
Acetone	Serum (red)	1
Acid hemolysis (PNH)	Plasma (blue)	3
Acid phosphatase	Serum (red)	2
Adenovirus antibody	Serum (red)	3
Adrenal cortical antibody	Serum (red)	3
Alcohol	Serum (red)	3
Aldolase	Serum (red)	2
Aldosterone	Serum (red) Plasma (purple or green) *Ice needed for transportation *Patient should be recumbent for at least 30 minutes prior to blood collection	3
Alkaline phosphatase	Serum (red)	2
Alkaline phosphatase isoenzymes	Serum (red)	2
Alpha$_1$-antitrypsin	Serum (red)	1
Alpha$_2$-macroglobulin	Serum (red)	1
Ammonia	Plasma (green)	3
Amoebiasis	Serum (red)	3
Ampicillin	Serum (red)	5
Amylase	Serum (red)	1
Antibody to hepatitis A virus	Serum (red)	3
Antibody to hepatitis B core antigen	Serum (red)	3
Antibody to hepatitis B surface antigen	Serum (red)	3
Antibody to hepatitis BE antigen	Serum (red)	3
Antibody identification	Whole blood (red)	7
Antibody screen and blood grouping	Whole blood (red)	5
Antibody titer	Whole blood (red)	5
Anticonvulsants (Dilantin, Mysoline, phenobarbital, carbamazepine, valproic acid)	Serum (red)	7
Antidiuretic hormone (ADH, Vasopressin)	Whole blood (purple)	3
Antinuclear antibodies, fluorescent	Whole blood (red)	5
Antithrombin III	Plasma (blue)	1
APTT	Plasma (blue)	1.8

(*continued*)

TABLE 3–6. (Continued)

Test Name	Specimen Type/ Stopper Color	Whole Blood Minimum Volume (mL)
Arboviruses	Serum (red)	3
Arsenic (As)	Whole blood (green, purple) *Use acid-washed syringes	2
ASO titer	Serum (red)	3
Australia antigen (HAA) (HB$_s$ Ag)	Serum (red)	3
Autologous blood	Whole blood (red)	5
B-Cell antigen	Whole blood (red)	3
Barbiturates	Serum (red)	2
Benzodiazepines	Serum (red)	2
Beta$_2$-microglobulin	Serum (red)	3
Bilirubin, total and direct	Serum (red)	1
Blastomycosis complement fixation (fungal serology)	Serum (red)	7
Bleeding time	Patient	Test performed on patient's arm
Blood cell count, survey (WBC, RBC, Hgb, Hct, MCV, MCH, MCHC)	Whole blood (purple)	3
Blood cell count, differential	Blood smear	Blood smear
Blood cell count, eosinophil	Whole blood (purple)	3
Blood cell count, erythrocyte (RBC)	Whole blood (purple)	3
Blood cell count, leukocyte (WBC)	Whole blood (purple)	3
Blood cell count, platelets	Whole blood (purple)	3
Blood cell count, reticulocyte	Whole blood (purple)	3
Blood, packed red blood cells	Whole blood (red)	5
Bordetella pertussis antibody (whooping cough)	Serum (red)	3
Borrelia burgdorferi antibody (Lyme disease)	Serum (red)	3
Bromide	Serum (red)	2
Brucella	Serum (red)	2
BUN (blood urea nitrogen)	Serum (red)	1
Cadium (Cd)	Whole blood (green, purple) *Use acid-washed syringes	2
Calcitonin	Serum (red) Plasma (green)	3
Calcium	Serum (red)	1

(continued)

TABLE 3–6. (*Continued*)

Test Name	Specimen Type/ Stopper Color	Whole Blood Minimum Volume (mL)
Calcium, ionized	Serum (red)	2
Candida serology, qualitative	Serum (red)	5
Carbon dioxide	Serum (red)	2
Carcinoembryonic antigon (CEA)	Serum (red)	3
Carotene	Serum (red)	3
Catecholamines	Plasma (gray) or	5
	Whole blood (purple)	3
Ceruloplasmin	Serum (red)	3
Chemistry screen (T. Protein, Alb, Ca, l Phos, Glu, BUN, Uric acid, Creat, T Bili, Alk P'tase, LDH, ALT)	Serum (red)	3
Chloramphenicol	Serum (red)	5
Chloride	Serum (red)	3
Cholesterol	Serum (red)	1
Cholinesterase	Serum (red)	3
Chromium (Cr)	Serum (royal blue) *Avoid chromium plated needles; use platinum needles and acid-washed syringes	2
Chromosome analysis	Whole blood (green) (Na heparin)	7
Circulating anticoagulants	Plasma (blue)	3
Clonazepham	Serum (red) or plasma (purple)	2
CMV, IFA serology	Serum (red)	5
Coccidioides immitis (San Joaquin Valley fever)	Serum (red)	3
Cold agglutinins	Whole blood (red)	3
Complement, total	Serum (red)	5
Complement-C_3	Serum (red)	5
Complement-C_4	Serum (red)	5
Coombs' test, direct (direct antiglobulin test)	Whole blood (red)	3
Coombs' test, indirect (indirect antiglobulin test)	Whole blood (red)	5
Copper	Plasma (blue)	3
Copper (Cu)	Whole blood (royal blue) Plasma, serum *Use acid-washed syringes	2

(*continued*)

TABLE 3–6. (*Continued*)

Test Name	Specimen Type/ Stopper Color	Whole Blood Minimum Volume (mL)
Cortisol	Plasma (purple)	2
Coxiella burnetii (Q Fever)	Serum (red)	3
Coxsackie virus (Bornholm's disease)	Serum (red)	3
C-Peptide	Serum (red)	7
CPK	Serum (red)	1
CPK isoenzymes	Serum (red)	5
C-reactive protein	Serum (red)	2
Creatinine	Serum (red)	1
Cross-match	Whole blood (red)	3
Cryofibrinogen	Plasma (green)	1
Cryoglobulin	Serum (red)	4
Cryptococcal antigen	Serum (red)	3
Cyclosporin A	Plasma (green)	7
Cysticercus collulosae (Pork tape worm)	Serum (red)	3
Cytomegalovirus (CMV), IFA serology	Serum (red)	5
Dengue virus antibody (Bonebreak fever)	Serum (red)	3
Deoxycorticosteroids	Serum (red) Plasma (green)	3
Digitoxin	Serum (red)	2
Digoxin	Serum (red)	2
Dilantin (phenytoin)	Serum (red)	2
Directogen for *Hemophilus influenzae, Streptococcus pneumoniae, Neisseria meningitides*	Serum (red)	3
DNA antibody (anti-DNA)	Serum (red)	3
E-Rosette	Whole blood (purple)	3
E-Rosette receptor	Whole blood (purple)	3
Echinococcus (Hydatid disease)	Serum (red)	3
Electrolytes (Na, K, Cl, HCO$_3$)	Plasma (green) or Whole blood (green)	2
Electophoresis (hemoglobin)	Whole blood (purple)	1
Electrophoresis (SPE)	Serum (red)	1
Electrophoresis, immuno	Serum (red)	3
Elution studies	Whole blood (purple)	2
Entamoeba histolytica	Serum (red)	3
Eosinophil count	Whole blood (purple)	1
Epstein-Barr virus (EBV)	Serum (red)	5
Erythrocyte fragility	Whole blood (purple)	1
Erythromycin	Serum (red)	5

(*continued*)

TABLE 3–6. (*Continued*)

Test Name	Specimen Type/ Stopper Color	Whole Blood Minimum Volume (mL)
ESR	Whole blood (purple)	2
Estradiol	Serum (red) or Plasma (green)	3
Estriol	Serum (red) or Plasma (green)	3
Estrogens, total	Serum (red)	7
Ethanol	Whole blood (gray) Plasma (gray)	2
Euglobulin lysis	Plasma (blue)	4.5
Factor assays	Plasma (blue)	4.5
Fasting blood glucose	Plasma (gray)	1
Febrile agglutinins	Serum (red)	7
Ferritin	Serum (red)	5
Fetal hemoglobin	Whole blood (purple)	2
Fibrinogen	Plasma (blue)	1.8
Fibrin degradation products (FDP)	Plasma (blue)	2
Fibrinopeptide A	Whole blood with special tube from hematology	5
Fluorescent antinuclear antibody	Serum (red)	3
Fluorescent treponemal antibody test (MHA-TP)	Serum (red)	3
Fluoride	Serum (red)	6
Folate, serum	Serum (red)	5
Folate, whole blood (RBC and serum)	Whole blood (purple)	3
Follicle-stimulating hormone (FSH)	Serum (red) or plasma (green)	3
Francisella tularensis antibody (Tularemia)	Serum (red)	3
Fragility, erythrocyte (RBC)	Whole blood (purple)	2
Fungal serology	Serum (red)	3
Gamma-glutamyl transpeptidase	Serum (red)	1
Gastrin	Serum (red)	7
Gentamicin	Serum (red)	5
Glucagon	Whole blood (purple)	3
Glucose (FBS and tolerance)	Plasma (gray) or Serum (red)	1
Glucose, 2-hr postprandial	Plasma (gray) or Serum (red)	1
Glucose-6-phosphate dehydrogenase (G6PD), quantitative	Whole blood (purple)	2

(*continued*)

TABLE 3–6. (*Continued*)

Test Name	Specimen Type/ Stopper Color	Whole Blood Minimum Volume (mL)
Gonadotrophin HCG-beta (immuno test)	Serum (red)	7
Ham's test (PNH) confirmation	Serum (red)	3
Haptoglobin	Serum (red)	1
HDL (high-density lipoprotein)	Serum (red)	5
Heinz body prep	Whole blood (purple)	3
Helper T	Whole blood (purple)	2
Hematocrit	Whole blood (purple)	1
Hematology survey (Hct, Hgb, WBC, RBC, MCV, MCH, MCHC)	Whole blood (purple)	1
Hemoglobin	Whole blood (purple)	1
Hemoglobin, plasma	Plasma (purple)	1
Heparin	Plasma (blue)	3
Hepatitis B surface antigen (HB_sAg)	Serum (red)	3
Hepatitis B core antibody (HB_cAb)	Serum (red)	3
Hepatitis delta antibody and antigen	Serum (red)	3
Herpes simplex, virus serology	Serum (red)	3
Heterophile antibody (Monospot)	Serum (red)	3
HI Titer—St. Louis encephalitis	Serum (red)	3
Histamine	Serum (red)	5
Histoplasmosis, complement fixation	Serum (red)	5
HIV antigen	Serum (red)	3
HLA typing (microcytotoxicity)	Whole blood (green)	5
Human T-lymphotropic virus type III antibody (HTLV-III)	Serum (red)	2
Hydroxybutyric dehydrogenase (HBD)	Serum (red)	5
IgA	Serum (red)	1
IgD	Serum (red)	1
IgG	Serum (red)	1
IgM	Serum (red)	1
Imipramine	Serum (red)	3
Inhibitor assay	Plasma (blue)	4.5
Insulin (on ice)	Plasma (purple)	4.5
Insulin tolerance	Serum (red)	3
Intrinsic factor antibody	Serum (red)	3
Iron profile (iron, TIBC, and saturation)	Serum (red)	3
Kanamycin	Serum (red)	5
Lactic acid (on ice)	Plasma (gray)	3
Lactate dehydrogenase (LDH)	Serum (red)	2
Lead, blood	Blood (dark blue)	10

(*continued*)

TABLE 3-6. (Continued)

Test Name	Specimen Type/ Stopper Color	Whole Blood Minimum Volume (mL)
LE cell test	Whole blood (green)	3
Legionnaires' serology	Serum (red)	3
Leishmania antibody	Serum (red)	3
Leptospira agglutination	Serum (red)	3
Leucine aminopeptidase (LAP)	Serum (red)	3
Leukocyte alkaline phosphatase stain (LAP)	Six fresh blood smears	
Lipase	Serum (red)	2
Lipids, total	Serum (red)	7
Lipoprotein phenotype	Serum (red)	1
Lithium	Serum (red)	2
Low-density lipoprotein (LDL)	Serum (red)	5
Luteinizing hormone	Serum (red)	3
Lymphocyte blastogenesis (LBR)	Whole blood (green)	7
Lymphogranuloma venereum	Serum (red)	3
Lysozyme, serum	Serum (red)	2
Magnesium, serum	Serum (red)	3
Malaria antibody	Serum (red)	3
Malaria smear	Blood smear	
Manganese (Mn)	Whole blood (royal blue) Serum *Use acid-washed syringes	5
Mercury (Hg)	Whole blood (royal blue) Serum (red)	5
Methemalbumin	Serum (red)	2
Methemoglobin	Serum (red)	3
Methicillin	Serum (red)	5
Methotrexate	Serum (red)	2
Monocyte antigens	Whole blood (purple)	2
Mumps serology	Serum (red)	3
Mycoplasma pneumoniae	Serum (red)	2
Myelin antibodies	Serum (red)	3
Nickel (Ni)	Plasma, serum, whole blood Must prepare collection vials by acid-washing syringes	5
5'-nucleotidase	Serum (red)	2
Opiates (methadone, codeine, morphine)	Serum (red)	3

(continued)

TABLE 3–6. (*Continued*)

Test Name	Specimen Type/ Stopper Color	Whole Blood Minimum Volume (mL)
Osmolality, serum	Serum (red)	2
Parathyroid hormone (PTH)	Serum (red)	3
Partial thromboplastin time (PTT)	Plasma (blue)	1
Penicillin	Serum (red)	5
Phenobarbital	Serum (red)	2
Phenylalanine	Whole blood Filter paper with low background fluorescence	Droplets used to saturate filter paper (<.5)
Phenytoin (Dilantin)	Serum (red)	2
Phospholipids	Serum (red)	5
Phosphorus	Serum (red)	2
Platelet function profile	Whole blood (purple) Whole blood (blue)	1 7
Pneumocystic serology	Serum (red)	3
Potassium	Plasma (green)	2
Precursor T	Whole blood (purple)	2
Primidone (Mycoline)	Serum (red)	2
Procainamide, *N*-acetylprocainamide	Serum (red)	2
Progesterone	Clotted whole blood (red) *Avoid serum separator tube	3
Prolactin	Serum (red)	2
Pronestyl (procainamide)	Serum (red)	2
Propranolol	Serum (red) or Plasma (purple)	3
Protein, total	Serum (red)	1
Protein, total A/G ratio	Serum (red)	1
Prothrombin consumption time	Serum (red)	3
Protime	Plasma (blue)	2
Proteus OX 19	Serum (red)	2
Pyruvate	Whole blood (special tube from chemistry)	5
Quinidine	Serum (red)	2
Rabies virus antibody	Serum (red)	3
Renin activity (on ice)	Plasma (purple)	2
Reticulocyte	Whole blood (purple)	5
Rheumatoid factor assay	Serum (red)	2
Rickettsial proteus antibodies (Proteus OX 19)	Serum (red)	3
RPR	Serum (red)	2

(*continued*)

TABLE 3–6. (*Continued*)

Test Name	Specimen Type/ Stopper Color	Whole Blood Minimum Volume (mL)
Rubella	Serum (red)	5
Rubeolla serology	Serum (red)	1
Russell viper venom time (Stypven time)	Plasma (blue)	2
Salicylate	Serum (red)	2
Salmonella	Serum (red)	5
Sedimentation rate (ESR)	Whole blood (purple)	3
Selenium (Se)	Plasma, whole blood, serum (royal blue with heparin or EDTA or no anticoagulant)	3
Sickling screen	Whole blood (purple)	2
SGOT (AST)	Serum (red)	6
SGPT (ALT)	Serum (red)	2
Sodium, serum	Serum (red)	3
SPE	Serum (red)	1
Special stains		
Acid phosphatase	Blood smear	
Alkaline phosphatase	Blood smear	
Lipid	Blood smear	
PAS for glycogen	Blood smear	
Peroxidase	Blood smear	
Toludine blue	Blood smear	
Sudan black	Blood smear	
Iron	Blood smear	
Esterases	Blood smear	
Heinz bodies	Blood smear	
Streptozyme	Serum (red)	2
Stypven time (RVV time)	Plasma (blue)	3
Sucrose presumptive (PNH)	Whole blood (blue)	3
Sulfa level	Plasma (gray)	5
Suppressor	Whole blood (purple)	3
Syphilis (RPR)	Serum (red)	2
Teichoic acid antibody	Serum (red)	5
Tegretol	Serum (red)	5
Testosterone	Serum (red)	7
Theophylline (aminophylline)	Serum (red)	2
Thiamine	Whole blood (green)	10
Thrombin time—Fibrindex	Plasma (blue)	3
Thyroglobulin	Serum (red)	5
Thyroid antibodies	Serum (red)	3
Thyroiditis, antithyroglobulin, and anti-microsomal fraction	Serum (red)	5

(*continued*)

TABLE 3–6. (Continued)

Test Name	Specimen Type/ Stopper Color	Whole Blood Minimum Volume (mL)
Thyroxine (T_4) free	Serum (red)	3
Thyroxine (T_4)	Serum (red)	3
Tobramycin	Serum (red)	3
Toxoplasmosis serologic test, IFA	Serum (red)	3
Transaminase (AST, SGOT)	Serum (red)	2
Transaminase (ALT, SGPT)	Serum (red)	2
Transferrin	Serum (red)	2
Transferrin receptor	Whole blood (purple)	5
	Serum (red)	2
Trichinella agglutination	Serum (red)	3
Tricyclic antidepressants (amitriptyline, nortriptyline)	Serum or plasma (red, green or purple) *Avoid gel separator	3
Triglycerides	Serum (red)	2
Thyroid-stimulating hormone (TSH)	Serum (red)	5
Urea nitrogen (BUN)	Serum (red)	1
Uric acid	Serum (red)	1
Valium (diazepam)	Serum (red)	2
Valproic acid (Depakene)	Serum (red)	2
Vancomycin	Serum (red)	2
Varicella-zoster immune status	Serum (red)	2
Varicella-zoster serology	Serum (red)	2
VDRL (RPR) syphilis	Serum (red)	2
Vitamin A	Serum (red)	3
Vitamin B_{12}	Serum (red)	2
Vitamin B_{12} binding capacity	Serum (red)	3
Vitamin B_6	Whole blood (purple)	10
Vitamin C	Serum (red)	7
Vitamin D (25-OH)	Whole blood (purple)	7
D-Xylose	Serum (red)	3
Zinc	Serum (red)	5

Abbreviations: A/G, albumin/globulin (ratio); Alb, albumin; Alk p'tase, alkaline phosphatase; ALT, alanine aminotransferase; APTT, activated thromboplastin time; AST, aspartate aminotransferase; Ca, calcium; CMV, cytomegalovirus; CPK, creatine phosphokinase; Creat, creatinine; ESR, erythrocyte sedimentation rate; FBS, fasting blood sugar; Glu, Glucose; HAA, hepatitis-associated antigen; HB_SAG, hepatitis B surface antigen; HCG, human chorionic gonadotropin; Hct, hematocrit; Hgb, hemoglobin; HI, hemaglutination inhibition; IFA, indirect fluorescent antibody (test); IgA, immunoglobulin A; IgD, immunoglobulin D; IgG, immunoglobulin G; IgM, immunoglobulin M; I phos, Inorganic phosphorus; LDH, lactate dehydrogenase; LE, lupus erythematosus; MCH, mean corpuscular hemoglobin; MCHC, mean corpuscular hemoglobin concentration; MCV, mean corpuscular volume; PAS, periodic acid–Schiff; PNH, paroxysmal nocturnal hemoglobinuria; RPR, rapid plasma reagin; RVV, Russell viper venom (time); SGOT, serum glutamic oxaloacetic transaminase; SGPT, serum glutamic pyruvic transaminase; SPE, serum protein electrophoresis; T bil, total bilirubin; TIBC, total iron-binding capacity; T protein, total protein; VDRL, Venereal Disease Research Laboratory.

the risk of accidental exposure to blood specimens, and (3) help contain blood and glass fragments in the highly improbable event of breakage during usage.

Syringes, Needles, and Safety Devices

Some patients' veins are too fragile to collect blood using the vacuum tubes. Thus, syringes must be used for the collection process. Syringes, as well as tubes, must be chemically clean in order to avoid any interfering effects with the constituents to be measured. In general, syringes and tubes do not have to be sterile to measure chemical constituents. The phlebotomist should know whether the tubes or syringes to be used in collection are sterile or chemically clean because a sterile tube or syringe does not indicate that the collecting device is also chemically clean. The syringe must be the correct size for the amount of blood to be collected. Disposable plastic syringes are most frequently used. Infrequently, a glass syringe is needed to collect blood for a special procedure, and, thus, the glass plunger and barrel should be inspected carefully before using.

The gauge and length of a needle used on a syringe or vacuum tube is selected according to the specific task. For example, larger needles (18 gauge) are used in collecting donor units of blood (up to 450 mL), whereas smaller needles (21 and 22 gauge) are used to collect specimens for laboratory assays. The *gauge number* indicates the diameter of the needle, and the smaller the number, the larger the needle. Needles are packaged by vendors in individual containers that are color-coded according to their respective gauge sizes.[30] When collecting blood from children, a 21- to 23-gauge needle is usually used with a tuberculin or 3-mL syringe. The length of the needle depends upon the depth of a vein. The tip of the needle should be checked for damage; a blunt or bent tip can be harmful to the patient's vein and may lead to failure of blood collection.

Different types of needles are used for single- or multiple-sample collections. *Multiple-sample needles* are used with vacuum collection tubes and the holder in order to allow for multiple tube changes without blood leakage within the plastic holder. The multiple-sample needle has a plastic cover over the stopper-puncturing portion of the needle to create the leakage barrier. The *single-sample needle* is usually used for collecting blood with a syringe.

One type of needle that has been introduced to help in the prevention of accidental needle sticks and transmission of AIDS and other infectious diseases to phlebotomists is the High Risk (HR) needle (ICU Medical, Inc., Mission Viejo, Calif. 92691). It covers the used needle permanently, at the point of injection, eliminating the hazard of recapping or disassembly and reducing the possibility of accidental needle sticks.

Another *protective needle device* is the SAF-T-CLIK shielded blood needle adapter that the company claims can prevent up to 80 percent of needle-stick injuries. Ryan Medical, Inc. (Brentwood, Tenn.) has developed this disposable adapter that is said to fit all standard blood needles and collection tubes. The

Sterimatic Safety Needle (SSN) (Abnash, Chalford Hill, STROUD, Gloucestershire) is a safety needle that automatically and permanently covers the needle point as it is withdrawn from the patient. Thus, no part of the needle, including the point, is ever exposed.

The B-D Safety Lok needle (Becton-Dickinson Vacutainer Systems, Rutherford, N.J.) is a device designed to encourage safer venipuncture technique. Following venipuncture, the protective shield slides and snaps into place, providing immediate containment of the used needle. Another protective needle device is the Pro-Ject 200 Safety blood needle holder. It can be used to safely eject the contaminated blood needle into a needle-puncture-proof device. It has a one-handed lever release that allows the needle hub to separate from the holder threads. The Pro-Ject 200 can be reused approximately two hundred times. The device can be used with blood needles made by all major manufacturers.

Medical Safety Products, Inc. (Denver, Colo.) has Acci-Guard Reusable Blood Collection Holders (Figure 3–5) that provide a self-sheathing process with a mechanical barrier for the needle. The blood collector can single-handedly retract a used blood collection needle and then safely recover the needle while it is enclosed and locked inside the holder. This holder system can provide disposal of the needle as it remains locked and enclosed with the Acci-Guard Holder (Figure 3–6). The holder is similar to existing vacuum holders, and, thus, standard blood collection techniques can be used. A companion biohazard container, used in combination with the Acci-Guard Holder,

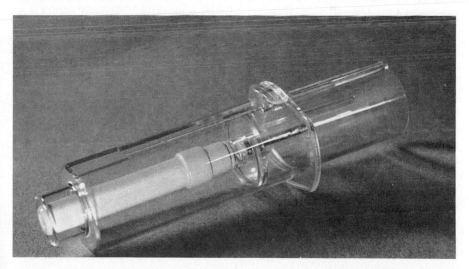

Figure 3–5. Acci-Guard Reusable Holder. *(Courtesy of Medical Safety Products, Inc., Denver, Colo.)*

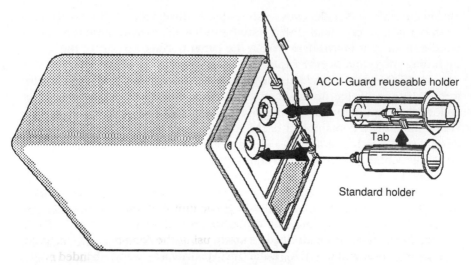

Figure 3–6. Acci-Guard Reusable Holder offers disposal of the needle in safe, locked system. *(Courtesy of Medical Safety Products, Inc., Denver, Colo.)*

is available. This system provides protection from needle sticks by removing used needles from the holder without user contact with the needle.

After blood collection, the phlebotomist or laboratorian must gain access to the blood in the vacuum tube for testing purposes. To protect against blood exposure during this hazardous step, different types of items have been recently developed by manufacturers. For example, the Saf De-Cap (Current Technologies, Inc., Crawfordsville, Ind.) can be placed over the tube stopper, the stopper is then gripped through the device, and is twisted and pulled out. This cap protects the phlebotomist or laboratorian by blockage of splashing and aerosol from the blood.

Another example is the B-D Vacutainer Brand Tubes with Hemogard. It is a vacuum blood collection tube with a plastic shield over the stopper. The shield protects the person from splattering blood when the stopper is removed from the tube.

The Pumpette (Helena Laboratories, Beaumont, Tex.) is a device that can provide access to the needed blood sample without ever uncapping the blood collection tube. The sample is aspirated by pressing the accordion-style pump on top of the stopper. Safety and efficiency are increased using this device.

Another device that has been developed to reduce the possibility of infection, contamination, and aerosol is the Aerotrap (Innovative Laboratory Products, Ltd., distributed by Fisher Scientific). It is used in laboratories to remove the stopper from vacuum tubes. Aerotrap allows the handling of vacuum tubes without ever touching their stoppers and reduces hand-carried contamination throughout the laboratory.

After the blood is drawn by syringe, it should be immediately transferred to a chemically clean, dry tube. The needle must be removed from the syringe to avoid hemolysis before transferring the blood. The blood should be allowed to clot for a minimum of 15 minutes at room temperature, and longer if it is refrigerated. If the clot is allowed to retract for a longer period of time, the chances for hemolysis are decreased and the yield of serum is enhanced. The longer the blood cells remain in contact with the serum, the greater the shift of substances from blood cells to serum through the metabolic process of glycolysis.

Needle Resheather and Disposal Containers

As shown in Figure 3–7, Datar, Inc. (Long Lake, Minn.) produces a phlebotomy resheather and tube holder. This system allows needles to be resheathed safely, and it acts as a holder for vacuum tubes. The unit is autoclavable so that it can be reused. Also, Datar, Inc. has a pocket resheather (see Figure 3–8) that allows the user to resheath needles safely using the "one-handed" technique. The IV Pole Resheather (IV-R) (Datar, Inc.) provides a safe one-handed method

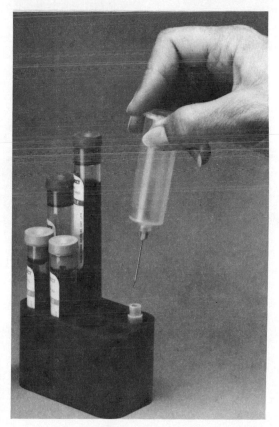

Figure 3–7. Phlebotomy resheather and tubeholder. *(Courtesy of Datar, Inc., Long Lake, Minn.)*

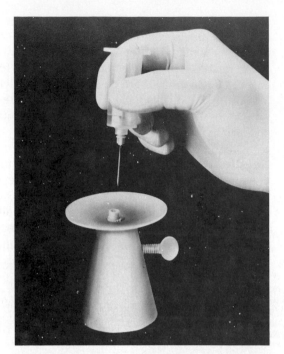

Figure 3–8. Pocket resheather.
(Courtesy of Datar, Inc., Long Lake, Minn.)

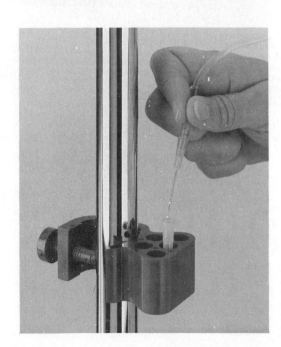

Figure 3–9. IV pole resheather.
(Courtesy of Datar, Inc., Long Lake, Minn.)

(see Figure 3–9) for recapping needles from intermediate IV tubing and sy-ringes. It can connect directly to an IV pole or be used as a portable stand-alone resheather. In addition, Datar, Inc. produces a no-cut needle disposal system (Fig. 3–10). This system consists of several sizes for bedside, cart, isolation, surgery, and so on. Needles and syringes can be discarded in these rigid plastic containers, which reduce the possibilities of needle sticks for the phlebotomist. The unit is completely disposable and no needle cutters are needed.

Separation Tubes

Another collection method is to draw blood into a serum separation tube such as the Monoject Corvac. Blood is collected in the vacuum Corvac tube using conventional blood collecting techniques. As illustrated in Figure 3–11, this tube contains a gel in a cup-shaped plastic "energizer" containing microscopic

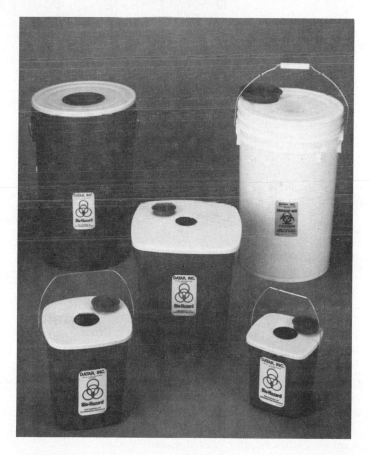

Figure 3–10. Needle disposal system. *(Courtesy of Datar, Inc., Long Lake, Minn.)*

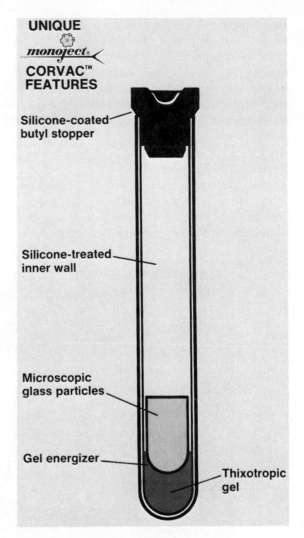

UNIQUE
monoject
CORVAC™ FEATURES

Silicone-coated butyl stopper

Silicone-treated inner wall

Microscopic glass particles

Gel energizer

Thixotropic gel

Figure 3–11. Corvac tube. *(Courtesy of Monoject Scientific, a Division of Sherwood Medical.)*

glass particles. As blood enters the tube, the glass particles go into suspension and accelerate clotting by providing increased surface area. As shown in Figure 3–12, when the blood in the Corvac tube is centrifuged, the energizer cup displaces the gel and forces it from the bottom to the sides of the tube. The gel's specific gravity is intermediate to serum and clotted blood. Thus, it stops moving when the equilibrium point is reached. At this point, the gel forms a positive, stable, chemical and physical barrier between the clotted blood and serum for up to 24 hours after centrifugation.

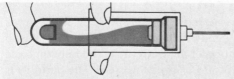

1. The CORVAC tube utilizes traditional phlebotomy techniques.

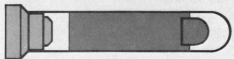

2. Powdered glass suspended throughout the sample accelerates coagulation.

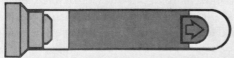

3. Centrifugal force drives the gel energizer into the silicone gel at the base of the tube.

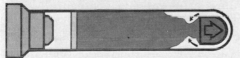

4. The energizer controls the flow of the gel up the sides of the tube.

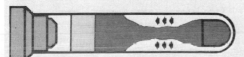

5. The gel continues to move up the sides of the tube, seeking an equilibrium between serum and coagulum.

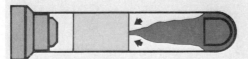

6. The gel reaches an equilibrium between serum and coagulum.

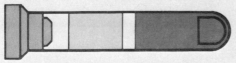

7. The gel forms a stable barrier between serum and coagulum.

Figure 3–12. How the Corvac works. *(Courtesy of Monoject Scientific, a Division of Sherwood Medical.)*

The Butterfly (Winged Infusion Set)

The butterfly (winged infusion set) is the most commonly used intravenous device. It is a stainless steel beveled needle and tube with attached plastic wings as shown in Figure 3–13. A variation of the butterfly is the heparin lock. The most common butterfly sizes are 20- and 23-gauge needles. The butterfly is sometimes used in the collection of blood from patients who are difficult to stick by conventional methods or in pediatric patients. MBO Laboratories, Inc. (North Chelmsford, Mass.) has developed the Angel Wing Safety Needle System (see Figure 3–14) that is equivalent to a butterfly needle apparatus but includes a stainless steel barrier to prevent needle-stick injuries.

Tourniquets

The tourniquet is a key to successful venipuncture: it provides a barrier against venous flow. Tourniquets that are usually used include: (1) pliable strap, (2) velcro-type, and (3) blood pressure cuff. The blood pressure cuff can be used very successfully when veins are difficult to find. The most efficient blood barrier provides a resistance that is less than systolic blood pressure, but greater than diastolic; or stated another way, blood flows in, but not out. The blood pressure cuff can determine these pressures, and consequently, is a perfect tourniquet.[19]

A new sophisticated tourniquet is the Seraket, which uses a seat-belt design. It allows the phlebotomist to partially release the venous pressure by using a lever that releases some pressure, but not all. Thus, if the phlebotomist

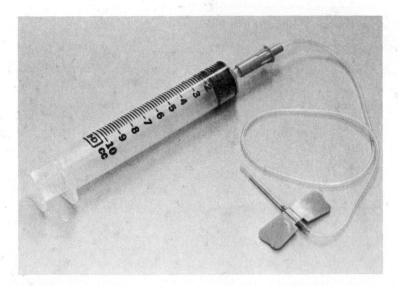

Figure 3–13. The butterfly. *(From Abbott Hospitals, Inc., North Chicago, Ill., and Becton-Dickinson and Company, Rutherford, N.J.)*

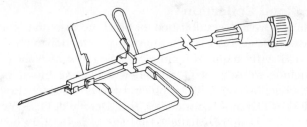

Figure 3–14. Angel wing safety needle system. *(Courtesy of MBO Laboratories, Inc., North Chelmsford, Mass.)*

needs to tighten the tourniquet again, the lever can be used to adjust the tourniquet. Since errors in laboratory test results can occur from prolonged tourniquet pressure, the Seraket provides a solution to this problem.

The Velcro-type tourniquets are popular because they are easy to apply and comfortable for the patient. With a major concern for infection control in health care institutions, many facilities are using disposable natural latex tourniquet strap (The Hygenic Corp., Akron, Ohio), to help prevent cross-contamination. If the tourniquets used in the health care facility are not disposable, it is extremely important to frequently wipe them with 70 percent isopropyl alcohol.

Testing Interference from Tourniquet Pressure

Laboratory test results can be falsely elevated or decreased if the tourniquet pressure is too tight or maintained too long. The pressure from the tourniquet causes biological analytes to leak out of the tissue cells into the blood or vice versa. For example, plasma cholesterol, iron, lipids, proteins, and potassium will be falsely elevated if the tourniquet pressure is too tight or prolonged on the arm. Significant elevations may be seen with as short as a 3-minute application of the tourniquet.[33] Some enzymes can be falsely elevated or decreased due to the tourniquet pressure that is too tight or prolonged.

Bleeding Time Equipment

Bleeding time is an assay used to assess the contributions of platelet function and blood vessel integrity to primary blood clotting abilities.[20] The test is performed by making a minor standardized incision in the forearm or earlobe and recording the length of time required for bleeding to stop. There have been many procedures used to measure the bleeding time. Recent advances have led to the development of mechanical devices to create uniform skin incisions for bleeding time. One such device is the Hemalet (Medprobe Laboratories, New York, N.Y.), which has an automatic blade retraction mechanism. Another such device is the Surgicutt (International Technidyne, Edison, N.J.), which provides a uniform, surgical incision. The procedure for bleeding time is provided in Chapter 5.

Gloves for Blood Collection

Safety guidelines have been established for phlebotomists and other laboratory workers to avoid the possibility of acquiring an infection such as hepatitis or those associated with acquired immunodeficiency syndrome (AIDS). These guidelines include the use of gloves when collecting blood from patients. Examples of gloves being used by phlebotomists include Ultraderm Sterile Surgeon's Gloves (Travenol Laboratories, Inc., Deerfield, Ill.); Talc Free Eudermic Surgical Gloves (Deseret Medical, Inc., Parke, Davis and Co., Sandy, Utah); Medi-Pak Latex Gloves (General Medical Corp., Richmond, Va.); and Non-Irritating Surgical Gloves—made without talc (Lab Safety Supply, Janesville, Wis.). It has been found that latex gloves have greater protection than vinyl gloves.[31] The Safeskin Hypo-Allergenic latex glove outperformed all other brands in the referenced study. If a phlebotomist develops allergenic dermatitis to gloves, he should try other brands of gloves or wear cotton gloves under the latex gloves. Also, glove liners have been developed that provide hand protection from cuts, nicks, and abrasions (Vigard Medical Products, Lovell-Schenck, Inc., Charlotte, N.C.). They are available in three styles—reusable, disposable, and clinical. It is recommended to avoid using gloves with a talc powder containing calcium since tubes of patients' blood may become contaminated with this powder, leading to falsely elevated calcium values.

Adhesive labels have been developed by Uarco Inc. that do not stick to gloves. These Glove-Free labels adhere firmly to glass, plastic, and paper, but will not stick to vinyl or latex gloves. The labels, coated with special adhesive, aid laboratory safety by eliminating the problems of torn gloves.

Antiseptics, Sterile Gauze Pads, and Bandages

The phlebotomist needs *antiseptics, sterile gauze pads,* and bandages for blood collection by either venipuncture or microcollection. Therefore, 70 percent isopropyl alcohol preps and povidone-iodine (Betadine) swab sticks or pads (for blood cultures) are essential items for blood collection. In addition, sterile gauze pads are needed to apply after blood collection. A new type of blood gauze has become available that is specifically designed to prevent hand contact with blood and other body fluids. The product, developed by Sealed Air Corporation (Fair Lawn, N.J.), consists of an absorbent material sandwiched between a fluid-permeable bottom layer and a fluid-barrier top layer. It can be used rather than sterile gauze pads for additional phlebotomy safety.

MICROCOLLECTION EQUIPMENT

Usually, skin-puncture blood collecting techniques are used on infants because venipuncture is excessively hazardous. Skin-puncture collection is indicated in adults for the following reasons: (1) severely burned, (2) veins that are difficult to stick due to their small size or location, (3) bedside clinical testing, (4) extreme obesity, or (5) home glucose testing.

The volume of plasma or serum that generally can be collected from a premature infant is approximately 100 to 150 μL, and about two times that amount from a full-term newborn. Larger volumes are obtained from older children and adults.[21]

A *disposable sterile lancet* should be used to puncture the skin for skin-puncture collection. In newborns, lancets with tips 2.4 mm or less in length, such as the B-D Microtainer Brand Safety Flow Lancet, are required to avoid penetrating bone.[22] Research indicates that for some infants (including premature infants) a puncturing depth of 2.4 mm may be excessive and needs more study.[32] The Monolet OPD Lancet (Sherwood Medical, St. Louis, Mo.) as shown in Figure 3–15 is a lancet available for safe skin puncture of neonates. In addition, Sherwood Medical manufactures Monolet Lancets for adults and children (see Figure 3–15).

International Technidyne Corp., Edison, N.J., has produced fully automated, single-use, automatically retracting, disposable devices that provide safety both for the neonate and for the phlebotomist. Tenderlett Jr. for children, Tenderlett for adults, and Tenderlett Toddler for infants and toddlers are

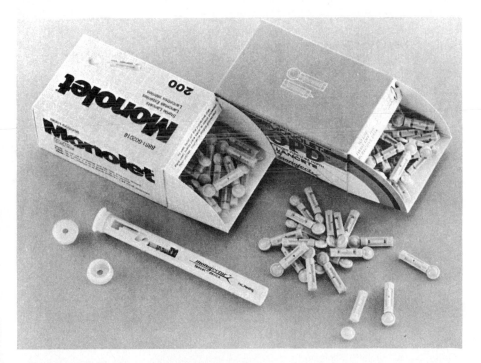

Figure 3–15. Monolet and Monojector lancet device. *(Courtesy of Sherwood Medical, St. Louis, Mo.)*

engineered to incise to the least invasive but effective depth for optimal blood flow. The Tenderlett incises 1.75 mm deep, Tenderlett Jr. incises 1.25 mm deep, and Tenderlett Toddler incises only 0.85 mm deep. The retracting blade eliminates potential injury from an exposed blade contaminated with blood.

Another method of microcollection is by the Autolet II Clinisafe (Figure 3–16) and the Autolet Lite Clinisafe (Figure 3–17). The Autolet II Clinisafe is a spring-activated puncture device that has easy ejection of the lancet and platform, providing safety for both patient and phlebotomist. The Autolet platform can be chosen for the patient's level of comfort and needed blood volume. These platforms are available in three (color-coded) depths; white (1.8 mm) for shallow penetration, yellow (2.4 mm) normal, and orange (3.0 mm) deeper (Figure 3–18).

The Autolet Lite Clinisafe features a new added safety mechanism that actually inhibits the use of the device unless first reloaded with a new lancet and platform. Complying with FDA/CDC guidelines, both lancet and platform can be used only *once,* and are simultaneously ejected at the touch of a button.

The Superfine lancets have been developed with a slimmer needle and a new bevel to allow for smooth and easy skin penetration, providing more comfort for the patient. Blades that do not have appropriate control of the cutting edge and depth of puncture should not be used.

Microcontainers used by the CPCC for blood gases, electrolytes, and general chemistry collections are shown in Table 3–7. Usually, microspecimens for blood gases are collected in heparinized glass Natelson tubes. These tubes may have a color band indicating the presence and type of anticoagulant. The band also identifies the top part of the pipet in reference to sample handling. A red band indicates ammonium heparin coated in the tube and green indicates sodium or lithium heparin. Since ammonium ions can falsely change the blood pH of the collected blood, sodium or lithium heparin should

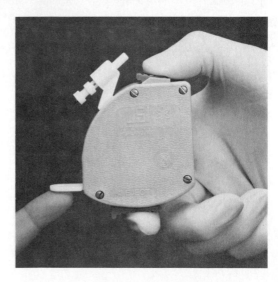

Figure 3–16. Autolet II Clinisafe blood drawing device. *(Courtesy of Ulster Scientific, Inc., New Paltz, N.Y.)*

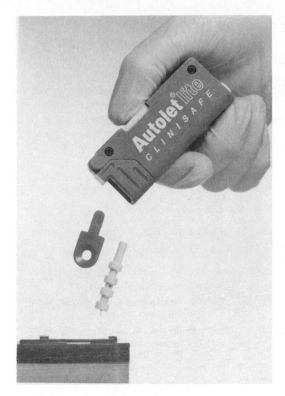

Figure 3–17. Autolet Lite Clinisafe blood drawing device. *(Courtesy of Ulster Scientific, Inc. New Paltz, N.Y.)*

be used in blood gas collections. The blood collected in these tubes must be mixed with the heparin by a small metal "flea" or bar with a magnet. After mixing, the ends are sealed with sealing wax or plastic caps.

AVL Scientific Corporation has recently developed the AVL microsampler for collection of two 120 µL arterial blood gas samples from children or adults.

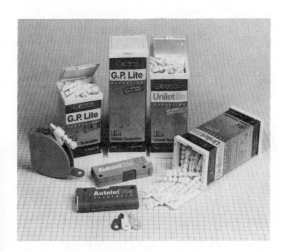

Figure 3–18. Ulster Scientific blood collection products. *(Courtesy of Ulster Scientific, Inc., New Paltz, N.Y.)*

TABLE 3–7. CONTAINERS FOR BLOOD COLLECTION

Container[a]	Remarks
Blood gases (pH, Pco_2, Po_2): Natelson glass collecting pipets, 250-μL volume, lithium heparin; heparinized glass capillary tubes, 100 to 250 μL.	To mix, insert metal "fleas" or mixing bars, after filling.[b] Seal with plastic caps or sealing wax. Mix by use of a magnet. Source: many laboratory suppliers.
Blood-collecting pipet kits and component parts, supplied by manufacturers of blood-gas apparatus.	Kits containing glass capillaries, sealing wax, metal mixing bars, and magnets. Source: laboratory suppliers of Corning, IL and Radiometer equipment.
Caraway glass tubes, 370-μL volume, ammonium heparin.	Mix and seal as above, or by inverison. Source: many laboratory suppliers.
Electrolytes (CO_2, Cl, K, Na) and general chemistry:	
Microhematocrit glass capillary tubes 1.1–1.2 mm i.d., 75 mm long, ammonium heparin; other sizes.	Plasma obtained. Mix and seal as above.
Microsample tubes, polyethylene, 300 μL, lithium heparin; larger sizes (400 to 550 μL) for general chemistry, with and without heparin.	Plasma obtained. Seal with attached cap. Mix by inversion.[c] Source: Kew Scientific and Beckman Instruments, Inc.
B-D Microtainer, polypropylene, 600 and 700 μL, silicone separator, with and without lithium heparin.	Serum obtained. Seal with accompanying cap. Centrifuge at 6000 $\times$ g. Source: Becton-Dickinson.

[a]Containers listed here are all commercially available.
[b]Mixing without a flea is also possible by gently inverting the capillary before sealing.
[c]Shake the first drop entering the tube to its bottom. All further drops should then flow along the path of the first drop if the tube is held in a nearly vertical position.
From Meites S (ed.): *Pediatric Clinical Chemistry*, 3rd ed. Washington, D.C., American Association of Clinical Chemistry, 1989, p. 10, with permission.

It has a 26 gauge microneedle, which reduces the chances of puncture pain and hematomas. The tubes are coated with heparin to prevent clotting. They automatically fill without any bubble formation. This microsampler is used on the radial, brachial, or femoral artery.

Microhematocrit *capillary tubes* are disposable narrow-bore pipets that are used for packed red cell volume in microcentrifugation. These tubes have colored bands in which a red band indicates heparin-coated and a blue band indicates no anticoagulant.

Plastic microcollection devices for general laboratory collections (e.g., chemistry, immunology) usually are color-coded according to the established protocol for blood collection vacuum tube stoppers. Thus, purple (lavender) tubes contain EDTA, green tubes contain heparin, red or pink tubes have no additive, and gray tubes have sodium fluoride to inhibit blood enzymes that destroy glucose.

Electrolytes and general chemistry microspecimens can be collected in the B-D Microtainer tube (Becton-Dickinson and Company, Rutherford, N.J.) that has its own capillary blood collector, self-contained serum separator, and red stopper, as shown in Figure 3–19. This system can collect up to 600 µL of blood. Alternately, two or more capillary tubes can be used for electrolyte and general chemistry collection. An advantage of these tubes is that if blood is hemolyzed in one capillary tube, another capillary tube containing the patient's sample can be used for the chemical analyses.

The Microvette Capillary Blood Collection system (Becton-Dickinson and Company, Rutherford, N.J.) is another microcollection system that has a full range of the anticoagulants and serum separation gel. This system can be used to collect, store, and separate samples in the same unbreakable, disposable container (Fig. 3–20).

Sherwood Medical (St. Louis, Mo.) manufactures the Samplette capillary blood collector. One of their collectors is an amber capillary blood separator that provides protection for light-sensitive analytes (i.e., bilirubin).

The RAM Scientific Co. (Princeton, N.J.) has developed an unbreakable plastic capillary/receptacle system. The device consists of a plastic capillary inserted in a microtube receptacle. With the attached receptacle, blood flows directly to the bottom of the tube. It makes the blood drawing safe and clean.

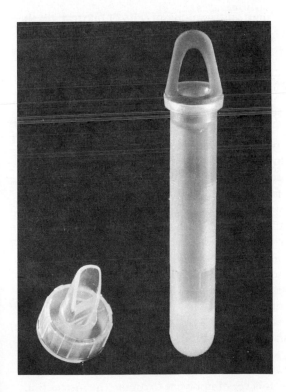

Figure 3–19. Microtainer tube. *(Courtesy of Becton-Dickinson and Company, Rutherford, N.J.)*

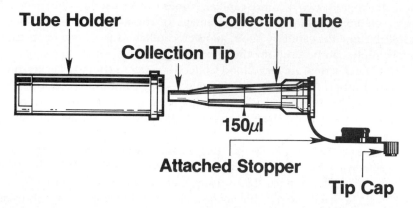

Figure 3–20. Microvette capillary blood collection system. *(Courtesy of Sarstedt, Inc., Princeton, N.J.)*

The capillary can then be removed and the tube is closed with the appropriate color-coded cap.

For most chemical assays, lithium and ammonium salts of heparin are the anticoagulants of choice for microcollections. They have rarely been reported to interfere with the determination of electrolytes and most other chemical assays.[23]

Another type of microcollection device is the B-D *Unopette* as shown in Figure 3–21. This device serves as a collection and dilution unit for blood samples, and thus increases the speed and simplicity of laboratory procedures. They are prefilled with specific amounts of diluents or reagents or both for different types of laboratory assays. Some of the more prevalent procedures in which Unopettes are used include WBC count, RBC count, platelet count, hemoglobin, RBC fragility test, sodium and potassium, and lead.

The standard Unopette test is comprised of (1) a disposable, self-filling diluting pipette consisting of a straight, thin-wall, uniform-bore glass capillary tube fitted into a plastic holder, and (2) a plastic reservoir containing a pre-measured volume of reagent for diluting.

Each capillary pipette is color-coded according to capacity for quick and easy visual identification. Color-coding for all disposable self-filling Unopette capillary pipettes is as follows: 3 μL—green, 3.3 μL—gray, 10 μL—pink, 20 μL—yellow, 25 μL—blue, and 44.7 μL—black.

Sealing Items for Microcollection Tubes

For capillary pipets and tubes, sealing wax or caps are necessary when the blood is drawn into the tube. Puttylike sealants and plastic closures are available from various manufacturers. It is very important to follow the instructions

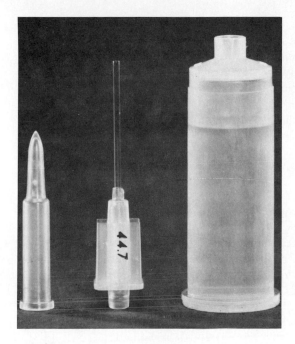

Figure 3–21. Unopette—a collection and dilution unit for blood samples. *(Courtesy of Becton-Dickinson and Company, Rutherford, N.J.)*

with the sealant in order to provide safe sealing during microcentrifugation. A capillary tube device that has been developed to reduce the opportunity for blowout of the sealant during microcentrifugation is the Safecap capillary and Safeplug (Safe-Tec, Inc.). Safecap capillary has a self-sealing plug called Safeplug that has been manufactured to permit a more accurate measurement of the packed cell volume and decrease biohazardous risk to blood splatters and aerosols during microcentrifugation.

Transporting Microspecimens

Glycolysis in RBCs and WBCs causes a decrease in blood pH that can be detected after a blood gas sample has been at room temperature for approximately 20 minutes. Therefore, blood gas microsamples should be immersed in ice water from time of collection until delivered to the clinical laboratory. Plastic containers that are small enough to hold these specimens with ice and water should be carried on the specimen collection tray. Ice is usually available on the patient ward. Other items to be carried on a microcollection tray include

1. 70% isopropyl alcohol and Betadine pads
2. Marking pens for labels
3. Microtainer blood serum separator tubes, 600 μL
4. Microtainer capillary whole blood cell collectors with 0.23 mg EDTA, 200 μL
5. Lancets for skin puncture

6. Sterile gauze pads
7. Unheparinized plastic microcentrifuge tubes
8. Heparinized plastic microcentrifuge tubes, 250, 400, and 500 μL
9. Heparinized Natelson tubes, 75 μL
10. Unopettes for collection and dilution procedures
11. Disposable gloves
12. Cloth towel or washcloth and thermometer

BLOOD-DRAWING CHAIR

For an outpatient clinic that requires blood collections, it is important to have a *blood-drawing chair* for these patients. The chair is designed for maximum safety and comfort of the patient plus the phlebotomist's easy accessibility to either arm of the patient. The chair should have a patient's arm rest for blood drawing. The arm rest should lock in place so that the patient cannot fall from the chair if he or she becomes faint. Also, the arm rest should adjust in an up and down position so that the best venipuncture position for each patient can be achieved.

SPECIMEN COLLECTION TRAYS

The phlebotomist needs a specimen tray (Fig. 3–22) to take on blood collecting rounds. The tray is usually made of plastic and must be sterilizable. The tray should include all necessary collection equipment and usually differs from one hospital or clinic to another depending upon the patient population. For example, if the phlebotomist works in a children's hospital, he or she needs micro-collection trays as described earlier.

Phlebotomists who collect blood from adults usually have the following equipment on their trays:

1. Marking pens
2. Vacuum tubes (sterile and nonsterile) with the anticoagulants designated in the clinical laboratory blood collection manual
3. Holders for vacuum tubes
4. Needles for vacuum tubes and syringes
5. Syringes
6. Tourniquet
7. 70% isopropyl alcohol, iodine, and Betadine pads or swab sticks
8. Sterile gauze pads
9. Bandages
10. Dispensers for needles

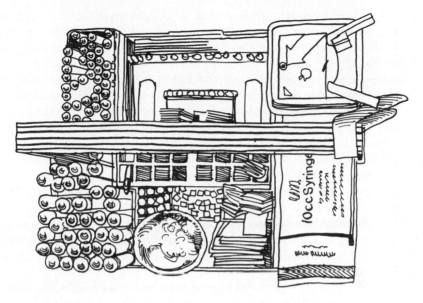

Figure 3–22. Specimen collection tray. *(Courtesy of College of American Pathologists [CAP], Skokie, Ill.)*

11. Lancets for skin puncture
12. Unopettes for finger-stick blood collection
13. Microtainer blood serum separator tubes, 600 μL
14. Microtainer capillary whole blood collectors with 0.23 mg EDTA, 200 μL
15. Disposable gloves
16. Cloth towel or washcloth and thermometer

TRANSPORTING AND PROCESSING PATIENT SPECIMENS

Every hospital or clinic has its specific protocol for specimen transport and process. Many institutions require the use of a leakproof plastic bag for insertion of the specimen container. This bag provides protection of the phlebotomist from pathogenic (disease-producing) organisms during transportation of the specimen. Usually, this special transport bag has a pouch to carry the laboratory request slip on the outside of the bag. Thus, the potential for contamination of the request slip is eliminated with the use of this outer pouch. For special types of specimens, the clinical laboratory has special handling steps. For example, if a phlebotomist is requested to transport to the laboratory an arterial specimen for blood gases, then he or she should be aware that the specimen must be transported in an airtight heparinized syringe and packed in ice with water. The airtight container and the ice water decreases the loss of gases from the specimen. Speed is essential to avoid loss of gases from the blood.

Because glycolytic action from the blood cells interferes in chemical analysis of various chemical analysis (e.g., glucose, calcitonin, aldosterone, phosphorus, enzymes), the blood samples should be transported to the clinical laboratory within 45 minutes from the time of collection so that the serum or plasma can be separated from the blood cells. The serum or plasma that is separated from the cells must be handled according to the laboratory procedure; therefore, it may remain at room temperature, be refrigerated, stored in a dark place, or be frozen depending upon the prescribed laboratory method.

Some chemical constituents in blood such as bilirubin are light sensitive and decrease in value if exposed to light. Thus, blood collected for chemical analysis should be protected from bright light with an aluminum foil wrapping around the tube.

Blood specimens for microbiology need to be transported to the laboratory as quickly as possible so that the blood can be transferred to culture media.

The blood vacuum tubes and microtainers should be maintained in a vertical position to (1) promote complete clot formation, if required, and (2) reduce the possibility of hemolysis. It is also imperative to transport the blood specimens in a gentle manner to avoid hemolyzing the specimens.

Processing specimens may occur in one location of the clinical laboratory or in each section (hematology, clinical chemistry, clinical immunology, blood bank, coagulation) dependent upon the organization of the laboratory. The phlebotomist must learn the processing requirements of the clinical laboratory so that specimens are transported and processed as quickly as possible. As discussed earlier in this chapter, safety devices should be used to gain access to the blood to avoid splashing and aerosol from the blood sample. Efficient and safe processing of the specimens leads to better clinical laboratory results and thus better patient care. In many laboratories, the specimen collection area has a medical technologist (clinical laboratory scientist) or medical laboratory technician who centrifuges the specimens and makes the appropriate aliquots for each section. These aliquots are then distributed to the clinical laboratory sections for testing. Some specimens must be prepared for shipping to referral laboratories. This preparation sometimes involves special packaging requirements such as freezing the specimen to maintain stability and packaging it in a styrofoam mailing container. (See Chapter 10 for more information on shipping laboratory specimens to reference laboratories.) The phlebotomist should learn the clinical laboratory tasks in which he or she can assist the technologist/ technician in enhancing the efficiency of specimen processing.

KEY TERMS

acid citrate dextrose	gastric secretions	separation tubes
amniotic fluid	gauge number	serum
anticoagulants	gloves	single-sample needle
antiseptics	heparin	sodium fluoride and
bleeding time	microcollection	thymol
equipment	equipment	specimen collection
blood-drawing chair	microcontainers	trays
capillary tubes	midstream specimens	specimen transport
cerebrospinal fluid	multiple sample	sterile gauze pads
citrates	needle	synovial fluid
citrate phosphate	needle resheather	tourniquet
dextrose	oxalates	24-hour urine
clean-catch urine	pericardial fluid	specimen
specimen	peritoneal fluid	Unopette
culture specimens	plasma	urine collections
disposable sterile	pleural fluid	vacuum tube
lancet	protective needle	(Vacutainer)
drug interferences	device	whole blood
ethylenediaminetetra-	sealing items	winged infusion set
acetate (EDTA)	seminal fluid	

STUDY QUESTIONS

The following questions may have one or more answers:

1. Which of the following anticoagulants prevents coagulation of blood by removing calcium through the formation of insoluble calcium salts?

   a. EDTA   c. sodium citrate
   b. ammonium oxalate   d. sodium heparin

2. Which of the following anticoagulants is found in a green-stoppered blood collecting vacuum tube?

   a. EDTA   c. sodium citrate
   b. ammonium oxalate   d. sodium heparin

3. Which of the following proteins is found in plasma, but not in serum?

   a. albumin   c. fibrin
   b. fibrinogen   d. globulins

4. Which of the following body fluids is extracted from joint cavities?

   a. pleural fluid
   b. peritoneal fluid

   c. synovial fluid
   d. pericardial fluid

5. When blood is collected from a patient with a syringe, the needle should be removed from the syringe before transferring the blood to a tube in order to prevent

   a. hemoconcentration
   b. hemolysis

   c. glycolysis
   d. hemostasis

6. For capillary collection from newborns, a lancet with which of the following lengths should be used to avoid penetrating bone?

   a. 2.50 mm
   b. 2.75 mm

   c. 3.00 mm
   d. 3.25 mm

7. Which of the following blood chemical constituents is light sensitive?

   a. glucose
   b. bilirubin

   c. phosphorus
   d. blood gases

8. When blood is collected from a patient, the serum should be separated from the blood cells as quickly as possible to avoid

   a. hemoconcentration
   b. hemolysis

   c. glycolysis
   d. hemostasis

REFERENCES

1. Garza D: Urine collection and preservation. In Ross DL, Neely AE (eds): *Textbook of Urinalysis and Body Fluids.* New York, Appleton-Century-Crofts, 1983, p 61.
2. Free AH, Free HM: *Urinalysis in Clinical Laboratory Practice.* Cleveland, CRC Press, 1975.
3. Tietz N (ed): *Fundamentals of Clinical Chemistry.* Philadelphia, WB Saunders, 1976.
4. National Committee for Clinical Laboratory Standards: *NCCLS Document EP7-P— Interference Testing in Clinical Chemistry.* NCCLS, 1986, Vol 6, no 13, 1986.
5. Sunderman FW: Drug interference in clinical biochemistry. *Crit Rev Clin Lab Sci* 1:427, 1970.
6. Meites S: Calcium (fluorometric). *Stand Methods Clin Chem* 6:207, 1970.
7. Sher PP: Drug interferences with clinical laboratory tests. *Drugs* 24:24, 1982.
8. Romano AT: Automated glucose methods: Evaluation of glucose oxidase– peroxidase procedure. *Clin Chem* 19:1152, 1973.

9. Neely WE: Simple automated determination of serum or plasma glucose by a hexo-kinase/G6PD method. *Clin Chem* 18:509, 1972.

10. Garb S: *Clinical Guide to Undesirable Drug Interactions and Interferences.* New York, Springer, 1971.

11. El-Dorry HF, Medina H, Bacila M: Interference of phenothiazine compounds in colorimetric determination of inorganic phosphate. *Anal Biochem* 47:329, 1972.

12. Hansten PD: *Drug Interactions.* Philadelphia, Lea & Febiger, 1981.

13. Lubran M: The effects of drugs on laboratory values. *Med Clin North Am* 53:211, 1969.

14. Sapira JD, Klaniecki T, Ratkin G: Nonpheochromocytoma. *JAMA* 212:2243, 1970.

15. Siest G (ed): *Drug Effects on Laboratory Test Results.* The Hague, Martinus Nijhoff, 1980.

16. Sherlock S: Progress report: Hepatic reaction to drugs. *Gut* 20:634, 1979.

17. Mettler FA: Manifestations of drug toxicity. *Curr Prob Diag Radiol* 13(4):1, 1979.

18. College of American Pathologists: *Standards for Accreditation of Medical Laboratories.* Skokie, Ill., 1974.

19. Scranton PE: *Practical Techniques in Venipuncture.* Baltimore, Williams & Wilkins, 1977, p 66.

20. Harker LA, Slichter SI: The bleeding time as a screening test for evaluation of platelet function. *N Engl J Med* 287:155, 1972.

21. *Procedures for the Collection of Diagnostic Blood Specimens by Skin Puncture: H4-A3.* Villanova, Penn., National Committee for Clinical Laboratory Standards (NCCLS), 1991.

22. Meites S (ed): *Pediatric Clinical Chemistry,* 3rd ed. Washington, D.C., American Association for Clinical Chemistry, 1989.

23. Young DS, Pestaner LC, Gibberman V: Effects of drugs on clinical laboratory tests. *Clin Chem* 21, ID-4320, 1975 (special issue).

24. Young DS: *Effects of Drugs on Clinical Laboratory Tests.* Washington, D.C.: AACC Press, 1990.

25. Routh J, Paul W: Assessment of interference by aspirin with some assays commonly done in the clinical laboratory. *Clin Chem,* 22:837, 1976.

26. Panek E, Young D, Bente J: Analytical interference of drugs in clinical chemistry. *Am J Med Technol* 44:217, 1978.

27. Siest G, Galteau M: *Drugs Effects on Laboratory Test Results.* Littleton, MA, PSG Pub. Co, 1988, p 433.

28. Letellier G, Desjarlais F: Analytical interference of drugs in clinical chemistry: I—study of twenty drugs on seven different instruments. *Clin Biochem* 18:345, 1985.

29. Elin RJ, Bloom JN, Herman DC, et al: Interference by intravenous fluorescein with laboratory tests. *Clin Chem* 35(6):1159, 1989.

30. National Committee for Clinical Laboratory Standards: *Procedures for the Collection of Diagnostic Blood Specimens by Venipuncture* (3rd ed). Approved Standard, NCCLS Document H3-A3. Villanova, Penn., NCCLS, 1991.

31. Brown JW, Backwell H: Putting on gloves in the fight against AIDS. *Med Lab Observ* Nov:47, 1990.

32. Reiner CB, Meites S, Hayes J: Optimal sites and depths for specimens by skin puncture of infants and children as assessed from anatomical measurements. *Clin Chem* 36:574, 1990.

33. Statland BE, Winkle P, Bokelund H: Factors contributing to intra-individual variation of serum constituents. 4. Effects of posture and tourniquet application on variation of serum constituents in healthy subjects. *Clin Chem* 20:1513, 1974.

34. Hyman D, Kaplan N: The difference between serum and plasma potassium (letter). *N Engl J Med* 313:642, 1985.

4 Collection Procedures and Physiologic Complications

BLOOD COLLECTION

In preparing for blood collection, each phlebotomist generally establishes a routine that is comfortable for him or her. However, several essential steps go into every successful collection procedure. This chapter discusses the following steps in the sequential manner in which one would progress through the blood collection process.

1. Assessing the patient's physical disposition
2. Identifying the patient and samples
3. Approaching the patient
4. Selecting and preparing equipment/supplies
5. Finding a puncture site
6. Preparing the puncture site
7. Skin or venipuncture methods
8. Collecting the sample in the appropriate tubes
9. Complications and special considerations associated with phlebotomy

10. Assessing criteria for sample recollection or rejection
11. Prioritizing patients and sample tubes

PHYSICAL DISPOSITION

Basal State

It is recommended that blood specimens for determining the concentration of body constituents such as glucose, cholesterol, triglycerides, electrolytes, and proteins be collected when the patient is in a *basal state,* that is, in the early morning approximately 12 hours after the last ingestion of food. Laboratory test results on basal state specimens are more reliable because normal values are most often determined from specimens collected during this time. Several factors such as diet, exercise, emotional stress, obesity, menstrual cycle, pregnancy, *diurnal variations,* posture, tourniquet application, and chemical constituents (alcohol or drugs), cause changes in the basal state. For information on chemical substances that interfere with laboratory results, see Chapter 3.

Diet

To ensure that the patient is in the basal state, an overnight fast is necessary. The term *fasting* refers to abstinence from food and beverages (except water). The required time period necessary for abstaining varies with test procedure(s) to be performed. Before collecting a specimen, it is recommended that the phlebotomist ask the patient if he or she has eaten. Blood composition is significantly altered after meals and consequently is not suitable for many clinical chemistry tests. If the patient has eaten, and the physician still needs the test, it is informative if the word "NONFASTING" is written on the requisition form.[1]

Inadequate patient instructions are often the cause of mistakes in specimen collection. The phlebotomist may be asked to explain diet restrictions to a patient. In such cases, it is necessary to explain the fasting restrictions clearly and in detail. Written instructions can be given, if available. Gaining the patient's understanding and cooperation is important and is determined by the professional behavior and degree of confidence displayed by the phlebotomist. Casual instructions are apt to be taken lightly by the patient or even forgotten. A phlebotomist who is organized, attentive, and skilled and who emphasizes important points of the procedure is more likely to get patient cooperation and an accurate test result and to make the patient more comfortable. If a procedure involves some discomfort or inconvenience, the patient should be so informed. For example, if timed blood glucose levels are to be drawn, the patient needs to fast for 12 to 14 hours. The phlebotomist can inform the patient that several specimens will be collected at timed intervals and that he or she may drink water but coffee and tea should be avoided because they cause a transitory fluctuation in the blood sugar level. Similarly, some patients assume that the term "fasting" refers to abstaining from food *and* water. Abstaining from water can result in dehydration which can also alter test results.

Normally, serum is clear, light yellow, or straw colored. *Turbid* serum appears cloudy or "milky" and can be due to bacterial contamination or high lipid levels in the blood. It is caused primarily by ingestion of fatty substances such as meat, butter, cream, and cheese. If a patient has recently eaten these substances, she may have a temporarily elevated lipid level and the serum will appear "lipemic" or cloudy. Lipemic serum does not represent a basal state and a note on the requisition form about the appearance may be useful to the physician. Some chemical abnormalities may be indicated by lipemic serum.[1]

Exercise

Muscular activity, as a result of moderate or excessive exercise, has a marked effect on laboratory results such as lactic acid, creatinine, fatty acids, some amino acids, proteins, and some enzymes. Most of these values, except for certain enzymes, return to baseline levels shortly after stopping the exercise. However, enzymes such as creatine phosphokinase (CPK), aspartate amino transferase (AST), and lactate dehydrogenase (LDH) can remain elevated even after 24 hours following 1 hour of moderate to strenuous exercise.[1]

There are also substantial data available to suggest that exercise has some effects on hemostasis. Some reports indicate that physical exercise activates coagulation, fibrinolysis, and platelets. Due to different types of exercise, other studies report conflicting results or no changes in measured hemostatic parameters. Most would conclude, however, that some hemostatic changes do occur after strenuous exercise.[2]

Stress

Patients are often frightened, nervous, and overly anxious. These emotional stresses can cause a transient elevation in white blood cells (WBCs), transient decrease in serum iron, and abnormal adrenal hormone values.[1,3] Newborn infants who have been crying violently will display WBC counts 140 percent above resting baseline counts. Even mild crying has been shown to increase WBC counts 113 percent. These elevated counts return to baseline values within 1 hour. It is recommended that blood samples for WBC counts be taken after approximately 1 hour has elapsed.[4] Anxiety that results in hyperventilation also causes acid–base imbalances, increased lactate, and increased fatty acids.[1]

Diurnal Rhythms and Posture

Diurnal rhythms are body fluid fluctuations during the day. Certain hormone levels are decreased in the afternoon, while eosinophil counts and serum iron levels are elevated.

Posture changes are known to vary laboratory results of some constituents. This is an important consideration when comparing inpatient and outpatient results. Changing from *supine* (lying) position to a sitting or standing position causes body water to shift from intravascular to interstitial compartments (in tissues). Certain larger molecules are not filterable into the tissue; therefore they become more concentrated in the blood. Enzymes, proteins, lipids, iron, and calcium are significantly increased with changes in position.[2]

Other Factors Affecting the Patient
Many other factors can affect laboratory results. Age, gender, and pregnancy have an influence on laboratory testing. Reference ranges are often noted according to age.

Geographical location, that is, altitude, temperature, and humidity, also affect normal baseline values. Therefore, it is important that each clinical laboratory establish normal reference values for their own population of patients and their location.

Medications may also alter laboratory results significantly. Therefore, physicians must work closely with pharmacy and laboratory staff to rule out falsely elevated laboratory results due to medications. (See Chapter 3 on Interference of Drugs and Other Substances in Blood.)

IDENTIFICATION

Patient Identification
Hospitalized patients should wear an identification bracelet indicating their name and designated hospital number (often called a "unit number"). Hospital identification numbers help distinguish patients with the same first or last names. Upon entering the room, the phlebotomist should ask the patient what his or her name is. If one asks, "Are you Ms. Doe?" an ill patient on medication may mistakenly answer yes, so it is best to ask "What is your name?" and let the patient reply. PRIOR TO ANY SPECIMEN COLLECTION, THE PATIENT *MUST* BE CORRECTLY IDENTIFIED BY HIS OR HER IDENTIFICATION BRACELET. Information on the bracelet may also include the patient's room number, bed assignment, and physician (Fig. 4–1). A three-way match should be made using the ID bracelet, the test requisition, and the patient's statement of his or her name. Never use the name card on the bed or door as these are frequently incorrect. If the patient does not have an identification bracelet, the nurse responsible for the patient must be asked to make the identification. Documentation of the situation and the nurse's name should be made on the requisition form. It is recommended that specimens *not be collected* until a positive identification can be made. Blood drawn from a misidentified patient can lead to serious consequences and is an action for which one may be counseled or dismissed.

Patient identification for ambulatory patients is usually more difficult to monitor. Most outpatient clinics distribute identification cards to patients prior

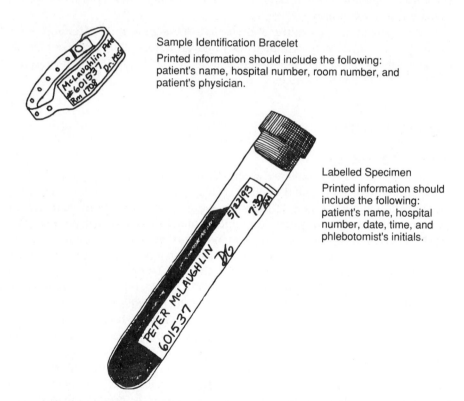

Sample Requisition Form

Sample Identification Bracelet

Printed information should include the following: patient's name, hospital number, room number, and patient's physician.

Labelled Specimen

Printed information should include the following: patient's name, hospital number, date, time, and phlebotomist's initials.

Figure 4–1. Identification bracelet, requisition, labeling.

to having any specimens collected. If this is the case, and the patient has it available, positive identification can occur in the same manner as with hospitalized patients. More recently, some ambulatory clinics have issued identification bracelets to patients. If the patient does not have a patient identification bracelet or card, it is *strongly recommended* that another form of identification be checked and documented prior to specimen collection. Sometimes the patient, for example, an infant or child, may not have any form of identification. It is *strongly recommended* that someone else, for example, the nurse or a parent, be asked to confirm the identification, verify the birth date, and document the incident prior to specimen collection. Misidentification of patients' specimens can result in serious medical consequences for the patient and disciplinary action or dismissal for the employee who collected the specimen.

Specimen Identification and Labeling
Specimens should be labeled immediately at the patient's bedside or ambulatory setting and consistently include the following information (see Fig. 4–1):

1. Patient's full name
2. Patient's ID number
3. Date of collection
4. Time of collection
5. Phlebotomist's initials
6. Patient's room number, bed assignment, or outpatient status is optional information

For hospitalized patients, the tubes should be labeled immediately after the specimen has been collected. It is recommended that tubes not be "prelabeled" because the tubes may end up not being used. They might then be erroneously picked up and used on another patient. Also, a different phlebotomist may complete the venipuncture after another phlebotomist was unsuccessful. In that case, the "prelabeled" tubes may contain the initials of the first phlebotomist, and therefore, be inaccurate. In addition, if the "prelabeled" tubes are not used, it may be difficult to tear off the old or unused label because of the adhesive; thus, one would either have to place a new label (from a different patient) onto the tube with a partially torn label, *or* discard the unused tube entirely. Either option is unsatisfactory, messy, and wasteful. For the ambulatory care setting, there are mixed opinions about when to label the blood collection tube. The *National Committee for Clinical Laboratory Standards (NCCLS)* suggests that the phlebotomist "must apply a label to each of the necessary tubes," prior to the actual collection process.[1] However, many phlebotomists (the authors included) believe that the same risks exist with "prelabeled" tubes in the outpatient setting as in the inpatient setting. Therefore, each laboratory procedure manual should contain explicit instructions on labeling requirements and supervisors should spend ample time training and observing new employees in their identification and labeling practices.

For unidentified or unconscious patients who come to the hospital through the emergency room or through unusual circumstances, a temporary identification number can be assigned. It is recommended that it be a multiple part form with the same ID number on each part. One part can be attached to the patient's arm and the other can be used for the specimens. When the hospital's permanent identification number is assigned to the patient, it can be cross-referenced to the "temporary" one.[1]

The phlebotomist should confirm all the information before leaving the patient's hospital room or before drawing another clinic outpatient. The date and time are necessary because requisition forms may indicate the date and time a laboratory test was *ordered,* rather than the date and time it was *collected.* In timed specimens, for example, glucose tolerance, the actual collection time is critical to the test. The phlebotomist's initials are necessary to help clarify questions about the specimen if any arise during laboratory processing or testing.

There is no foolproof method for labeling specimens. The phlebotomist may write directly on the container. Many commercial collection tubes have an affixed blank label for this purpose. In addition, many hospitals use computer-generated labels for collection tubes. However, capillary tubes, microcollection tubes and vials, or other containers without labels must be identified either by labeling them directly with a permanent felt-tip pen, by wrapping an adhesive label around them, or by placing them into a larger labeled test tube for transport. In some cases, small computerized adhesive labels with printed information are available with and detachable from the requisition form.

Laboratory requisition forms must contain the following information (see Fig. 4–1):

1. Patient's full name
2. Patient's identification number
3. Date of collection
4. Time of collection
5. Collector's initials
6. Room number
7. Physician's name and code

PERFORMING THE PHLEBOTOMY

Phlebotomist Preparation

Prior to performing any type of specimen collection it is important to have all equipment, supplies, forms, and so forth ready for the procedure. If patient information is incomplete, the phlebotomist will not be able to correctly identify the patient. Assistance from a nurse will be required. Also, if the phlebotomist does not understand the test ordered, a supervisor or laboratory technologist should be consulted prior to the phlebotomy procedure. All phlebotomists must be familiar with current recommendations and hospital policies on precautions for handling blood and body fluids. In general, ALL SPECIMENS SHOULD BE TREATED AS IF THEY ARE HAZARDOUS AND INFECTIOUS. Hands should be washed before and after specimen collection procedures. A clean pair of gloves should be put on in the presence of the patient. This is a safety conscious, reassuring gesture for the patient and the phlebotomist. A clean, pressed uniform with a laboratory coat also instills a sense of commitment to safety and cleanliness, which is gratifying to patients and promotes a safer work environment for phlebotomists. Changing, wearing, and discarding gloves appropriately are all vital aspects in the safety and well-being of patients and phlebotomists. According to the Centers for Disease Control (CDC), "blood and other body fluids from *all* patients should be considered infective."[7] Among other recommendations, CDC states that "gloves should be worn for touching blood and body fluids, mucous membranes, or nonintact skin of all patients, for handling items or surfaces soiled with blood or body fluids, and for performing venipuncture and other vascular access procedures."[7] If the phlebotomist's skin or clothing is contaminated with a specimen, the contaminated site must be decontaminated before moving to the next patient. In the case of a blood spill on a laboratory coat, the coat should be removed and washed properly. A clean lab coat should be worn. If a phlebotomist accidently sustains a needle injury, it should be reported to supervisory personnel immediately for appropriate action. After it is reported, employers are responsible for notifying appropriate people within the hospital (the patient's physician, employee health physician, Infection Control staff, etc.). Appropriate infection control policies and procedures must be followed for the phlebotomist's protection. All other supplies should be regularly checked for expiration dates, and availability should be easily accessible during the procedure.

In addition to being prepared with the proper equipment and supplies, it is also important to be emotionally prepared. This involves professional appearance and behavior, and exercising good communication skills. These topics are discussed in greater detail in Chapter 8.

Approaching the Patient

There are several professional and courteous behaviors and phrases that can help ease into the patient–phlebotomist interaction. The first of these is a polite knock on the patient's door prior to entering her room. The phlebotomist should introduce himself and state that he is from the laboratory and has come to collect a blood sample. As stated above, it is vitally important that a correct identification be made. Once this has occurred, the process may continue. Sometimes, it is necessary to explain to the patient that the physician ordered the laboratory test(s). The phlebotomist may need to explain the procedure as supplies are being set up. The specimen collecting tray should *not be placed on the patient's bed or eating table!* As supplies are being readied and the vein is being palpated, the phlebotomist may try to alleviate some of the fears the patient may have. Chapter 8 covers verbal and nonverbal cues for detecting apprehension in patients.

A typical, professional patient approach and conversation may progress as follows:

Phlebotomist knocks on patient's door.

Phlebotomist:	"Good morning, I am Ms. Smith from the laboratory. I have come to collect a blood sample." Pause to give patient an opportunity to speak. If the lights are off or dimmed, explain that you need to turn the lights on. This gives the patient a moment to adjust to the idea of bright lights if she has been asleep.
	"What is your name please?"
Patient responds:	"I am Jenny Jones."
Phlebotomist:	"May I see your identification (ID) armband?" Armband is checked in conjunction with laboratory requisitions, and patient's verbal identification. If all match, the process continues.
Phlebotomist:	"This will only take a few minutes."
Patient:	"Will it hurt?"
Phlebotomist:	"It will hurt a little but it will be over soon. Please allow me to look at your arm veins."

The remainder of the procedure can then take place keeping a highly professional and respectful atmosphere.

In general, it is not wise to ask a patient "How are you?" since most patients in the hospital do not feel well. Also, for certain tests the phlebotomist may need to ascertain whether or not the patient has been fasting. In this case the following question can be used: "Ms. Jones, when was the last time you ate or drank anything?" Use of this question avoids the term "fast" since some patients may not understand it completely. Also, when the phlebotomist is finished with the procedure it is nice to say, "Thank you, Ms. Jones."

EQUIPMENT SELECTION AND PREPARATION

The major categories of equipment and supplies used in specimen collection (Fig. 4–2) are as follows:

- Supplies for venipuncture
- Supplies for skin (capillary) puncture

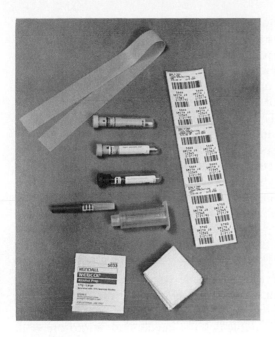

Figure 4–2. Supplies for venipuncture and skin puncture.

Supplies for Venipuncture

Supplies for venipuncture are different based on which method is used, i.e., *syringe method* or the *evacuated tube system.* Both methods of venipuncture involve the use of gloves, a *tourniquet,* alcohol pads or disinfectants, cotton balls, bandages or gauze pads, glass microscope slides, needles, syringes, or evacuated tube holders, capillary tubes, tube sealer, blood collection tubes, laboratory request slips or labels, marking pens, and discard buckets. These supplies are discussed in more detail in Chapter 3.

Tourniquets.   Tourniquets are used in specimen collection to apply enough pressure to the arm to slow the return of venous blood to the heart. This causes pooling of blood in the veins, which makes the veins more visible and easier to feel and find. A tourniquet should *not* restrict arterial blood flowing into the arm. Blood should enter the arm at a normal rate and, with the use of a tourniquet, return to the heart at a slower rate. Many tourniquets are available commercially worldwide. However, the most common one, which has been used for many years, consists of a 1-in. wide strip of rubber or rubber tubing. It is typically 12 to 15 in. long, which is long enough to go around the upper arm. Widths narrower than 1" can be very uncomfortable to the patient when tightened. Some of the more elaborate tourniquets have Velcro pads at the ends that adhere to each other, or a seat-belt type of fastener, which is released by lifting up on the buckle.[5]

Syringes.   Syringes may be various sizes and used for a variety of purposes such as withdrawing medications from a bottle, injections, and venipuncture procedures (Fig. 4–3). A syringe, without the needle, consists of the barrel, the plunger, and the tip. The barrel and plunger are made to fit together tightly so that when the plunger is in the barrel and drawn back, a vacuum is created. Thus, this vacuum allows blood or other fluids to be aspirated, or sucked into, the barrel as the plunger is pulled back. The barrel of the syringe has graduated measurements in milliliter (mL) increments. Sizes range from approximately 0.2 mL to 50 mL; however, for specimen collection purposes, syringes most often used are 5 to 20 mL. Most syringes used for phlebotomy are made of plastic and are disposable. Glass syringes are reusable, but are rarely used because they must be washed and sterilized prior to each use.

Needles are usually attached directly on the smooth tip of the syringe. Some glass syringes have "luer-lok" tips, which lock the needle onto the tip for a firm hold.

Evacuated Tube System.   The evacuated tube system requires three components: the evacuated sample tube, the double-pointed needle, and a special plastic holder (adapter) (Figure 4–4). Since the tube contains no air, a vacuum is created inside. One end of the double-pointed needle enters into the vein, then the other end pierces the tube's rubber stopper and the vacuum aspirates in the blood.

Needles for the evacuated tube system are pointed at both ends. The

Plunger   Barrel

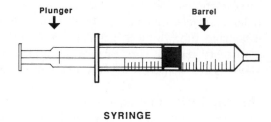

SYRINGE

Hub

Shaft   Bevel

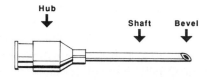

Figure 4–3. Syringe and needle.   NEEDLE

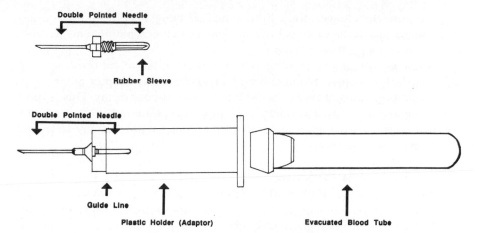

Figure 4–4. Evacuated tube system.

longer end is used for the vein puncture and the shorter end extends into the barrel to pierce the cap (or rubber stopper) of the sample tube. The needle typically screws or slips tightly onto the tip of the adapter, depending on which manufacturer is used. The needle also has a rubber "sleeve," which covers the short end and prevents blood leakage as multiple tubes are filled then removed. The needles are commercially available in various lengths and guages.

The evacuated tubes themselves are also available in a variety of sizes and with or without additives. The type of additive contained in the tube is depicted by the color of the rubber stopper or tube cap. Additives may be anticoagulants (to prevent blood clotting), clot activators (to speed up blood clotting), or separation media (to form a barrier between the cellular and liquid portions of the blood). Chapter 3 reviews specific additives in greater detail.

Many tubes are specifically designed to be used directly on chemistry, hematology, or microbiology instrumentation. In these cases, the tube of blood is identified by its bar code and pierced by the instrument probe, and some sample is aspirated into the instrument for analyses. Use of these "closed systems" minimizes the risk for exposure to blood. In addition, some tubes have plastic "screw-on" enclosures around the rubber stopper to minimize exposure to blood left on the top of the cap or blood splatters during cap removal. One example of this is the Labco Exetainer System, which was invented and is widely used in Great Britain. It is approved for use in the United States and numerous other countries.

Evacuated tubes are also used for transferring blood from a syringe into the tubes. The syringe needle is simply pushed through the rubber stopper and blood is automatically pulled into the tube because of the vacuum. There is no need to push the plunger down if the tubes are being filled from the syringe. This would hasten the process but may damage cellular components because of the forceful expulsion of blood.

There are also specialized tubes and bottles for blood culture collection that may fit the adapter. Blood cultures are discussed in Chapter 5.

Expiration dates of tubes should be monitored continually. This is most easily accomplished by a computerized inventory system; however, routine rotation of stocked supplies and careful checking of phlebotomy trays and carts can also accomplish this.

Supplies for Skin Puncture

Supplies for skin puncture would include the following: gloves, lancets or automatic puncture devices, capillary tubes or micropipets, disinfectant pads, cotton balls, bandages, or gauze pads, glass microscope slides, microcollection tubes or capillary tubes, capillary tube sealer, laboratory request slips or labels, a marking pen, and a discard bucket.

Skin punctures are particularly useful for pediatric patients when small amounts of blood can be obtained and adequately tested. In contrast, venipuncture in children can be hazardous and difficult because of the risk of complications such as anemia, cardiac arrest, hemorrhage, venous thrombosis, reflex arteriospasm, gangrene of an extremity, danger to surrounding tissues or organs, infections, and injuries from restraining the child during the procedure.[5] It is particularly important to withdraw only the smallest amounts of blood necessary from neonates, infants, and children so the effects of blood volume reduction are minimal. A 10-mL sample from a premature or newborn infant can represent 5 to 10 percent of the total blood volume in the entire body.

Skin punctures may also be more useful in adult patients who are severely burned or obese or have thrombotic tendencies, oncology patients whose veins are being "saved" for therapy, geriatric patients, or those who have fragile veins, and patients doing home testing (e.g., blood glucose screening).[6] There are also times when skin puncture cannot be used, i.e., if a patient has poor peripheral circulation.

Lancets.   *Lancets* have sharp metal points that are used for piercing skin and cutting the capillaries to allow blood flow and collection. They are made of sterilized metal, some are surrounded by plastic, and all are packaged individually. They are disposable and should BE USED ONLY ONCE! The distance that the lancet penetrates the skin is predefined by the manufacturers and ranges from 2.4 to 3.0 mm. This ensures a free flow of blood but minimizes the risk of bone puncture and damage. Some are color coded according to the depth of the puncture such that the pediatric devices are different from the adult ones.

Skin Puncture Devices.   Other automated puncture devices such as the Autolet are also available commercially and are typically designed to give a faster, more uniform puncture at the specified depth. These are reviewed more thoroughly in Chapter 3. They are easy to use and are particularly helpful for patients who must do blood glucose screening at home.

Collection Tubes.   *Micropipets* and *capillary tubes* for collecting skin punc-ture blood are manufactured in a variety of bore sizes, volume capacities, and shapes. They may be heparinized or nonheparinized, contain additives, be conical, cylindrical, straight-walled with open ends, and be made from glass or plastic.[6] They are also discussed in more detail in Chapter 3.

Positioning of the Patient and Venipuncture Sites

It is important to choose the least hazardous site for blood collection by skin puncture or venipuncture. Several techniques can facilitate the selection of a suitable site.

Proper positioning is important to both the phlebotomist and the patient for a successful venipuncture or skin puncture. Efforts to make sure that the patient is comfortable are worthwhile. Patients should *not* stand or sit on high stools during the procedure because of the possibility of fainting. A reclining position is preferred; however, sitting in a sturdy, comfortable chair with arm supports is also acceptable (Fig. 4–5). The phlebotomist can position herself in

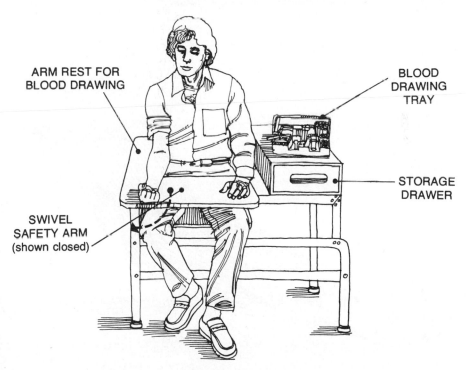

ARM REST FOR
BLOOD DRAWING

BLOOD
DRAWING
TRAY

SWIVEL
SAFETY ARM
(shown closed)

STORAGE
DRAWER

Figure 4–5. Equipment and patient positioning. *(Courtesy of College of American Pathologists, Skokie, Ill.)*

front of the chair to protect the patient from falling forward if he faints. A slight rotation of the arm or hand may help expose a vein and keep it from rolling as the needle is inserted. A pillow may be used for arm support of a bedridden patient. Equipment should be placed in an accessible spot where it is not likely to be disturbed by the patient.

Wrist, hand, ankle, and foot veins should be used only after arm veins have been determined unsuitable (Figs. 4–6, 4–7, 4–8). Reasons for not using arm veins include the following: the patient has IVs in both arms, is burned, has casts, thrombosed veins, or edematous arms. Hand and foot veins have a tendency to move or "roll" aside as the needle is inserted; therefore, it may be helpful to have the patient extend the foot or hand into a position that helps hold the vein taut. However, veins of the extremities should be avoided if they are edematous. Some hospitals do not allow phlebotomists to use the lower extremities for blood sampling sites at all. Others allow it after permission is granted from the patient's physician. Venipuncture in small veins may be facilitated by the use of a 19- to 21-gauge butterfly needle.

Skin Puncture Sites

Skin puncture in adults most often involves one of the fingers. The fleshy surface of the distal portion of the second, third, or fourth fingers can be used for puncture. The "middle finger" is recommended.

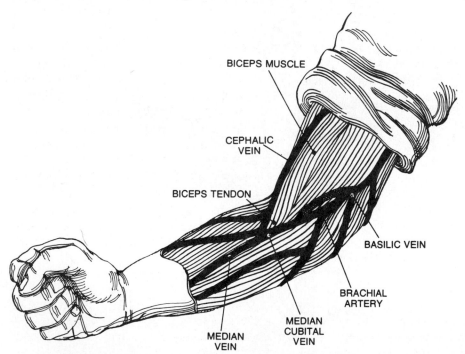

Figure 4–6. Veins of the anterior surface of the arm. *(Courtesy of American College of Pathologists, Skokie, Ill.)*

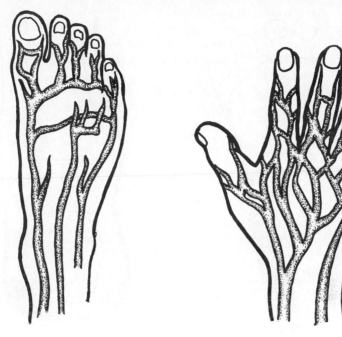

Figure 4–7. Foot and ankle veins.   **Figure 4–8.** Hand and wrist veins.

The heels of infants and neonates are good sites for skin puncture if properly performed. The most medial or lateral sections of the plantar or bottom surface of the heel should be used. If one draws an imaginary line from the outside edge of the great toe to the heel and from the outside edge of the fifth toe to the heel, the area outside these lines is least hazardous for skin puncture (Figs. 4–9 and 4–10).[8] If areas inside this region are punctured, the possibility of hitting bone is increased. If the bone is punctured, it may become infected, resulting in osteomyelitis.[9] Previously punctured sites should not be repunctured; the posterior curve of the heel should not be used; and the puncture should not be deeper than 2.4 mm to avoid hitting the bone.[10]

The thumb, great toe, or earlobe are rarely used as sites for skin puncture. Swollen or edematous areas should not be used for venipuncture or skin puncture because body fluids can contaminate the specimen. Fingers that are cyanotic, swollen, or inflamed should be avoided.[8]

Warming the Site

Warming the site helps facilitate phlebotomy by increasing arterial blood flow to the area. Although several methods for warming are available, surgical towels or a wash cloth heated with warm water to 42°C will not burn the skin. When wrapped around the site for 3 to 10 min, the skin temperature can increase several degrees. The wrap can be encased in a plastic bag to help retain heat and keep the patient's bed dry. The phlebotomist may leave the

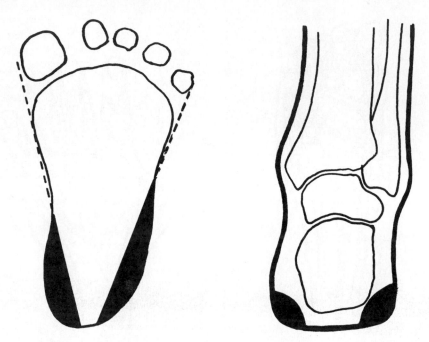

Figure 4–9. Heel puncture sites. **A.** The least hazardous areas for skin puncture are outside the *dotted lines.* **B.** Posterior view of heel and bones.

warm wrap on the patient while she collects specimens from other patients, and then can return to the original patient after several minutes.

Tourniquet Application

A tourniquet or blood pressure cuff may be used to help find a site for venipuncture. As mentioned previously, a soft rubber tourniquet about 1 in. (2.5 cm) wide and about 15 to 18 in. (45 cm) long is most comfortable. To apply it the ends should be stretched around the arm; both ends can be held in one hand while the other hand grasps the area next to the skin and makes a partial loop with the tourniquet. It should be tight but not painful to the patient (Fig. 4–11E). The partially looped tourniquet should allow for easy release during the venipuncture procedure. It should not be left on for more than 2 minutes because it becomes uncomfortable and causes hemoconcentration, that is, increased blood concentration of large molecules such as proteins, cells, and coagulation factors.[8] Patients may be asked to clench and unclench their fist a *few* times. Excessive clenching also results in hemoconcentration. If no vein surfaces, the patient may be asked to dangle the arm for 1 to 2 minutes, and then the tourniquet may be reapplied and the area palpated again. The phlebotomist should *never* stick a vein unless it can be seen or felt. It is better to defer the

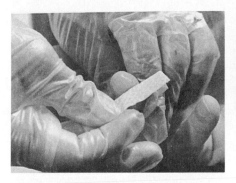

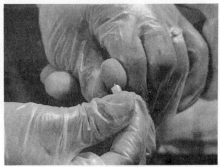

A. Decontamination of skin puncture site.

B. Performing the skin puncture using a quick continuous movement. The lancet should be perpendicular to the site and puncture across the fingerprint.

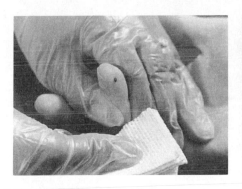

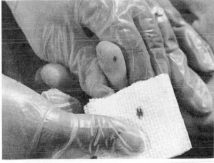

C. The first drop of blood comes out.

D. The first drop of blood is wiped off with a sterile gauze.

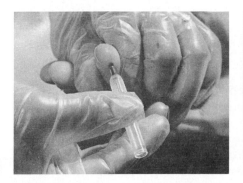

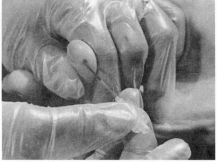

E. Blood is collected into a microcollection tube.

F. Blood is collected into a Unopette capillary tube.

Figure 4–10. Performing a skin puncture.

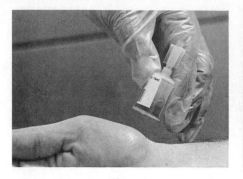

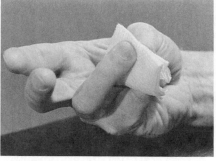

G. The Unopette capillary tube is inserted into the vial and mixed thoroughly.

H. The patient presses sterile gauze on finger to stop the bleeding.

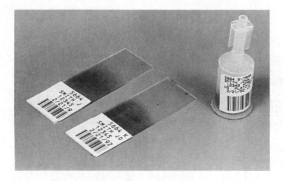

I. Slides are also made and all specimens are appropriately labelled.

Figure 4–10. (Continued).

patient to someone else who can search for the vein than to take a "blind" chance.[5]

Decontamination of the Site

Once the site has been selected, it should be decontaminated with a sterile swab or sponge soaked in alcohol; 70 percent isopropanol is recommended (see Fig. 4–11G).

The site should be rubbed vigorously with the alcohol sponge. Some recommend rubbing in concentric circles working from the inside out. The phlebotomist should decontaminate his or her own gloved finger if he or she intends to palpate the site again. The decontaminated area should never be touched with any nonsterile object. Alcohol should be allowed to dry or wiped off with sterile gauze or cotton after preparing the site; otherwise it will sting at the puncture site and can interfere with test results, for example, blood

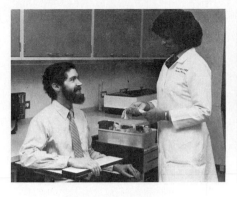

A. Greeting the patient.

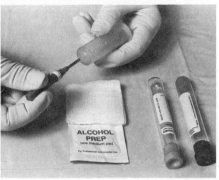

B. Equipment preparation.

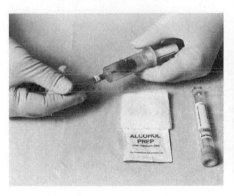

C. Needle preparation.

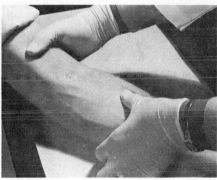

D. Site selection: inspecting the site.

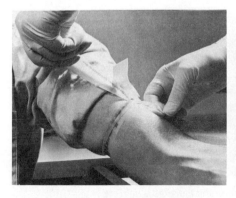

E. Tourniquet application.

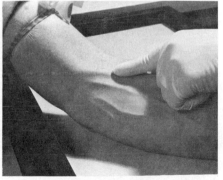

F. Palpating the site.

Figure 4–11. Performing a venipuncture using the evacuated tube system.

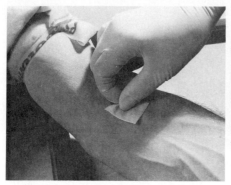

G. Decontamination with alcohol.

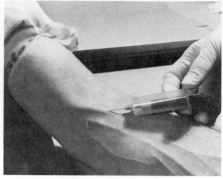

H. The venipuncture procedure.

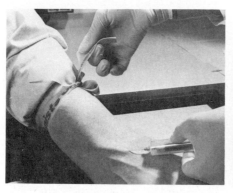

I. Removal of tourniquet.

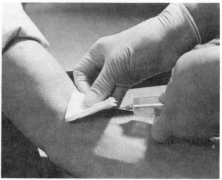

J. Tube and needle removal.

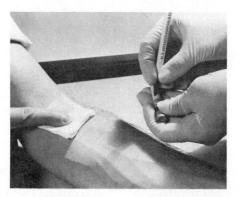

K. Application of pressure and immediate labeling of tubes.

Figure 4–11. (Continued).

alcohol levels. When doing a finger stick, if alcohol is not wiped dry with sterile gauze, the blood will not form a round drop, therefore making micro-collection more difficult. It also causes misleading cell counts because red blood cells are hemolyzed.

Povidone-iodine (Betadine) preparations are primarily used for drawing blood gases and blood cultures (refer to Chapter 5). For some patients, iodine causes skin irritations. Efforts should be made to remove iodine from the skin with sterile gauze after decontamination because excess iodine can interfere with some laboratory tests.

METHOD OF VENIPUNCTURE AND SKIN PUNCTURE

Venipuncture

Once the area has been cleansed, the patient's arm may be held below the site, pulling the skin tightly with the thumb. A syringe, butterfly, or Vacutainer assembly can be used for venipuncture. (Before inserting the needle, if a syringe is used, the plunger should be moved back and forth to allow for free movement and to expel all air.) The whole assembly can be held between the thumb and the third or fourth finger. (The index finger may rest on the hub of the needle to guide the needle entry.) The needle should run in the same direction as the vein and should be inserted quickly and smoothly at approximately a 15 degree angle with the skin. The needle should be inserted with the bevel side upward and directly above a prominent vein or slightly below the palpable vein. It may be necessary to palpate with one hand after needle insertion if the vein has not been hit. Often the phlebotomist can feel a slight "pop" when the needle enters the vein. As the blood begins to flow, the patient may open her fist. The tourniquet can be released immediately or after the blood has been collected, but before needle withdrawal.

Collection Tubes

If the evacuated tube system, e.g., Vacutainer, system is used, the test tube should be pushed *carefully* into the holder, thereby puncturing the test tube cap with the inside needle and allowing blood to enter the evacuated tube (see Fig. 4–11). If multiple sample tubes are to be collected, each tube should be *gently* removed from the Vacutainer holder and replaced with another tube. Experienced phlebotomists are able to mix a full tube in one hand while waiting for another tube to fill. It is recommended that tubes for coagulation studies be filled last to avoid contamination by tissue coagulation factors released during needle insertion. (See Chapter 5 for further discussion.) Figure 4–12 demonstrates a venipuncture using a combination butterfly and evacuated tube system.

If a syringe is used, the plunger can be drawn back slowly until the

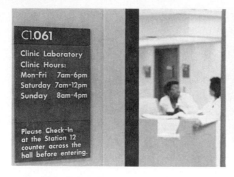

A. The outpatient specimen collection area.

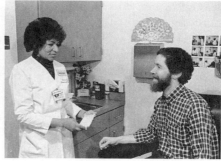

B. Greeting the patient, explaining the specimen collection process, and confirming identification.

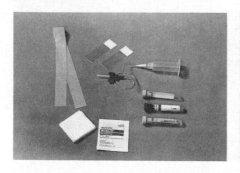

C. Preparation of supplies.

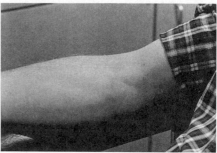

D. Visual inspection of potential puncture sites.

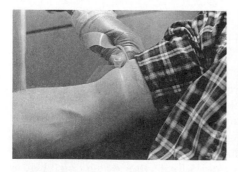

E. Selection of site using tourniquet.

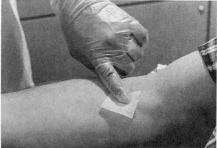

F. Decontamination of site.

Figure 4–12. Performing a venipuncture using a combination butterfly needle (double-pointed) and evacuated tube system.

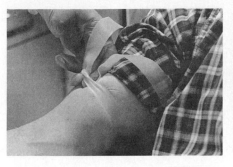

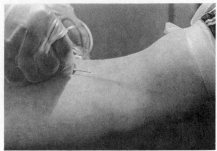

G. Reapplication of tourniquet as alcohol is drying.

H. Needle insertion in a steady, smooth fashion.

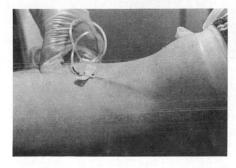

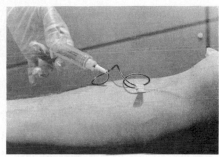

I. Needle insertion and blood begins to flow.

J. Collection tube is inserted into barrel and blood enters the tube.

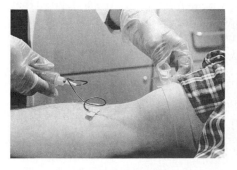

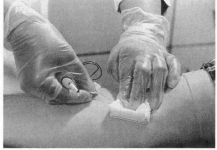

K. Tourniquet is released.

L. Collection is completed and the needle is withdrawn.

Figure 4–12. (Continued).

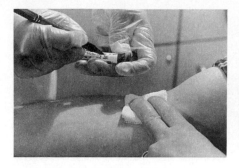

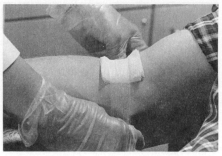

M. Patient presses sterile gauze on puncture site to stop bleeding. Phlebotomist labels and initials the specimen.

N. Phlebotomist assures that bleeding has stopped and puts bandage on.

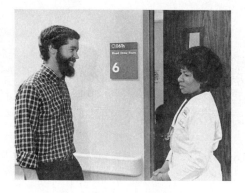

O. Thanking the patient.

Figure 4–12. (Continued).

required amount of blood is drawn. It may be helpful to turn the syringe so that the graduated markings are facing upward for easier visibility. Care must be taken not to accidentally withdraw the needle while pulling back on the plunger, or not to pull hard enough to cause hemolysis or collapse of the vein.

After tourniquet release and collection of the appropriate amount of blood, the entire needle assembly should be withdrawn quickly. A sterile, dry gauze or cotton ball should be applied with pressure to the puncture site for several minutes or *until bleeding has ceased.* If the patient has a free hand, he may apply the pressure. The arm may be kept straight, slightly bent at the elbow, or elevated above the heart.

If a syringe has been used, the blood should be quickly transferred to the appropriate test tubes to avoid clotting in the syringe barrel. This can be accomplished by using evacuated test tubes. The needle may be inserted into the tube allowing blood to be suctioned into the tube. Blood forced into the tube may cause damage to or hemolysis of cells. It is often recommended that the needle and the tube cap be removed before transferring the blood from the syringe to the test tube to avoid hemolysis. All anticoagulated specimens should be *gently* mixed by inverting 10 to 12 times.

Figures 4–13 through 4–16 describe specific laboratory procedures used to do venipuncture, finger puncture, and nursery collection. All laboratories should have phlebotomy procedures that have been approved by both the clinical laboratory supervisor and the laboratory director. These procedure manuals are subject to inspection by accrediting and regulating agencies.

Performance of a Venipuncture

1. Greet the patient in a friendly, professional manner.

   In an outpatient setting:

   Ask the patient a direct question, "What is your name, sir/madam?" "What is your date of birth?" Compare the name and date of birth stated by the patient with information on the identification card, computer labels, and laboratory request slips. When a blood specimen is required for blood components, an identification bracelet must be worn by the patient.

   In a hospital setting (inpatients):

   Knock on the patient's door and enter the room. Compare your request slip or computer labels with the patient's name and hospital number found on the door of the patient's room. Identify yourself to the patient, stating that you have come to draw blood for some laboratory tests ordered by his physician. Compare information on the patient's identification bracelet with that on your computer labels and laboratory request slips. This information must be identical. Request a nurse to identify a patient who does not have an identification bracelet. The nurse should also place a bracelet on the patient's wrist except in cases when this is not feasible. Some patients cannot wear ID bracelets because their wrist is irritated or too edematous for an ID bracelet to fit.

   If this is the case, make a note on the requisition of the nurse who identified the patient.

2. The phlebotomist must gain the patient's confidence and remind the patient that the venipuncture may be slightly painful. Patients should never be told "This will not hurt."

3. Position the patient:

   Procedure for seating the patient (usually outpatients):
   The patient should be seated comfortably in a chair and should position his or her arm on an armrest, extending the arm so as to form a relatively straight line from the shoulder to the wrist. The arm is supported firmly by the armrest and should only be slightly bent at the elbow.   *(continued)*

Figure 4–13. Sample procedure for performance of a routine venipuncture.

Procedure for having the patient lie down (usually inpatients):

The patient lies comfortably on his back. If additional support is needed, a pillow may be placed under the arm from which the specimen is to be drawn. The patient extends the arm so as to form a relatively straight line from the shoulder to the wrist.

4. Assemble the following supplies for collecting a blood specimen: gloves, blood collecting tubes, needles, syringe, or Vacutainer holder, tourniquet, alcohol 70 percent isopropyl, and gauze pads or alcohol prep pads, povidone-iodine and acetone alcohol swab sticks (if blood cultures are to be drawn), gauze bandage rolls or paper tape and cotton balls.

5. Select a vein site. Place a tourniquet on the patient's arm. Choose the vein that feels fullest. Look at both arms. Ask the patient to make a fist that makes the veins more prominent and easier to enter. Vigorous hand exercise "pumping" should be avoided because it may affect some test values. Use the index finger to palpate and trace the path of the vein. Thrombosed veins lack resilience, feel cordlike, and roll easily. Feel firmly, but do not tap or rub finger lightly over skin because you may feel only small surface veins. Always feel for the median cubital vein first; it is usually bigger, anchored better, and bruises less. The cephalic vein (depending on size) is the second choice over the basilic vein because it does not roll and bruise as easily. The bend of the elbow is the best place to make a puncture. When this is not possible other sites include the surface of the forearm, wrist area above the thumb, volar area of the wrist, knuckle of the thumb or index finger, back of the hand, and back of the lower arm. If a "good" vein cannot be found, try the following:

   - Try the other arm unless otherwise instructed.
   - Ask the patient to make a fist again.
   - Apply the tourniquet, remembering that the tourniquet should never be left on the arm for more than 2 min.
   - Massage the arm from wrist to elbow.
   - Tap a few times at the vein site with your index finger.
   - Apply heat to the vein site.
   - Lower the arm over the bedside or venipuncture chair.

6. Cleanse the venipuncture site. Using an alcohol prep or cotton ball saturated with alcohol, cleanse the area by moving the pad in a circular motion from the center of the vein site outward. The area must be allowed to dry. NEVER touch the skin after the site is cleansed unless you have prepped your gloved finger.

7. Inspect the needle, syringe, or evacuated tube before performing the venipuncture. The appropriate needle is attached to the syringe or evacuated tube holder and threaded into the holder until it is secure, using the needle sheath as a wrench. The cover of the needle must not be removed until the phlebotomist is ready to draw blood, thus avoiding needle contamination. If the needle touches anything but the sterile site, it should be changed.

Figure 4–13. (Continued).

8. Perform the venipuncture:

Evacuated tube method:

The phlebotomist should grasp the patient's arm firmly, using the thumb to draw the skin taut. The vein is entered with the bevel of the needle upward. One hand should hold the evacuated tube while the other depresses the tube to the end of the holder.

The tube should be filled until the vacuum is exhausted and the blood flow ceases, thus ensuring a correct ratio of anticoagulant to blood. After drawing each tube, an additive should be mixed immediately by inverting the tube at least five times. Gentle inversion will avoid hemolysis. *Never* shake a tube of blood after collecting a blood specimen.

Occasionally a faulty tube will have no vacuum. If a tube is not filling and the needle is inside the vein, another tube should be used. If a tube starts to fill but then stops, the needle should be moved slightly forward or backward. Usually this adjustment will increase the blood flow. The needle can then be rotated half a turn, and the tourniquet, which may have been applied too tightly, is loosened. Probing is not recommended because it is painful to the patient. If none of these procedures is helpful, the needle should be removed and an alternate site used.

Syringe method:

A syringe and needle should be used to collect blood from patients with more difficult veins. If the puncture has been made and the blood is not flowing, the phlebotomist should determine if he is pulling too hard on the plunger and collapsing the vein. The needle should be drawn back while the plunger is being pulled slightly. The phlebotomist must make sure the bevel is covered by the skin. With the syringe in the right hand, the phlebotomist uses the index finger of the left hand to feel for the vein. After the vein is relocated, the finger is kept gently on the vein and the needle guided to that point. The phlebotomist then pulls gently on the plunger. As soon as the blood starts to flow into the syringe, the needle should not be moved.

Other methods:

A winged infusion set with leur adapters can be used instead of a syringe and needle for very difficult veins. The winged collection set is a "closed" system. Blood flows from the vein through the set directly into a Vacutainer brand tube.

If all possibilities have been exhausted, and you have not successfully performed a venipuncture on a patient after two attempts, enlist the aid of a co-worker or supervisor. Inform the nurse caring for the patient that you have made two unsuccessful attempts to draw blood from the patient. Make a notation of the circumstances on a worksheet.

9. The tourniquet is released after the blood is drawn and the patient has opened her hand. Releasing the tourniquet allows for normal blood circulation and a reduction in the amount of bleeding at the venipuncture site. The phlebotomist folds a gauze pad or places a cotton ball over the needle, which is then gently removed. The gauze pad or cotton ball is held firmly over the venipuncture site.

Figure 4–13. (Continued).

10. All tubes should be appropriately mixed and labeled at the patient's bedside. Labels must include patient's first and last name, ID number, date, time of collection, and initials of the phlebotomist.

11. Dispose of contaminated materials/supplies in designated containers.

12. Specimens must be delivered to the appropriate laboratory.

   Summary of steps in performing a venipuncture:

   - Ensure identification of patient.
   - Reassure patient and assure that the patient is properly positioned.
   - Assemble supplies.
   - Verify paperwork and tube identification.
   - Select vein site.
   - Apply tourniquet.
   - Cleanse venipuncture site.
   - Perform venipuncture.
   - Release tourniquet.
   - Remove needle.
   - Bandage arm.
   - Fill tubes (when syringe and needle are used).
   - Label tubes.
   - Dispose of contaminated supplies.
   - Chill specimen, if necessary.
   - Distribute specimen(s) to the appropriate laboratory section(s).

Figure 4–13. (Continued).

Skin Puncture

Microcollection by skin puncture involves many of the same steps as venipuncture. The site should be cleansed as was indicated. If performing a heel stick, the infant's heel should be held with a firm grip, forefinger at the arch of the foot and thumb below and away from the puncture site. (See Fig. 4–9 for appropriate sites for heel puncture.) If doing a finger stick, the finger should be held firmly with the thumb away from the puncture site (see Fig. 4–10). The puncture should be done in one sharp continuous movement almost perpendicular to the site and across the fingerprint. If the puncture is made along the lines of the fingerprint, blood has a tendency to run down the finger. Average depth of a skin puncture should be 2 to 3 mm. In heel sticks on infants, the depth should not exceed 2.4 mm.[9,10] Special lancets, which control the depth of the puncture, are available commercially. Pressure from the phlebotomist's thumb may be eased and reapplied as the drops of blood appear. Massaging or milking the area should not be done because it causes hemolysis and contamination of tissue and intracellular fluids into the blood specimen.[9]

Procedure for Finger Puncture

1. Remember the following supplies: gloves, sterile cotton balls or gauze sponges (2 × 2), alcohol swabs, sterile lancets, pipets, capillary tubes, microcollection tubes, glass tubes, diluting fluids, marking pen/pencil, and bandages.
2. Choose a finger that is not cold, cyanotic, or swollen. If possible, the stick should be at the tip of the fourth or ring finger of the nondominant hand.
3. Gently massage the finger five or six times from base to tip to aid blood flow.
4. With an alcohol swab, cleanse the ball of the finger. Allow to air-dry.
5. Remove the lancet from its protective paper without touching the tip.
6. Hold the patient's finger firmly with one hand and make a swift, deep puncture with the lancet halfway between the center of the ball of the finger and its side.
7. The cut should be made across the fingerprints to produce a large, round drop of blood.
8. Wipe the first drop of blood away with a clean gauze.
9. Gently massage the finger from base to tip to obtain the proper amount of blood for the tests requested.
10. Each type of micro sample has different collection tube and blood volume requirements.

Notes

If the patient's hands are cold, wrap one of them in a warm to hot towel 10 to 15 min before the puncture is performed.

A free-flowing puncture is essential to obtain accurate test results. *Do not use excessive squeezing to obtain blood.*

Figure 4–14. Sample procedure for performance of a finger puncture.

The first drop of blood should be removed with a sterile dry pad. Capillary tubes, for example, Unopette, and blood smears can then be made from subsequent drops of blood.

Figures 4–17 and 4–18 indicate methods for making blood smears and blood dilutions with capillary pipets. Figure 4–19 demonstrates types of microcollection tubes. The phlebotomist should remember that alcohol prevents

THIS   **NOT THIS**

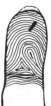   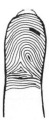

Figure 4–15. The finger puncture should involve a quick, deep puncture across the fingerprints, not parallel to the fingerprint.

Obtaining Blood Specimens from Infants (Heel Stick)
Principle
To obtain blood specimens from infants with the least amount of trauma while maintaining good isolation techniques.

Procedure
1. The entrance to the nurseries (intensive care, intermediate care, and low risk) is located on _____ _____.
2. Place blood collection tray on the table near the scrub sinks outside the nurseries.
3. Remove rings, watches, and lab coat.
4. Wash hands with regular soap. The water is controlled using foot pedals.
5. Put on a gown with ties in the back. If your clothes have long sleeves, wear a yellow paper gown. With short sleeves, wear a short-sleeved cotton gown.
6. Wear sterile gloves.
7. Pick up tray with two clean paper towels and enter nursery area.
8. Find the small metal cart and place tray on a clean diaper on the cart.
9. Discard paper towels.
10. Identify the baby by making sure the request slip is identical to the baby's armband.
11. After ensuring the skin is warm, perform a heel puncture to obtain the proper blood specimen for the tests requested.
12. Hold a clean cotton gauze over the puncture site until bleeding stops. Do not put adhesive strips on the baby's feet.
13. Remove all collection equipment from the crib to avoid harming the baby.
14. Before collecting blood from the next baby, wash hands at the sink inside the nursery proper and change gloves.
15. Initial the log book for all work completed.
16. Remove gown and gloves and discard in proper receptacle.
17. Wash hands.
18. When moving from one nursery area to the other, the blood collector must repeat the complete procedure and put on a clean gown and gloves.

Notes
1. The baby's heel may be punctured a maximum of two times. Do not stick a baby more than twice to obtain a specimen at any given time. If a particular baby must always be punctured the maximum number of times, notify the phlebotomy supervisor and the baby's primary nurse.
2. Do not puncture a foot if there are bruises, abrasions, or sloughing skin present. Call this to the attention of the baby's nurse.
3. To help obtain a free-flowing puncture wound from a baby who doesn't bleed freely, have a nurse wrap the baby's heel in a warm towel 10 to 15 min before the puncture is made. This is also necessary for collection of all capillary blood gases.
4. Use only gentle massage when obtaining blood. Excessive massaging dilutes the blood with tissue fluids and may also cause hemolysis. It is sufficient to massage with your thumb and forefinger.
5. Never repuncture old puncture wounds.
6. *Never* remove a baby from its crib or change its position in any way without the approval of a nurse.

Figure 4–16. Sample nursery procedure for a heel stick on an infant.

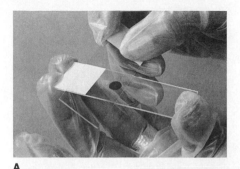

A

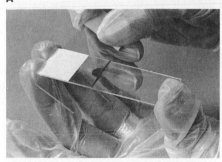

B

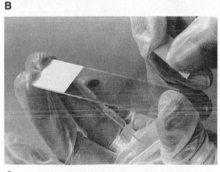

C

Figure 4–17. The blood smear. Blood smears can be made from venous or capillary blood. In both cases, it is preferred that smears be made from fresh blood. With the capillary method the finger puncture should be made in the usual way by wiping away the first drop of blood. The slide can be touched to the second drop. It should be touched approximately 1/2 to 1 in. from the end of the slide. As depicted in **A,** a second spreader slide should be placed in front of the drop of blood. The spreader slide should be pulled into the drop, allowing blood to spread along the width of the slide, as indicated in **B.** When the blood spreads almost to the edges, the spreader slide should be quickly and evenly pushed forward at an angle of approximately 30 degrees. The only downward pressure should be the weight of the spreader slide. Allow the slide to air-dry. DO NOT BLOW ON IT. If using the venous method, the needle should be touched immediately to the slide after it has been withdrawn. A drop about 1 to 2 mm in diameter will suffice. Then the procedure is the same as for capillary blood. **C.** Good smears should cover approximately half of the surface of the glass slide. There should be no ridges, lines, or holes in the smear. Errors are often the result of too large a drop, too long a delay in making the smear, or using a chipped slide. **D.** Allow blood smears to air-dry after labeling.

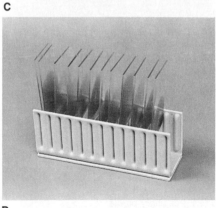

D

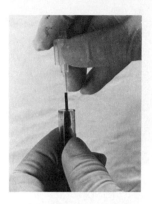

A. Using the shield on the capillary pipet, puncture the diaphragm of the vial. Fill the capillary pipet with the blood sample. It will fill by capillary action if held almost horizontally. When filling is complete it will stop automatically. Excess blood should be wiped gently from the pipet, making sure that no sample is removed.

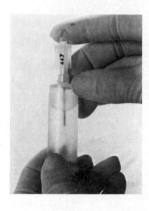

B. Cover the upper opening of the pipet with index finger and insert into the vial. With the other hand, slight pressure can be added to the vial to facilitate release of the blood inside. Negative pressure will then draw the blood into the diluent when the index finger is removed from the pipet.

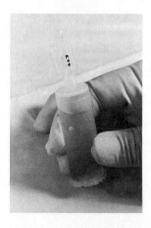

C. The vial must then be squeezed *gently* to rinse the capillary bore. Caution must be used not to force diluent out of the chamber by excessive squeezing. The index finger can then be again placed on top for further mixing.

Figure 4–18. Blood dilutions using capillary pipets.

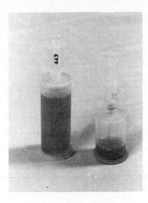

D. The vials are ready for testing or can be stored if the capillary shield is used to cover the vial opening.

Figure 4–18. (Continued).

round drops from forming. Care must be taken when filling capillary tubes not to get air bubbles into the tube. This leads to erroneous results for many laboratory tests.

All disposable equipment should be discarded in appropriate containers. Paper and plastic wrappers can be thrown in a waste basket. Needles and lancets should *not* be thrown in a waste basket, but in a sturdy, puncture-proof disposable container to be autoclaved or incinerated. Any items that have been contaminated with blood should be disposed of in biohazard disposal containers. Key guidelines from the Occupational Safety and Health Administration (OSHA) pertain to phlebotomists and include the following:[11]

- Needles should not be recapped, broken, bent, or removed unless the action is required for a specific procedure, e.g., blood gas analyses.

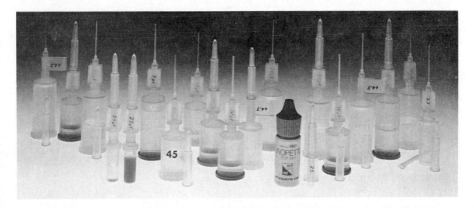

Figure 4–19. Microcollection tubes. *(Courtesy of Becton-Dickinson and Company, Rutherford, N.J.)*

- All specimens should be handled with universal precautions. All employees who have or may have contact with specimens and containers must be knowledgeable and trained in the use of universal precautions.
- Employers must provide personal protective equipment for minimizing contact between specimens and skin, eyes, mucous membranes, or parenteral areas. Employers must ensure proper use. Laboratory coats are viewed as personal protective equipment if used to prevent employees' work clothes or uniform from being contaminated with blood. They must be provided. Employees should not wash contaminated personal protective equipment at home.
- Gloves should be worn anytime an employee risks contact with blood or infectious materials or when performing vascular access procedures such as venipunctures or skin punctures.
- If there is potential for splattering or spraying of blood, masks, eye protection, and face shields must be worn.
- Hands should be washed after contact with each patient (Fig. 4–20).

Before leaving the patient's side, the phlebotomist must check the site to make sure that the bleeding has stopped. All tubes must be appropriately labeled and confirmed. All supplies and equipment brought in should be removed or discarded, and the phlebotomist should thank the patient.

An adhesive bandage may be applied. However, they are not recommended for infants or young children because of possible irritation and the potential of swallowing or aspirating a bandage.[9]

Dorsal Hand Vein Procedure

An alternative technique for blood collection, which has been reported recently but is not yet widely practiced, is the *"dorsal hand vein technique."*[12,13] It is used for collecting blood on infants, children, and individuals with extremely small or difficult veins. The preferred needle is 21 or 23 gauge, $3/4$ to 1 in., with a translucent hub. No tourniquet is necessary as the phlebotomist's finger is used to apply pressure. Use the hand that has the most visible veins. The phlebotomist can use her middle and index fingers in the shape of a "V." The baby's arm or wrist area can be placed in the "V," and pressure can be applied gently using the phlebotomist's 2 fingers. The baby's wrist can be bent over the phlebotomist's middle finger and held in place gently by the phlebotomist's thumb. By bending the baby's wrist and applying gentle pressure, veins become more visible and easy to palpate. The wrist should not be flexed so tightly that it causes the veins to collapse. The back of the baby's hand can be lightly touched or brushed with the phlebotomist's index finger to locate the vein and establish its direction.

Once the vein is located, pressure should be released and blood allowed to circulate freely again. The baby should be wrapped snugly in a blanket to minimize the amount of movement during the procedure. Cleanse the site as usual and reapply the finger tourniquet. Once the site is dried, puncture the

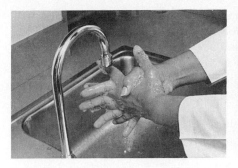

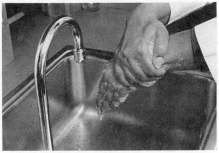

A. Handwashing technique should involve soap lather, friction between hands, and thorough washing between fingers. Foot pedals are preferable for controlling flow of water.

B. Washing should include the wrist areas also.

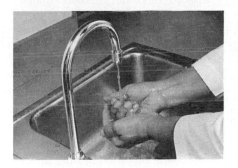

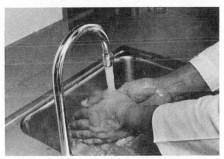

C. Lather should be rinsed.

D. Rinsing should continue until all soap is removed. If the water must be turned off by hand, it is recommended that a clean paper towel be used to grab the faucet.

Figure 4–20. Handwashing technique.

vein carefully with the small needle. Just as the blood appears in the hub of the needle, the appropriate microcollection tubes can be placed under the free-flowing droplets. *Blood is collected directly from the hub of the inserted needle into the microcollection tubes or capillary tubes.* Caution must be taken not to push the needle through the vein with the collection tubes. A steady flow of blood can be sustained by applying gentle periodic pressure to the arm using the finger tourniquet. Pressure must be released periodically to allow the vein to refill. If the blood flow stops, the needle should be rotated slightly without moving it in or out. When blood specimens have been collected, a clean dry gauze should be placed over the puncture site and the needle withdrawn in a swift, quick manner. The gauze should be held on the site until all bleeding has stopped. Careful evaluation of bleeding stoppage is essential to the prevention of bruising and hematoma. Use of this technique has reportedly resulted in decreased hemolysis, decreased sample dilution with tissue fluid, fewer multiple punctures, and decreased technologist stress. Based on observations of those who are familiar with the procedure, the dorsal hand vein technique seems to be less painful.[12,13]

COMPLICATIONS AND SPECIAL CONSIDERATIONS IN BLOOD COLLECTION

Fainting (Syncope)

Many patients become dizzy and faint at the thought or sight of blood. It is important to be aware of the patient's condition throughout the collection procedure. This can be done by verbally asking ambulatory patients if they have a tendency to faint or if they have previously fainted during blood collections. If so, it is recommended that they be moved from a seated position to a lying position. If a seated patient feels faint, the needle should be removed and the head lowered between the legs, and the patient should breathe deeply. If possible, the phlebotomist should ask for help and move the patient to a lying position. Talking to patients can often reassure them and divert their attention from the collection procedure. Patients in bed rarely feel faint. In both cases, however, the phlebotomist should stay with the patient till he recovers. A wet towel gently applied to the forehead or a glass of juice or water may help the patient feel better.

If a patient faints during or after the procedure, the phlebotomist should try to terminate the venipuncture procedure immediately and make sure the patient does not fall or become injured. It is sometimes difficult to control the situation because of physical size of the patient; however, the phlebotomist should use common sense about the safest position for a patient. If a patient has fainted and is in a secure position, the phlebotomist should quickly request assistance from the nursing staff or a physician. A patient who has fainted should recover fully before being allowed to leave.

Failure to Draw Blood

Several factors may cause one to "miss the vein," such as not inserting the needle deep enough, inserting the needle all the way through the vein, holding the needle bevel against the vein wall, or losing the vacuum in the tube (Fig. 4–21). The phlebotomist's index finger can help locate the vein while the needle is inserted. It may be necessary to move or withdraw the needle somewhat, and redirect it. On occasion, a test tube will have no vacuum because of a manufacturer's error or tube leakage after a puncture. It behooves the phlebotomist to carry an extra set of tubes in her pocket in case this happens during venipuncture. Also, needles for evacuated tube systems have been known to unscrew

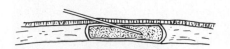

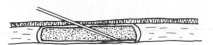

A. Correct insertion technique; blood flows freely into needle.

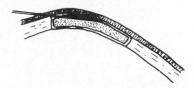

B. Bevel on vein upper wall does not allow blood to flow.

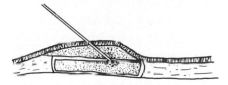

C. Bevel on vein lower wall does not allow blood to flow.

D. Needle inserted too far.

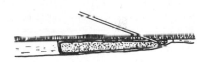

E. Needle partially inserted and causes blood leakage into tissue.

F. Collapsed.

Figure 4–21. Needle positioning and failure to draw blood.

from the barrel during venipuncture. If this happens, the tourniquet should be released immediately and the needle removed.

Hematomas

When the area around the puncture site starts to swell, this usually indicates that blood is leaking into the tissues causing a hematoma. This can happen when the needle has gone completely through the vein, the bevel opening is partially in the vein, or not enough pressure is applied to the site after puncture. This results in a large bruise after several days (Fig. 4–22). If a hematoma begins to form, the tourniquet and needle should be *removed immediately* and pressure applied to the area for approximately 2 minutes. If the bleeding continues, a nurse should be notified.

Petechiae

These are small red spots appearing on a patient's skin that indicate that minute amounts of blood have escaped into skin epithelium. This may be a result of coagulation problems, that is, platelet defects, and should caution the phlebotomist that the patient's puncture site may bleed excessively.

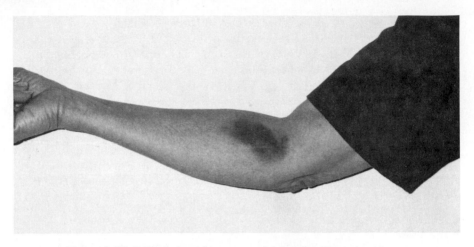

Figure 4–22. Patient's hematoma several days after the venipuncture.

Edema

Some patients develop an abnormal accumulation of fluid in the intercellular spaces of the body. This swelling can be localized or diffused over a larger area of the body. The phlebotomist should avoid collecting blood from these sites because veins are difficult to palpate or stick, and the specimen may be contaminated with fluid.

Obesity

Obese patients generally have veins that are difficult to visualize and palpate. If the vein is missed, the phlebotomist must be careful not to probe excessively with the needle because it causes rupture of RBCs, increases concentration of intracellular contents, and releases some tissue clotting factors.

IV Therapy

Patients on IV therapy for extended periods of time often have veins that are palpable and visible but are damaged or occluded (blocked). Every time a catheter is used, vein damage occurs. Circulatory blood is rerouted to collateral veins and can result in hemoconcentration.

In cases where a patient has an IV line, that arm should not be used for venipuncture because the specimen will be diluted with IV fluid. The other arm, or another site, should be considered. It is sometimes possible for the nurse or physician to disconnect the IV line and draw blood from the needle that is already inserted. The first few milliliters of the specimen should be discarded to remove the IV fluid. A note should be made on the laboratory requisition if this step is performed.

Damaged, Sclerosed, or Occluded Veins

Veins that are obstructed or occluded do not allow blood to flow through. Sclerosed or hardened veins are a result of inflammation and disease of the interstitial substances. Patients' veins that have been repeatedly punctured often become scarred and feel very hard when palpated. Blood is not easily collected from these sites; therefore they should be avoided.

Hemoconcentration

An increased concentration of larger molecules and formed elements in the blood is called hemoconcentration. Several factors can cause this to happen including tourniquet application, massaging, squeezing or probing a site, long-term IV therapy, and sclerosed or occluded veins.

Hemolysis

When RBCs are lysed, hemoglobin is released and serum (normally straw colored) becomes tinged with pink or red. If a specimen is grossly hemolyzed, the serum appears very dark red. Hemolysis can be caused by improper phlebotomy techniques such as using a needle that is too small, pulling a syringe plunger back too fast, expelling the blood vigorously into a tube, and shaking or mixing tubes vigorously. These problems can easily be prevented by appropriate handling. Hemolysis may also be the result of physiologic abnormalities. The phlebotomist should make a note on the requisition form when she notices that a specimen is hemolyzed.

Collapsed Veins

If a syringe plunger is withdrawn too quickly during venipuncture, it may cause the vein to collapse This is especially true when collecting blood from the smaller veins (see Fig. 4–21).

Allergies

Some patients are allergic to iodine or other solutions used to disinfect a site. If a patient indicates that he is allergic to a solution, all efforts should be made to use an alternative method.

Thrombosis

Thrombi are solid masses derived from blood constituents that reside in the blood vessels. A thrombus may partially or fully occlude a vein (or artery), making venipuncture more difficult.

Burned or Scarred Areas

Areas that have been burned or scarred should be avoided during phlebotomy. Burned areas are very sensitive and susceptible to infection. Veins under scarred areas are difficult to palpate.

Infections

The phlebotomist should remember at all times that many patients have transmittable diseases, for example, hepatitis. A phlebotomist, in turn, can pass an infection to a patient. (For precautionary techniques, see Chapter 6.)

Other Considerations

Since the health care team (including doctors, medical technologists, clerks, secretaries, and nurses) are all working for the welfare of the patient, they should strive to reduce the number of phlebotomies. Several suggestions for doctors, nurses, ward clerks, and laboratory personnel have been given to do this.

Doctors could write orders on the same line on the chart rather than scattered throughout a page. Orders can be coordinated among all the staff physicians working with the patient. Notification to the laboratory of multiple timed tests ordered would be helpful. If a patient needs a hemoglobin at 2 PM and a glucose at 3 PM, it may be possible to coordinate the times and draw both specimens with one venipuncture.[14] Lab testing for therapeutic drug monitoring could be coordinated among laboratory, nursing, and pharmacy personnel.

Nurses and ward secretaries could organize laboratory orders as much as possible to avoid sending frequent requests minutes apart. When transcribing orders, all of them should be requested at the same time. The laboratory should be notified of patient transfers. An up-to-date log of room numbers and patients' names should be available on the ward as a resource for laboratory personnel.

Laboratory personnel should organize requisition forms by patient and by floor. Any identification discrepancies should be communicated to a nurse.[14]

One hospital has suggested several slogans for their health care personnel regarding phlebotomy:[14]

- A stick in time saves nine.
- We care—several pokes are no joke.
- For their sake, let's stick together.

Other items that should be considered for inclusion in policies and procedures are as follows:

1. The number of times a patient can be punctured by the same phlebotomist. Generally, a phlebotomist should not puncture a patient more than twice before calling for a second opinion.
2. The number of times a patient can be punctured in one day. It is recommended that staff physicians, nurses, and phlebotomists coordinate their efforts to minimize patient venipunctures.
3. The volume of blood that can be drawn daily from a patient, especially in pediatrics and the nursery (see Table 4–1).

4. The type of information a phlebotomist may provide to the patient about the lab tests ordered. In general, the use of good judgment is required. Basic information about the tests ordered is acceptable *if* a phlebotomist is knowledgeable. However, it should always be emphasized that the patient's physician ordered the tests.
5. The steps to take if a patient refuses to have blood collected. All patients have a right to refuse treatment. In these cases, the phlebotomist should use good, sound judgment in explaining to the patient that laboratory results are used to help the physician make an accurate diagnosis, establish proper treatment, and monitor health status. The phlebotomist should explain that the patient's cooperation would be greatly appreciated. If the patient continues to refuse, the phlebotomist must remain very professional and acknowledge the right to refuse. The phlebotomist should indicate to the patient that he or she will make a note of the refusal and notify the patient's physician.

TABLE 4–1. MAXIMUM AMOUNTS OF BLOOD TO BE DRAWN ON PATIENTS UNDER 14 YEARS

Patient's Weight		Maximum Amount to Be Drawn at Any One Time (mL)	Maximum Amount of Blood (Cumulative) During a Given Hospital Stay (1 Month or Under) (mL)
lb	kg (approx)		
6–8	2.7–3.6	2.5	23
8–10	3.6–4.5	3.5	30
10–15	4.5–6.8	5	40
16–20	7.3–9.1	10	60
21–25	9.5–11.4	10	70
26–30	11.8–13.6	10	80
31–35	14.1–15.9	10	100
36–40	16.4–18.2	10	130
41–45	18.6–20.5	20	140
46–50	20.9–22.7	20	160
51–55	23.2–25.0	20	180
56–60	25.5–27.3	20	200
61–65	27.7–29.5	25	220
66–70	30.0–31.8	30	240
71–75	32.3–34.1	30	250
76–80	34.5–36.4	30	270
81–85	36.8–38.6	30	290
86–90	39.1–40.9	30	310
91–95	41.4–43.2	30	330
96–100	43.6–45.5	30	350

Adapted from Becan-McBride K: *Textbook of Clinical Laboratory Supervision.* New York, Appleton-Century-Crofts, 1982.

SPECIMEN REJECTION

Each department or section in the clinical laboratory should establish its own guidelines for rejection of a specimen. Generally speaking, the following factors should be considered: discrepancies between requisition forms and labeled tubes (names, dates, times), unlabeled tubes, hemolyzed specimens (except in tests where it does not interfere), specimens in the wrong collection tubes, use of outdated equipment, supplies, or reagents, and contaminated specimens.

When a problem arises, the appropriate investigational channels should be followed. The phlebotomist who drew the specimen and his or her supervisor should try to solve the problem initially. Other personnel may be involved as needed. Communication and honesty are the keys to an efficient and reliable health care environment.

PRIORITIZING PATIENTS AND SAMPLE TUBES

In the course of a day's work at a busy hospital or clinic, a phlebotomist may have to make decisions about the order in which blood work is obtained. Priorities must be set and adhered to whether they concern the order in which certain blood tests are drawn on a particular patient or which patients are to be drawn first among a group. If these distinctions are not made properly, test results can be affected and interpretation of the results may be very difficult.

Patient Priorities

Timed Specimens.   Whenever a test is ordered to be drawn at a particular time, it is the responsibility of the phlebotomist to see that blood is drawn as near to the requested time as is possible. The most common requests for timed specimens are glucose levels, drawn 2 hours after a meal. The glucose value in the blood is constantly changing, and it is most important that the blood not be drawn too early, which gives falsely elevated results, or too late, which gives a falsely normal result.

Other timed specimens may be for peak and trough levels of certain drugs. Often patients on drug therapy must be monitored to check if effective therapeutic levels are being given. If the trough level is too high, the drug may be discontinued for a period until the blood drug level returns to lower and safer levels. Again, the timing of the blood drawn on these patients can be critical and must be scheduled as close as possible to the time ordered. If a time delay is unavoidable, the actual time of the collection must be indicated on the requisition form.

Certain natural hormone levels, such as cortisol, rise and fall with the time of the day. A sample of blood taken at 8:00 AM shows the highest value for cortisol during the day. A sample taken at 8:00 PM is usually approximately two-thirds of the morning sample. Therefore if a phlebotomist has difficulty obtaining a blood specimen on a patient at 8:00 AM, someone else should try as soon as possible afterwards, or the test may be canceled until the following day at the discretion of the attending physician. Obtaining a specimen for cortisol at noon may give the doctor little information upon which to base her treatment. Another hormone, aldosterone, requires another type of timing for blood collection and analysis. The patient must be in a recumbent position for at least 30 minutes prior to blood collection. Serum or plasma can be used in the analyte determination, but heparin or EDTA should be the anticoagulant if plasma is preferred. Since glass interferes in the aldosterone determination, the collecting container should be made of plastic.

To collect for renin-activity, an anticoagulated blood specimen should be collected from the patient after a 3-day special diet. In addition, it is important to note if the patient is in an upright or supine position when blood is drawn. For this analyte, the blood should be collected from a peripheral vein (e.g., antecubital vein).

Fasting Specimens.   When a phlebotomist works at an institution that treats inpatients, care should be taken that the patient is not unduly inconvenienced by an order for fasting blood tests. The phlebotomist should arrange the order that he or she collects blood from neighboring patients such that a patient's meal is not kept waiting because his or her blood has not been drawn yet. Fasting levels of glucose, cholesterol, and triglycerides can be very important in diagnosis of patients and monitoring their progress during the hospital stay. If a patient is found not to be fasting when the phlebotomist reaches him or her, the phlebotomist should consult with the physician to determine if a nonfasting level will be of any benefit. The requisition should then indicate that the patient is nonfasting.

"STAT" Specimen.   The term "STAT," which means "immediately," has come to indicate a patient whose medical condition suddenly may become very critical and must be treated or responded to as a medical emergency. When blood work is ordered STAT, it generally means that a specimen should be drawn and analyzed *immediately* in order to properly handle a critically ill patient. This requires an immediate response and effective technique from the phlebotomy team and constant availability of personnel for STAT blood collections. The phlebotomist should not only draw the blood quickly and properly but should ensure its timely delivery to the laboratory for STAT analysis. However, regardless of the physical state of the patient, the phlebotomist must adhere to the proper procedure for obtaining the best possible specimen from the patient. No shortcuts can be allowed in spite of the emergency situation that may be in progress. The phlebotomist has a responsibility to the patient to obtain a properly labeled, correct specimen for the test that is ordered. Anything less than that may lose precious time for the patient being treated while another specimen is being collected.

Test Collection Priorities

Very often, multiple blood assays are ordered on patients. Whether the phlebotomist chooses to use a multiple-draw evacuated tube collection system or a plastic syringe, there are certain guidelines for delivery of blood into the proper collection tubes.

Evacuated Tube Collection System. Sterile blood culture specimens should be collected first to decrease the possibility of bacterial contamination. Whenever coagulation studies are ordered, at least one other tube of blood should be drawn before the coagulation test specimen. This diminishes contamination with tissue fluids, which may initiate the clotting sequence. Any tube that has an anticoagulant in it should be drawn last so that it can be mixed as soon after collection as possible. Care should be taken that the anticoagulant present in the tube does not come into contact with the multisample needle when changing tubes, as some may be carried into the next tube and cause erroneous test results. For example, it is recommended that blood for serum iron be drawn *before* other specimens collected in tubes with chelating anticoagulants [e.g., ethylenediaminetetraacetate (EDTA)] to avoid interference in testing the serum iron level. Also, since the chelating anticoagulant EDTA is usually bound to potassium as EDTA (K_3) or bound to sodium as EDTA (Na_2), it is important to collect specimens requiring this anticoagulant *after* a specimen is collected in heparin for electrolytes. The electrolyte determinations include measurement of potassium and sodium. If the EDTA (K_3) or EDTA (Na_2) is used for a blood collection prior to the electrolyte collected specimen, the K_3 or Na_2 may falsely elevate the patient's potassium value or sodium value, respectively. Generally, if the tube is held horizontally or slightly down during blood collection, transfer of anticoagulants from tube to tube will be minimal.

Syringe Collection. When a phlebotomist chooses to use a syringe, the order of delivery of blood to the tubes changes considerably. If coagulation studies are ordered, the blood should be delivered to the sodium citrate tube first and mixed; next, blood should be delivered to any other anticoagulated tube and mixed. Finally, tubes without anticoagulant may be filled from the syringe. If a large volume of blood (at least 20 mL) has been drawn and there is a possibility that part of the blood may be clotted, the needle should be removed from the hub of the syringe, the stopper removed from the tube and the blood expelled into the tube along the side.

When blood cultures are ordered, the procedure should be followed as described in the section of Chapter 5 on Blood Cultures. The blood should be

Evacuated tube method

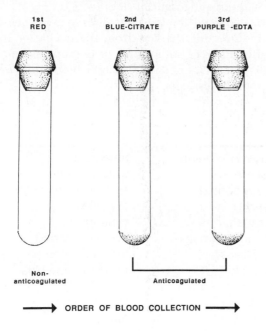

Syringe deposit method

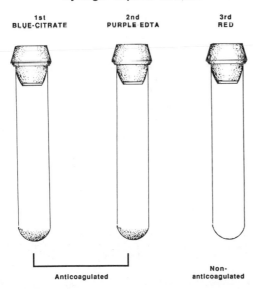

Figure 4–23. Collection priority. Based on which method is used, the order of tube collection is changed. Using the evacuated tube method, the plain red top tube is first, followed by the blue, purple, and any others that are needed. Using the syringe deposit method, the blood should be expelled into the blue top tube first, followed by other anticoagulated tubes, then the plain red top tube last.

delivered first aseptically into the culture bottle(s), then to the anticoagulated tubes, and finally to the tubes without anticoagulant (Fig. 4–23).

The blood should always be delivered gently to the tubes to avoid hemolyzing the cells. This is done by directing the flow from the needle or the syringe hub along the side of the tube without foaming or extra pressure on the plunger. Evacuated tubes fill themselves, and therefore the blood does *not* need to be forcefully ejected from the syringe.

KEY TERMS

basal state	hemoconcentration	petechiae
capillary pipets	hemolysis	skin puncture sites
decontamination	infection control	specimen rejection
diurnal variations	lancets	supine
dorsal hand vein	micropipets	syncope
technique	National Committee	syringe method
edema	for Clinical	test collection priority
evacuated tube	Laboratory	thrombosed veins
method	Standards (NCCLS)	thrombosis
fasting	occluded veins	tourniquets
hematoma	patient priority	turbid

STUDY QUESTIONS
Choose one or more of the following answers.

1. Laboratory reference values are calculated from which type of specimen?

   a. basal state   **c.** random samples during the day
   b. early morning   **d.** evening

2. A patient may be identified by which of the following means:

   a. patient's chart   **c.** patient's armband
   b. nurse   **d.** ward clerk

3. Which of the following is *not* a site for skin puncture:

   a. wrist   **c.** ankle
   b. vein   **d.** heel

4. When is it beneficial to use a "butterfly needle"? For

   a. heel puncture   **c.** veins in the ankle
   b. veins in the wrist or hand   **d.** fingerstick

5. What effect does warming the site have on venipuncture?

a. it keeps veins from rolling   c. it causes hemoconcentration
b. it makes veins stand out   d. it increases localized blood flow

6. What is the best angle for needle insertion during venipuncture?

a. 15 degrees   c. 45 degrees
b. 30 degrees   d. 80 degrees

7. Why is it necessary to control the depth of lancet insertion during skin puncture? To avoid

a. puncturing a vein   c. excessive bleeding
b. bacterial contamination   d. osteomyelitis

8. Which of the following factors result in failure to draw blood during venipuncture?

a. losing the vacuum in the tube
b. tourniquet is on too tight
c. needle was inserted through the vein
d. veins are sclerosed

9. Hematomas during venipuncture result from which of the following:

a. needle bevel is against the vein wall
b. needle bevel is partially inserted in the vein
c. needle is occluded
d. patient has coagulation problems

10. Hemoconcentration can be caused by which of the following:

a. long-term IV therapy   c. excessive needle probing
b. lengthy tourniquet application d. sclerosed or occluded veins

REFERENCES

1. Henry JB: *Todd, Sanford, Davidsohn—Clinical Diagnosis and Management by Laboratory Methods.* 18th ed., Philadelphia, W.B. Saunders, 1991.
2. Rudmann SV: The effects of exercise on hemostasis: A review of the literature and implications for research. *J Med Technol* 4(5): 215, 1987.
3. Damon Corporation: *Handbook of Specimen Collection and Preparation,* Damon Co., 1977.
4. Becton-Dickinson: *Blood Specimen Collection by Skin Puncture in Infants.* Becton-Dickinson Vacutainer Systems, Rutherford, N.J., 1982.

5. CACMLE, *Intro. to Phlebotomy*, Self-Study Course. Colorado Assn. for Continuing Med. Lab. Education, 925 S. Niagara St., Suite 220, Denver, Colorado 80224, 1988.

6. NCCLS: *Procedures for the Collection of Diagnostic Blood Specimens by Skin Puncture*, 3rd ed. 11(11), National Committee for Clin Lab Stds, Villanova, Pa., 1991.

7. Centers for Disease Control. Update: Universal Precautions for Prevention of Transmission of Human Immunodeficiency Virus, Hepatitis B Virus, and Other Bloodborne Pathogens in Health Care Settings. *MMWR,* 1988, 37(24), 377–382.

8. CAP: "So You're Going to Collect a Blood Specimen, An Introduction to Phlebotomy," 4th ed. Northfield, Ill, College of American Pathologists, 1989.

9. Meites S, Levitt MJ: Skin puncture and blood collecting techniques for infants. *Clin Chem* 25:183, 1979.

10. Lilien LD, Harris VJ, Ramamurthy RS, Pildes RS: Neonatal osteomyelitis of the calcaneus: Complications of heel puncture. *J Pediatr* 88:478, 1976.

11. Pailet JL: OSHA Publishes Final Regulations Governing Bloodborne Pathogens. *ASMT Today,* VII(1): 1992.

12. Clagg ME, Jamieson B: Pediatric Phlebotomy, *ASCP* Fall, Teleconference Series, No. 9434, Sept. 6, 1990.

13. Clagg ME: Venous Sample Collection from Neonates Using Dorsal Hand Veins. *Lab Medicine,* April 1989.

14. Larson JM: A stick in time saves nine. *MLO* April, 109, 1981.

5 Special Collection Procedures

SPECIAL TESTS

Depending on the specific needs of individual clinical settings, phlebotomists may be required to perform a variety of special tests or procedures in addition to routine skin tests and venipuncture. The following section presents basic techniques and precautions for various "special" tests. It is suggested that extensive training sessions and supervision accompany the student phlebotomist in these procedures because they can harm the patient if performed incorrectly.

Capillary Blood Gases

Arterial blood is the specimen of choice for testing the pH, O_2, and CO_2 content of the blood. As discussed in a preceding chapter, skin puncture blood is less desirable as a specimen source because it contains blood from capillaries, venules, arterioles, and fluids from the surrounding tissue. In addition, common collection methods for "capillary" blood gases employ an open collection system in which the specimen is temporarily exposed to room air, theoretically allowing for a brief exchange of gases (both O_2 and CO_2) before sealing the specimen from the air.

Capillary blood gases are often collected from small children and babies for whom arterial punctures can be too dangerous. They are collected from the same areas of the body as other capillary samples such as the lateral posterior area of the heel, the great toe, or the ball of the finger. (See Chapter 4 for microcollection procedures.)

When a capillary blood gas is ordered, the phlebotomist should warm the area ahead of time to ensure that a good blood flow is obtained and that blood can be quickly collected, anticoagulated, and sealed from contact with room air. To do this procedure, a site is chosen and a cloth or towel is saturated with warm water and wrapped around the foot or hand for 5 to 10 min. Care should be taken that the warming cloth is not too hot; if the warmed cloth can be held comfortably in the hand, it is not too warm for the patient. When the phlebotomist is prepared to collect the blood gas, the towel should be removed and the area dried. The puncture site should be cleaned and entered in the usual manner for all skin punctures (as discussed in Chapter 4). A heparinized capillary (Fig. 5–1) tube with a volume of at least 100 μL should be used to collect the specimen. A metal filing may be inserted into the tube before collecting to help mix the specimen while it is entering the tube. It is extremely important that the specimen be collected with *no air bubbles,* which can distort the values obtained from the specimen. When the tube is full, the ends should be sealed with plastic caps or clay (according to the individual laboratory protocol) and a magnet should be used to draw the metal filing back and forth across the length of the tube to completely mix the specimen. The tube should then be labeled and submerged in an ice water bath for transfer to the laboratory. The sample should be analyzed immediately in the laboratory. However, if

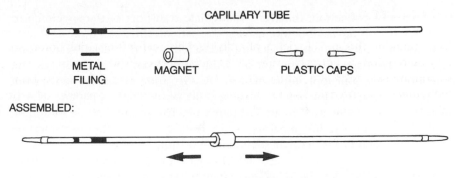

Figure 5–1. Capillary blood gas tubes.

it is stored horizontally, capped, and on ice water, it can be kept up to 2 hours without serious degradation. The skin puncture site should be pressed with a clean gauze sponge until bleeding stops and a bandage may be left over the spot.

Arterial Blood Gases

When an *arterial blood gas* is ordered, the experienced phlebotomist, nurse, or physician should palpate the areas of the forearm where the artery is typically close to the surface, namely, the brachial artery in the cubital fossa and the radial artery in the radial sulcus of the forearm. If the arms of the patient cannot be used, the femoral artery in the groin may be used. With the forefinger or first two fingers, the phlebotomist should press at these sites to find the artery. The thumb should never be used for palpating because there is a pulse in the thumb that may be confused for the patient's own pulse.

Once the site is decided upon, the area should be cleaned well with povidone-iodine solution (Betadine). No tourniquet is required as the artery has its own strong blood pressure. As in venipuncture, a syringe with needle can be used to withdraw the sample. However, the syringe should be small (5 mL or 10 mL) and made of glass. The addition of lithium liquid heparin to coat the syringe barrel will anticoagulate the blood. Using too much liquid heparin is probably the most common preanalytical error in blood gas measurements.[20] Therefore, the amount of anticoagulant should be 0.05 mL of liquid heparin (1000 IU/mL) for each milliliter of blood. The phlebotomist should pull the skin taut and enter the pulsating artery at a high angle, usually no less than 45 degrees. Little or no suction is needed as the blood flows quickly into the syringe under its own pressure. When enough sample has been drawn (usually about 1 mL), the phlebotomist withdraws the needle and applies gauze and direct manual pressure on the site for at least 15 minutes. The syringe should be quickly capped, mixed with the anticoagulant, labeled, and placed in ice water *immediately* in an effort to keep the blood gases from escaping into the atmosphere. Ideally the specimen should be analyzed within

10 minutes of collection; therefore, immediate transport of the specimen to the laboratory is advised. Before leaving the patient, the phlebotomist should clean the puncture site with an alcohol pad to remove the excess Betadine and a pressure bandage should be left on. If bleeding from the site persists, the phlebotomist should apply more manual pressure and ring for assistance from the patient's nurse. The phlebotomist should never leave a patient who is bleeding, particularly after an arterial puncture. The primary nurse should be notified after an arterial puncture is performed so that the area may be checked frequently for deep or superficial bleeding.

It should be noted that arterial blood results for some analytes (e.g., ammonia, glucose, lactic acid, alcohol) may differ from venous blood results because of metabolic activities. Therefore, arterial blood samples should be collected for the blood gas measurements only when specifically requested by the attending physician. In such situations, the request slip must indicate that arterial blood was collected for the analytes.

Bleeding Time Test

The *bleeding time test* is a useful tool for testing platelet plug formation in the capillaries. It is generally used in conjunction with other coagulation tests for diagnosing coagulopathies or problems in hemostasis, such as thrombocytopenia, qualitative platelet defects, vascular abnormalities, and von Willebrand's disease. It is most frequently used as a preoperative screening test.

The test is performed by making a minor standardized incision in either the earlobe or forearm and recording the length of time required for bleeding to cease. The duration of bleeding from a punctured capillary depends upon the quantity and quality of platelets and the ability of the blood vessel wall to constrict.

There have been many methods used to measure the bleeding time, dating back to 1910 when Duke originally described a method in which a lancet was used to make a puncture wound in the earlobe. This test was difficult to standardize, did not allow space for repeat testing, and often caused undue apprehension in the patient. Ivy improved the bleeding time test in 1941 by using a lancet to make puncture wounds on the forearm while maintaining a constant venous pressure with a blood pressure cuff. Both of these methods are difficult to reproduce due to several variables (i.e., depth of puncture, length of puncture).

Clinical research has led to the development of automated incision-making instruments for bleeding times. One is called Surgicutt.[2] It is a sterile, standardized, easy-to-use, disposable instrument that makes a uniform, surgical incision. This instrument is a spring-activated surgical steel blade housed in a self-containing plastic unit from which the blade protracts and retracts automatically, eliminating the variable of blade incision. The following steps provide the procedure for the Surgicutt Bleeding Time Test.[3]

1. Prior to beginning the procedure, patients should be advised that there is an occasional scarring problem inherent in the bleeding time test. Butterfly-type bandages can reduce the potential scarring by applying one to the incision area for a 24-hour period. If there is ooze from the incision as may be encountered in severe primary hemostatic disorders, then a pressure-type dressing should be used in conjunction with the butterfly-type bandage. If the puncture site is still bleeding beyond 15 minutes, the test should be discontinued by applying pressure to the area. A physician should be notified. The patient can also be asked if he or she has taken aspirin or other salicylates within the previous 2 weeks. These drugs interfere with the test.

2. Materials and supplies should be prepared before beginning the procedure. The following items are needed:
   - Surgicutt instrument. Each self-containing unit is sufficient for a single bleeding time determination. If package has been broken, do not use.
   - Gloves
   - Antiseptic swab
   - Blood pressure cuff (sphygmomanometer)
   - Filter paper disk (one to two Whatman's no. 1 filter paper disks per bleeding time test)
   - Butterfly-type bandage

3. Place the patient's arm on a steady support with the volar surface exposed. The incision is best performed over the lateral aspect, volar surface of the forearm approximately 5 cm below the antecubital crease. Avoid surface veins, scars, bruises, and edematous areas. Lightly shave the area if body hair will interfere with the test.

4. Place the blood pressure cuff on the upper arm. Inflate the cuff to 40 mm Hg. The time between inflation of the cuff and the incision should be 30 to 60 seconds. Hold at this exact pressure for the duration of the test.

5. Cleanse the area with an antiseptic swab and allow to air-dry. Remove the Surgicutt device from the package, being careful not to contaminate the instrument by touching or resting the blade-slot end on any unsterile surface.

6. Remove the safety clip. (Safety clip may be replaced if the test is momentarily delayed; however, prolonged exposure of Surgicutt to uncontrolled environmental conditions prior to use may affect its sterility.) Once safety clip is removed, DO NOT push the trigger or touch the blade slot.

7. Hold the device securely between the thumb and the middle finger. Gently rest it on the patient's forearm and apply minimal pressure so that both ends of the instrument are lightly touching the skin. A

horizontal incision parallel to the antecubital crease is the most sensitive technique for the bleeding time.

8. Gently push the trigger, starting the stopwatch simultaneously. The blade will make an incision 5 mm long by 1 mm deep. Remove the device from the patient's forearm immediately after triggering. After 30 seconds, wick the flow of blood with filter paper. Bring the filter paper close to the incision, but DO NOT touch the paper directly to the incision, so as not to disturb the formation of a platelet plug.

9. Wick the blood every 30 seconds thereafter until blood no longer stains the paper. Stop the timer. Bleeding time is determined to the nearest 30 seconds. Normal ranges vary from one health care facility to another. However, most are in the approximate range of 2.0 to 8.0 minutes.

10. Remove the blood pressure cuff and cleanse the incision site with an antiseptic swab. Apply the nonallergenic butterfly-type bandage for 24 hours.

The Simplate R (Retractable) and Simplate II R are sterile, disposable devices (Fig. 5−2) used to make uniform incisions for the bleeding time test. The spring-loaded blades are contained in a plastic housing. When triggered on the forearm, Simplate R and Simplate II R are designed to provide one to two incisions, respectively 5-mm long by 1-mm deep. Simplate II R is used for duplicate determinations. These devices standardize bleeding time testing by producing a uniform incision that provides reliable and reproducible results.

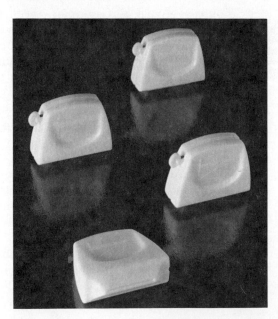

Figure 5−2. Simplate R (Retractable) bleeding device. *(Courtesy of Organon Teknika Corp., Durham, N.C.)*

Possible Interfering Factors.   This bleeding time test is a screening test and results of this test alone are not sufficient to diagnose specific conditions. A prolonged bleeding time may indicate the need for further testing (e.g., platelet count). In addition, the following items should be considered:

- The ingestion of aspirin-containing products up to 7 to 10 days prior to testing may affect results.
- Other drugs (e.g., dextran, streptokinase, streptodornase, ethyl alcohol, mithramycin) may cause a prolonged bleeding time.

There are other variations of this same procedure using different devices. For reproducible results, it is important to follow the manufacturer's instructions and to teach all phlebotomists in the same manner.

Lee-White Clotting Time

This manual test is poorly reproducible, insensitive to significant coagulation factor deficiencies, and time-consuming. The *Lee-White clotting time* can easily be replaced by automated methods for prothrombin (PT) and activated partial thromboplastin time (PTT). For monitoring heparin therapy, it is considered obsolete at many institutions because other routine coagulation will suffice.

Microbiologic Cultures

Specimens for microbial culture are often transported to the laboratory by phlebotomists. Most of them have been collected using sterile equipment and procedures. These specimens are screened in the microbiology laboratory for the presence of infectious agents such as bacteria, parasites, fungi, and viruses. The phlebotomist should recognize the potential hazards in handling these specimens and the need for maintaining them in sterile containers. If a phlebotomist inadvertently contaminates one of these specimens, it may lead to false-positive results, which can be harmful to the patient. Microbial specimens should be transported promptly to the laboratory.

Phlebotomists are asked most often to collect blood cultures. Occasionally, a phlebotomist may be asked to collect other specimens for culture such as swabs of the throat or nasopharynx, and urine. Regardless of the source, the phlebotomist should check hospital policies before practicing such procedures. If a health care facility does allow phlebotomists to collect these specimens, he or she should be thoroughly familiar with the procedures before attempting them on a patient.

Blood Cultures

Blood cultures are often collected on patients who have fevers of unknown origin (FUO). Sometimes, during the course of a bacterial infection, bacteremia may result and become the dominant clinical feature. In the case of a patient who experiences fever spikes, it is generally recommended that blood cultures be drawn before and after the spike, when bacteria may be most likely present in the peripheral circulation. It is best to draw one set of aerobic and anaerobic cultures at the time the order is given. Thirty minutes later, a second set of anaerobic and aerobic cultures should be obtained. A request for "second site" blood cultures that are obtained concurrently on opposite arms is useful when the physician suspects bacteremia due to a local internal infection. However, a "second site" culture is *not* a very effective tool for *routine* blood culture orders and provides relatively little information that properly spaced, timed blood cultures cannot provide.[4]

Prior to beginning the procedure, the phlebotomist may briefly explain the test to the patient. The following steps should then occur for blood culture collection:

1. Materials should be gathered and prepared next to the patient. The following items are needed: gloves, iodine scrub swabstick (10% povidone-iodine solution with lathering agents), acetone-alcohol swabstick, iodine prep swabstick (10% povidone-iodine solution), alcohol preps, two blood culture bottles: one aerobe, one anaerobe, two needles, and a syringe.

2. Scrub the site of the venipuncture with the iodine scrub swabstick for at least 2 minutes. The excess foam should be removed with the acetone-alcohol swabstick. The phlebotomist's gloved forefinger should also be cleaned in the same manner.

3. Prep the area of the venipuncture with the iodine swabstick by beginning in the center and rubbing the swab outward in concentric circles. Do not go back over any area that has been prepped (Fig. 5–3). Allow the area to dry for 1 minute. While the area is drying, prep the tops of the blood culture bottles with the iodine scrub swabstick and prepare the needle and syringe. A syringe and needle or evacuated tube assembly must be prepared cautiously so as not to exercise the plunger, destroy the sterility, or eliminate the anaerobic conditions of the syringe. A second needle should be readily available.

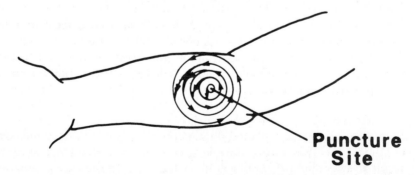

Puncture Site

Figure 5–3. Arm preparation for blood cultures.

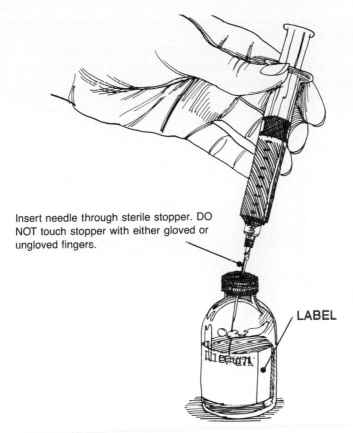

Insert needle through sterile stopper. DO NOT touch stopper with either gloved or ungloved fingers.

LABEL

Figure 5–4 Inoculating blood culture bottles. *(Courtesy of College of American Pathologists, Skokie, Ill.)*

4. The venipuncture is performed in the same manner as described in Chapter 4. Most blood culture bottles require 3 to 5 mL of blood per bottle. Some culture bottles contain resin beads that neutralize antibiotics in the patient's blood specimen. If not neutralized, the antibiotics can inhibit bacterial growth and give erroneously false-negative results. For inoculating the bottles use a clean needle. This eliminates bacterial contamination from the pores and deep recesses of the tissue that may be picked up as the needle is removed. Replace the iodine from the tops of the bottles with an alcohol prep. Place 3 to 5 mL of blood in the *anaerobic bottle first* and then 3 to 5 mL in the *aerobic bottle*. (See Fig. 5–4.) If only 3 mL (or less) was obtained, place the entire amount in the aerobic bottle. Some bottles are shaped to fit into the barrel apparatus just as an evacuated tube would, thereby eliminating one step (Fig. 5–5). Also, evacuated tubes containing *sodium polyanethole sulfonate (SPS)* may be used to collect specimens for blood culture

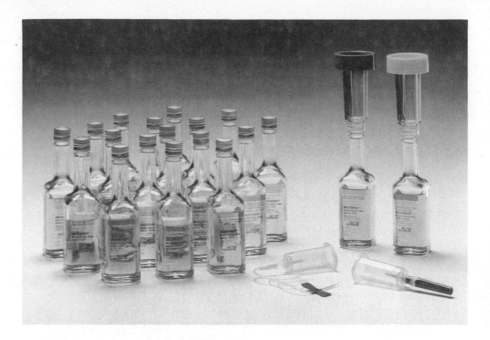

Figure 5–5. Vacutainer blood culture bottles. *(Courtesy of Becton-Dickinson and Company, Rutherford, N.J.)*

determinations. These tubes have yellow stoppers. After drawing blood, remove the iodine from the patient's skin with an alcohol prep. The phlebotomist must initial patient identification labels and attach them to each bottle.

Two studies have shown that the practice of changing needles after collecting blood for culture and inoculating the blood specimen into culture bottles has little if any effect on the contamination of blood cultures.[17,18] It was shown that careful skin cleansing is a more important factor in minimizing the contamination rate of blood cultures than is the common practice of replacing the needle used for venipuncture with a fresh, sterile needle before inoculating the blood into culture media. If a laboratory decides to discontinue the practice of changing needles during blood culture collection, the contamination rate of blood cultures should be compared before and after the procedural change to confirm that the contamination rate has not increased.

Blood drawn for culture must not be obtained through central venous catheter (CVC) lines if it cannot be obtained by venipuncture. Contamination rates may be increased if the indwelling catheter is used to obtain the culture specimen.

Another source of error may involve failure to follow the sterile procedure, resulting in contamination of the blood culture and misinformation to the clinician. Palpation of the venipuncture site after the site has been prepared without first cleaning the gloved finger can also result in contamination to the culture. Failure to wipe the iodine from the tops of the bottle with alcohol can result in a false-negative culture. Using too little blood for the culture can also result in a false-negative culture. Injection of air into the anaerobe bottle can cause death of some anaerobic microorganisms and result in a false-negative culture. For this reason, the anaerobe bottle must be inoculated first. Removal of the entire metal ring on some manufacturer's bottles introduces air into the bottles and could cause contamination.[5]

The Isostat System (Isolator microbial tubes) manufactured by Wampole Laboratories (Cranbury, N.J.) is a special blood culture tube system (see Figures 5–6 and 5–7). Isolator microbial tube has (1) a stopper that fits standard blood collection vacuum holders, (2) lysing and anticoagulating agents, (3) reagents in the tube that inactivate HIV within the normal 60 minute transport and processing time, and (4) containment adapters that help protect the phlebotomists/laboratorians against infection due to aerosols or breakage during centrifugation. Using this tube affords the advantage of faster microbial test results. It also helps safeguard the phlebotomist and laboratorian since the reagents in the Isolator tube inactivate HIV within the normal 60 minute transport and processing time. Also, the tube decreases the many

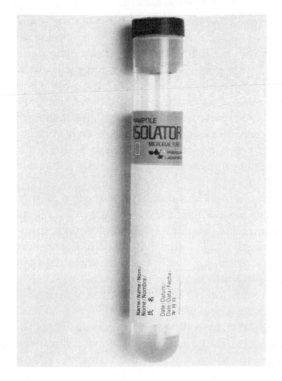

Figure 5–6. Wampole Isolator adult microbial tube. *(Courtesy of Wampole Laboratories, Cranbury, N.J.)*

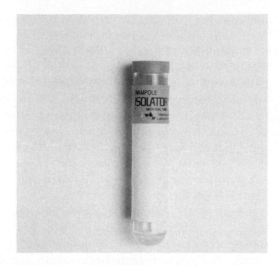

Figure 5–7. Wampole Isolator pediatric microbial tube. *(Courtesy of Wampole Laboratories, Cranbury, N.J.)*

procedural manipulations required during conventional blood culture collections.

Throat and Nasopharyngeal Culture Collections

Nasopharyngeal cultures are often performed to detect carrier states of *Neisseria meningitidis, Corynebacterium diphtheriae, Streptococcus pyogenes, Haemophilus influenzae,* and *Staphylococcus aureus.* In children and infants, from whom significant sputum cultures are difficult to obtain, nasopharyngeal cultures may be used to diagnose whooping cough, croup, and pneumonia. *Throat cultures* are most commonly obtained to determine the presence of streptococcal infections. As mentioned previously, phlebotomists should be fully taught this procedure prior to allowing them to acquire a specimen from a patient. Because coughing may force organisms from the lower respiratory tract into the nasopharynx, it may be best to perform a throat culture on a child or infant and stimulate coughing in order to obtain a more significant nasopharyngeal culture.

When a throat culture is ordered, the patient should be instructed to open the mouth wide, as if to yawn. A light source should be directed into the mouth and throat so that areas of inflammation, ulceration, exudation, or capsule formation can be readily seen. A tongue blade or spoon is used to depress the tongue and prevent contamination with organisms from the oral cavity. A sterile cotton swab should be used to brush both tonsillar areas, the posterior pharynx, and all other areas of possible infection.

The swab can then be placed in a special transport media or used to inoculate directly onto agar in a petri dish by rolling it across a small area of the media. It can then be transported to the laboratory, where it may be spread out or "streaked" for distribution of the microorganisms. A Gram-stained smear is often useful to provide preliminary indications of infection and should be made with the swab by rolling it across a sterile slide before placing it in transport media or inoculating plate agar. The slide, swab, and any inoculating media should be brought to the laboratory and processed as soon as possible after collection. The culture should be placed under optimal growth conditions for suspected pathogens. This is accomplished by incubating the culture. Timely processing of the specimen helps prevent overgrowth of normal flora, which can inhibit or mask any pathogenic organisms present.

Nasopharyngeal specimens should be obtained with a Dacron- or cotton-tipped flexible wire that can be easily sterilized prior to use. Commercially packaged sterilized swabs are also available. The swab is passed gently through the nose and into the nasopharynx where it is rotated, carefully removed, and then placed into transport media or inoculated onto media for isolation. Again, stress should be placed on the importance of timely processing of all specimens for very best results.

Skin Tests

On occasion, a phlebotomist may be asked to perform a skin test. Again, the phlebotomist should check the policies of the hospital prior to performing the procedure. Skin tests are simple and relatively inexpensive. They determine if a patient has ever had contact with a particular antigen and has produced antibodies to that antigen. A wide range of disease states stimulate antibody responses in individuals. Tests range from detection of ragweed and milk allergies in hypersensitive individuals, to tuberculosis and fungal infections in persons who have had contact with these organisms.

The skin test is administered by pulling in 0.1 mL of diluted antigen into a tuberculin syringe. All air bubbles should be expelled by holding the syringe straight up and tapping the sides of the barrel. The volar surface of the forearm should be cleaned with alcohol and prepared in the same manner as for a venipuncture. (See Chapter 4 on venipuncture collection.) The area should be devoid of scars, skin eruptions, or excessive hair. Holding the syringe at a small angle (approximately 20 degrees), the needle should be slipped just under the skin. The plunger should be pulled back to ensure that a blood vessel has not been entered. The fluid may be slowly expelled into the site. The needle should be promptly removed and only *slight* pressure is applied with gauze over the site. Care should be taken that the fluid does not leak out onto the gauze or run out of the injection site. It is best that the patient remain with the arm extended until the site has had time to close and retain the fluid. A bandage should not be used over the site as it may absorb some of the fluid and may distort the results of the skin tests by causing skin irritation from the adhesive. The patient should report any reaction whatsoever to the physician. Also, a return visit for proper interpretation of the skin reaction should be scheduled with the physician. Some health care agencies ask the patient to note the exact size of the reaction site and indicated it on a prelabeled card that can be mailed back to the institution. Patients should be fully informed of how to read these reactions if this is the case.

Glucose Tolerance Test

In patients who have symptoms suggesting problems in carbohydrate metabolism, such as diabetes mellitus, the *glucose tolerance test* can be an effective diagnostic tool. The test is performed by first obtaining fasting blood and urine specimens, giving the fasting patient a standard load of glucose, and obtaining subsequent blood and urine samples at intervals usually over a 5-hour period. Each specimen is then analyzed for glucose content. In general, glucose levels should return to normal within 2 hours after ingesting the glucose. In diabetic patients, it is necessary to carry out the test for 4 to 5 hours to observe how the patient metabolizes the glucose.

When a glucose tolerance test is to be performed, the patient should be given complete instructions about the procedure so his or her cooperation can be ensured (Fig. 5–8). For best results, the patient should eat normal, balanced meals for at least 3 days prior to the test. Twelve hours prior to the beginning of the test, the patient should fast completely. Water intake is strongly encouraged as frequent urine specimens are required throughout the procedure. Other beverages, including unsweetened tea or coffee, are not allowed. Cigarette smoking and gum chewing (including sugarless gum) should be discouraged until the completion of the test as they may stimulate digestion and interfere with the interpretation of the results. If a patient is chewing gum prior to or during the test, note this on the requisition slip.[5]

During the test, the patient drinks a standard dose of glucose, usually 75 or 100 g in adults or approximately 1 g/kg of body weight in children and small adults. A dose of 100 g is recommended for diagnosis of gestational diabetes.[16] Commercial preparations are available as flavored drinks to make the glucose more palatable. The patient must start and finish the drink within 5 minutes. Water intake is encouraged throughout the procedure. If the patient should vomit at any point in the procedure, the physician should be notified immediately to decide whether the test should be continued or stopped.[5]

When the patient has finished drinking the solution, the time is noted and 30-minute, 60-minute, 120-minute, and 180-minute blood and urine specimens are obtained. Thus, if the glucose is administered to the patient at 7:30 AM, then at 8:00 AM the 30-minute blood and urine specimens are obtained from the patient. This is followed by collections of blood and urine specimens at 8:30 AM (60 minutes), 9:30 AM (120 minutes) and 10:30 AM (180 minutes). In addition to the time, the tubes should be labeled "30 minutes," "1st hour," and so on (Fig. 5–9). If blood is obtained initially by venipuncture, all succeeding specimens must also be venous blood. Similarly, if capillary blood is used, all specimens should be collected by microtechnique because values and methods of analysis may vary between the two types of samples. If serum samples are used instead of plasma samples with a preservative, the tubes should be centrifuged

GLUCOSE TOLERANCE TEST

Introduction

A glucose tolerance test (GTT) has been ordered by your physician. The purpose of a GTT is to test the efficiency of your body's insulin-releasing mechanism and glucose-disposing system.

You must prepare your body for the GTT by changing your eating and medication routines slightly for 3 days before the test. It is very important that you follow the instructions below in order for accurate results to be obtained.

Basically, you will need to follow these 3 guidelines to prepare for your GTT test:
1. Your carbohydrate intake must be at least 150 grams per day for 3 days prior to the GTT.
2. Do not eat anything for 12 hours before the GTT, but do not fast for more than 16 hours before the test.
3. Do not exercise for 12 hours before the GTT.

Preparation: Medication

You must tell your physician if you are currently using any of the following medications before proceeding with the GTT, because they may interfere with test results:
- Alcohol
- Anticonvulsants (seizure medication)
- Blood pressure medication
- Clofibrate
- Corticosteroids
- Diuretics (fluid pills)
- Estrogens (birth control pills/estrogen replacement pills)
- Salicylates (aspirin, pain killers)—only if taken in high doses, such as for rheumatoid arthritis

Preparation: Diet and Exercise

Remember that for 3 days prior to your test, your diet must contain at least 150 grams of carbohydrate per day. The following is a list of high-carbohydrate foods:
- Milk and milk products—12 grams of carbohydrate per serving. One serving is equal to 8 ounces of milk (whole, skim, or buttermilk), 4 ounces of evaporated milk, or 1 cup of plain yogurt.
- Vegetables—5 grams of carbohydrate per serving. One serving is equal to ½ cup of any vegetables excluding starches (e.g., potatoes, corn, or peas).

(continued)

Figure 5–8. Example of a patient information card. *(Courtesy of Division of Laboratory Medicine, M.D. Anderson Hospital and Tumor Institute, Houston, Tex.)*

- Fruits and fruit juices—10 grams of carbohydrate per serving. One serving is equal to ½ cup of juice, 1 small piece of fresh fruit, or ½ cup of unsweetened canned fruit, with the following exceptions:

Apple juice	⅓ cup
Grape juice	¼ cup
Raisins	2 tablespoons
Watermelon	1 cup
Prunes	2 medium
Banana	½ small
Dates	2
Cantaloupe	¼ 6″ melon
Honeydew melon	⅛ 7″ melon

- Breads and Starches—15 grams of carbohydrate per serving. One serving is equal to 1 slice of bread or small roll. Other one-serving sizes are:

Bagel, English muffin	½
Tortilla	1
Cooked cereal	½ cup
Dry cereal	¾ cup
Cooked rice, noodles, pasta	½ cup
White potatoes, dried beans and peas	½ cup
Yams	¼ cup
Corn	⅓ cup
Crackers	5–6

- Meats, cheeses, and fats—contain few or no carbohydrate
- Miscellaneous

Ice cream	½ cup	15 grams of carbohydrate
Sherbet	½ cup	30 grams of carbohydrate
Gelatin	½ cup	30 grams of carbohydrate
Jams, jellies	1 tbsp	15 grams of carbohydrate
Sugar	1 tsp	4 grams of carbohydrate
Carbonated beverage	6 oz.	20 grams of carbohydrate
Hard candy	2 pieces	10 grams of carbohydrate
Fruit pie	⅙	60 grams of carbohydrate
Cream pie	⅙	50 grams of carbohydrate
Plain cake	¹⁄₁₀	30 grams of carbohydrate
Frosted cake	¹⁄₁₀	38 grams of carbohydrate

Preparation: General Health

The following physical conditions should be reported to your doctor, because they too may affect the results of your test:
- Acute pancreatitis
- Adrenal insufficiency
- Diabetes mellitus
- Hyperinsulinism (excess insulin secretion, resulting in hypoglycemia)
- Hyperthyroidism
- Hypopituitarism (decreased function of pituitary gland)
- Pregnancy
- Stress

If you have any difficulty making the necessary alterations in your diet or medication schedule, please inform your doctor. For accurate test results, the instructions on this card must be followed.

Figure 5–8. (Continued).

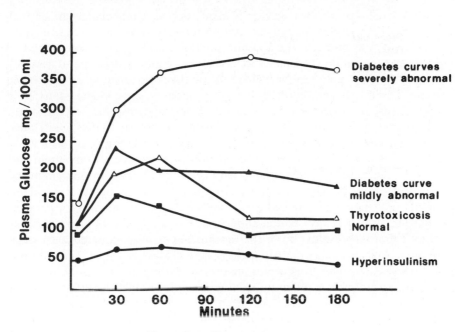

Figure 5–9. Glucose tolerance test.

immediately after collection, and then the serum should be separated from the blood cells and placed in the refrigerator to inhibit glucose utilization by white blood cells.

Postprandial Glucose Test

The 2-hour *postprandial glucose test* can be used to screen patients for diabetes because glucose levels in serum specimens drawn 2 hours after a meal are rarely elevated in normal patients. In contrast, diabetic patients will usually have increased values 2 hours after a meal.

For this test, the patient should be placed on a high carbohydrate diet 2 to 3 days before the test. The day of the test, the patient should eat a breakfast of orange juice, cereal with sugar, toast, and milk to provide an approximate equivalent of 100 g of glucose. A blood specimen is taken 2 hours after the patient has finished eating breakfast. The glucose level on this specimen is then determined. The physician can decide if further carbohydrate metabolism tests are needed (such as a glucose tolerance test).

"Rapid" Methods for Glucose Testing

In recent years there has been much emphasis on screening tests for detecting glucose metabolic abnormalities. Most of these "rapid" skin puncture methods are either visual, for example, a color change on a dipstick is compared to a preprinted color chart; or a device is used such as a reflectance meter that measures a color change as glucose in the specimen reacts with reagents on a dipstick pad. In both cases, the amount of color change is proportional to the glucose concentration. These "rapid" methods require whole blood samples collected by skin puncture from the finger, heel (in infants), or a flushed heparin line. As for any blood collection procedure, appropriate safety procedures must be followed (e.g., wearing gloves) and disposal of potentially contaminated waste must be part of the quality control and safety guidelines. These "bedside" procedures are handy for quick screening in a hospital or outpatient setting. However, *extreme caution* must be taken to maintain and provide a rigid quality control and training program prior to implementing these procedures. Variance in methodology and lack of quality control on reagents and equipment can lead to serious medical consequences for patients being tested.[6,7] Therefore, careful adherence to manufacturer's instructions as well as a thorough evaluation of the monitoring devices, coupled with strict adherence to daily quality control procedures, will ensure a more accurate and precise screening tool. In addition, careful recording of the results must include the date, time, and phlebotomist identification as well as verification that the results are from the bedside rather than the clinical laboratory. Some health care facilities have bedside test results recorded on special bedside testing forms or in a separate section of the patient's medical record.

Epinephrine and Glucagon Tolerance Tests

Epinephrine increases blood sugar by accelerating glycogenolysis (breakdown of glycogen). This tolerance test is used to determine availability and quantity of liver glycogen by stimulating an increase in blood sugar by epinephrine injection.

A fasting blood sugar is obtained. The physician or other qualified professional should inject 10 minims of a 1:1000 solution of epinephrine hydrochloride intravenously. Thirty minutes after the injection, another blood sample should be taken for glucose level determination. The blood sugar should rise at least 30 mg/dL at the 30-minute sample. The blood sugar level should return to the fasting level in about 2 hours. If the patient's blood sugar level does not respond or rises only slightly, several disease states may be responsible. If glycogen storage is depleted, the epinephrine has little effect and the blood sugar may rise only slightly. Such conditions exist in hepatocellular damage, such as cirrhosis and fatty liver. If glycogen stores are not readily available, though they may be present, the epinephrine has little effect on blood sugar. Von Gierke's disease is known to interfere with the availability of glycogen for conversion to sugar.

Because several disease states and possibilities exist for a low response to an epinephrine injection, this test is not considered a diagnostic tool, but used in combination with other carbohydrate metabolism studies.

The *glucagon tolerance test* is conducted in a similar manner as the *epinephrine tolerance test.* In fact, often the two stimulants may be given in combination to test liver glycogen stores. The amount of the stimulants given should be determined by the ordering physician and administered by a qualified professional or physician. The phlebotomist may be involved in drawing the blood samples for glucose determinations and may be responsible for labeling and delivering the specimens to the laboratory.

Lactose Tolerance Test

Some otherwise healthy adults experience difficulty in digesting lactose, a milk sugar. They appear to lack a mucosal lactase enzyme that breaks down the lactose into the simple sugars, glucose and galactose. Instead, gastrointestinal discomfort may result, followed by diarrhea. These patients usually show no further symptoms if milk is removed from their diet.

To determine if a patient suffers from lactose intolerance, a physician may order a *lactose tolerance test.* A 3-hour glucose tolerance test should be performed 1 day in advance to determine the patient's normal glucose curve. A lactose tolerance test should be performed the next day in the same manner as the glucose tolerance, substituting the same amount of lactose for the glucose given the previous day. Fasting, 1-hour, 2-hour, and 3-hour blood samples are drawn and tested for glucose. The curve should be similar to that obtained in the glucose tolerance if the patient has mucosal lactase and digests the sugar properly. If the patient is intolerant to lactose, his or her blood sugar will increase by no more than 20 mg/dL from the fasting sample.

The phlebotomist should be sure that a bathroom is conveniently located to the patient testing area because patients who are lactose intolerant may experience severe discomfort during the testing.

False-positive results have been known to occur in 25 to 33 percent of the patients tested who had normal lactase activity in small intestine biopsy specimens. This has been attributed to slow gastric emptying and not the absence of the lactase enzyme.

D-Xylose Tolerance Test

The D-xylose absorption test is commonly used for the diagnosis of malabsorption states. D-Xylose is a pentose found in certain fruits, such as plums, but does not normally occur in the blood or urine. Therefore, a patient should be fasting before the test and instructed not to eat fruits high in D-xylose for up to 3 days before the test. A measured load of D-xylose is given to the patient (25 g is recommended) and then his or her urine and blood are collected to determine concentrations of D-xylose. The patient should drink at least 250 mL of water during the next hour. However, the patient should not drink other fluids or eat during this next hour.

A 2-hour blood sample is taken and a pooled sample of urine is taken over the 5-hour period after dose administration. Both samples are analyzed for D-xylose and reported in mg/dL. Because xylose is not normally present in significant amounts in the blood, it is an excellent indicator of small intestine absorption as it passes unchanged through the liver and is excreted by the kidneys. Low values are seen in intestinal malabsorption, but are normal in pancreatic malabsorption. Low values are often obtained in cases where bacteria have overgrown in the small intestine and affected absorption in the jejunum.

Gastric Analysis and Hollander Tests

Gastric analysis and *Hollander tests* determine gastric function in terms of stomach acid production. The gastric analysis measures gastric acid secretion in response to stimulation from histamine or pentagastrin, whereas the Hollander test uses insulin to stimulate gastric secretions. Both tests involve passing a tube through the patient's nose and into the stomach. Both tests require intravenous administration of either histamine or insulin. Therefore, although the phlebotomist may be asked to assist and to draw specimens as required, the responsibility for properly intubating the patient (using fluoroscopic examination) and administering the stimulant intravenously should rest with the physician or nurse. The phlebotomist can be present to assist in patient care and to draw any required blood specimens, but should under no circumstances be expected to carry out the procedure. There is high risk to the patient if the tube is improperly placed and could puncture a lung if it enters the bronchial system instead of the esophagus. The phlebotomist can and should be responsible for proper labeling of gastric and blood samples when he or she is present and assisting during the procedure.

Sweat Chloride by Iontophoresis

The *sweat chloride test* is used in the diagnosis of cystic fibrosis. Patients with cystic fibrosis produce chloride in their sweat at 2 to 5 times the level produced by healthy individuals. Cystic fibrosis is a disorder of the exocrine glands, generally thought to be enzymatic in nature, which exhibits changes in mucous-producing glands in the body. Primarily affected are the lungs, upper respiratory tract, liver, and pancreas.

For the laboratory evaluation, pilocarpine hydrochloric acid (HCl) is iontophoresed into the skin of the patient to stimulate sweat production. The sweat is absorbed onto preweighed gauze pads and then the weight of the sweat is obtained. The pad is then diluted with deionized water and the chloride is generally read by titration with a chloridometer.

When a phlebotomist receives an order to perform a sweat chloride test on a patient, he or she should properly prepare for the procedure under the supervision of a medical technologist. Four cups and lids should be preweighed with two 2-in. square gauze pads in each cup. Only two cups are normally used, but the other two can be used as backups, if needed.

Choosing a site with the largest surface area (in children and infants, the leg is best suited), the phlebotomist should wipe the surface of the skin with a gauze pad soaked in deionized water. The area is wiped dry. Another 2-in. square, eight-ply gauze pad is soaked in 0.07 M sodium bicarbonate and placed on the cleaned area. The negative electrode is placed on the gauze and taped securely to the skin. The electrode should not be in direct contact with the skin at any time when the current is on.

Another gauze square is soaked in 0.33 percent pilocarpine-HCl and placed on the skin next to the sodium bicarbonate square, but not touching it. The positive electrode should be placed on that gauze and taped securely in place. Again, care should be taken that the electrode does not make direct contact with the skin at any time throughout the procedure. The area between and around the secured gauze squares should be wiped dry before the current is on. The current is turned on and very slowly raised to 1 mA. It is important that the current be increased slowly because a sudden increase may cause a shock to the patient.

After 10 minutes, the current is decreased to zero. The switch is turned off and the electrodes and gauze squares are removed. Reagent grade water is used to wipe off the pilocarpine-HCl area, which is then wiped dry.

A 2×2-in. square of thin waxed film, such as Parafilm,* should be cut out and handled with clean forceps. Using the forceps, the film can be placed against the cleaned area and taped securely on the skin on adjacent sides. Using forceps, two gauze pads from a preweighed cup are removed and placed between the Parafilm and the skin. The remaining side can be taped securely. Tape may also be applied across the top of the parafilm to prevent it from tearing. A timer should be started for 1 hour. During that period, the procedure should be repeated on the other arm or leg.

After 1 hour, the tape should be carefully removed and the gauze sponges removed with forceps and returned to the original cup. The lid must be tightly on the cup and then weighed again. After weighing, 200 µL of deionized water should be added to the cup. The lid should be replaced and wrapped securely with parafilm. The sponges should equilibrate for 2 to 3 hours or overnight. The phlebotomist should bring the cups and the weights measured during the procedure to the laboratory, where a medical technologist will measure the chloride on the chloridometer and calculate the results.

Therapeutic Drug Monitoring (TDM)

Laboratory drug monitoring of therapeutic agents is a complex endeavor that requires a great amount of coordination between laboratory, nursing, and pharmacy personnel. A basic understanding of the variables, information needed, and definitions of terms is important to accurate laboratory results.

To adequately evaluate the appropriate dosage levels of many drugs, the collection and evaluation of specimens for trough and peak levels is necessary. The trough level is the lowest concentration in the patient's serum, that is, the

*Brafilm, American Can Company, Dixie/Marathon, Greenwich, Conn.

specimen should be collected immediately prior to the administration of the drug. The peak level is the highest concentration of a drug in the patient's serum. The time it takes to reach the highest concentration varies with the mode of administration (intramuscular injection vs. intravenous infusion) and the rate at which the drug is infused. In addition, "random" levels may be appropriate for monitoring drug dosage if administered by continuous infusion and enough time has elapsed for the drug to reach equilibrium. Time of collection is much more critical for drugs with shorter half-lives (i.e., gentamicin, tobramycin, or procainamide) than for those with longer half-lives (phenobarbital or digoxin). Specimens for TDM should *not* be collected immediately following dosing.[14]

As a result of these factors, laboratory personnel must acquire and document additional information when performing these tests. A phlebotomist may be asked to acquire the following information: patient's name, identification number, location, test ordered, requesting physician, collection time and date, whether the order is for a peak, trough, or continuous infusion random level, time and date of last dose, time and date of next dose, and a nurse's verification that the dose was administered. Specific specimen guidelines for each drug should be established by pharmacy and laboratory staff and strictly adhered to.

It has been found that evacuated blood collection tubes without the plasticizer tris (butoxyethyl) phosphate (TBEP) on the tube stopper are suitable for most drugs.[10] However, to avoid the possibility of the blood coming into contact with an interfering stopper, blood specimens should be maintained in an upright position after collection. In addition, since falsely low levels of lidocaine, phenytoin, and pentobarbital occur with the use of gel serum separator tubes, this type of evacuated blood collection tube should be avoided in therapeutic drug monitoring.[11]

Most TDM assays should be performed on clotted blood. The National Committee for Clinical Laboratory Standards (NCCLS) has toxicology/drug monitoring requirements for blood collection containers that can be helpful to the health care institution in establishing specific specimen guidelines for each drug.[13]

Collection for Trace Metals

Testing for *trace metals* involves the use of specially prepared trace metal evacuated blood collection tubes. Also, special acid-washed plastic syringes are usually suitable for trace metal testing. For aluminum level determinations, a needle free of aluminum metal must be used. For lead levels, lead-free heparinized evacuated blood tubes equipped with sterilized stainless-steel needles should be used in blood collection.[12]

Specific specimen collection guidelines for trace metals should be established in the clinical laboratory's technical procedures on trace metal testing.

Blood Specimens for Toxicological Analysis/Forensic Specimens

In toxicological analysis, very small amounts of analytes are usually found in the blood, urine, or other specimen obtained for analysis. Thus, the type of specimen (e.g., venous blood, arterial blood), materials, and equipment used for collecting specimens for toxicological analysis can greatly affect the analytical results. The type of glass for the evacuated vacuum collection tube, stopper, or both may contain materials that will react with the analytes or absorb the analytes. Thus, for toxicological specimens, the phlebotomist must strictly adhere to the laboratory's guidelines for collection of these types of specimens. For example, since the source of blood analyzed (venous or capillary) must be considered in clinical laboratory test results for ethanol, the phlebotomist must be alert to collection requirements for this toxicological analyte and others that are tested.[19] In addition, when a specimen is collected for toxicology studies involving drug abuse testing, or other medical application related to civil or criminal law, these specimens are referred to as *forensic specimens*. They require a *chain-of-custody* form (Fig. 5–10) that must be completed showing specific identification, who obtained and processed the specimen, date, location, and the signature of the subject documenting that the specimen in the container is the one that was obtained on the person identified on the label. The specimen must be placed in a specimen transfer bag that permanently seals the specimen bag until it is cut open for analysis. The seal assures tamper-evident transfer of contents until it reaches its destination for analysis.[15]

Drawing Blood Through Central Venous Catheters (CVC)

Drawing blood specimens through *central venous catheter* (CVC) lines requires special techniques, training, and experience. Some hospitals require specialized training courses prior to allowing nursing or laboratory personnel to perform this function. The intravenous line is a direct pathway into the patient's bloodstream. Each time this intravenous system is entered, the possibility for contamination and infection exists. However, if strict adherence to aseptic technique is followed, this procedure can provide a relatively safe means of access to the CVC, thereby saving the patient some of the trauma of frequent venipuncture for laboratory studies. It is recommended that the CVC line be used only one time daily unless ordered otherwise by a physician. Specific criteria must be established at each hospital for obtaining blood through a CVC.

A 20-mL syringe is the largest syringe that is recommended with a soft-wall catheter because larger sizes may collapse the catheter wall. The patient should be placed in a position with the catheter hub at or below the level of the patient's heart to prevent possible air emboli when CVC is entered. Nursing or medical staff should be consulted before opening the CVC line to avoid interrupting medication, which is extremely vital to the maintenance of the

Name of subject: _____
Subject's SS#: _____-_____-_____
Specimen type: Blood___(Specify if venous, arterial, or capillary and if any additives
                       in container)
             Urine___
             Other (Specify) _____
Amount of specimen in mL: _____mL
Collected by (please print name here): _____
Signature of collector: _____
Date, time, and location of collection: _____
_____
Witness(es) _____
          _____

Signature of courier: _____ Date or time: _____

Received in lab by (please print) _____
Date & time: _____ (signature) _____

Condition of seals:
             1. Outside container sealed: _____Yes _____No
             2. Specimen sealed: _____Yes _____No
Seals broken and tested by: _____
             Date: _____ Time: _____
Additional transfers
From: _____ Date: _____ Time: _____
Reason: _____
To: _____ Date: _____ Time: _____

Figure 5–10. Chain of custody form

patient's care. At no time is it permissible for a phlebotomist to disconnect or reconnect an infusor or autosyringe pump. When drawing blood from multilumen catheters, the lumen(s) not being drawn should be clamped during the procedure to prevent dilution of the blood sample being drawn.

The following equipment and supplies should be prepared prior to beginning the procedure: lab requisitions, tubes, and labels for specimen, sterile gloves, two or three 20-mL disposable syringes, one 20-mL disposable syringe (optional), 10 mL normal saline for flushing the catheter, two or three sterile needles, sterile 4×4 gauze, linen protector to provide clean work area, plastic or paper container for waste or soiled items, adhesive tape, sterile heparin cap, alcohol wipe, and 100 U/mL heparin (optional).

The procedure may involve the following steps but is subject to differences among hospitals and must be performed by *authorized personnel only.*[5]

1. Check patient's chart for physician's order to draw blood through CVC.
2. Obtain laboratory requisitions and labels that reflect patient location and tests for which blood is needed.
3. Check labels against slips and patient's identification bracelet as described in Chapter 4.
4. Determine amount of blood to be drawn so that correct size syringe(s) can be used.
5. Assemble equipment, wash hands, and put sterile gloves on.
6. Aseptically draw up to 10-mL injectable normal saline and cap with sterile needle cover to maintain sterility. Take all supplies to bedside. Note: Take *only* tubes for the patient, no others.
7. Identify patient by armband ID, noting full name and hospital number. Check against preprinted labels.
8. Explain procedure to patient.
9. Provide adequate room and light for procedure.
10. Position patient by elevating the bed to a comfortable working level and making the bed flat, or have catheter hub at or below the level of the patient's heart.
11. Place linen protector with supplies on bed. Place sterile 4×4 in. gauze under connection site.
12. If IV is infusing, clamp off mainline IV tubing. Close slide clamp on short microbore tubing.
13. Loosen IV tubing connection or heparin cap. Aseptically disconnect IV tubing or injection cap from short microbore tubing, holding short microbore tubing and IV tubing "up" to avoid contamination.
14. Cap IV tubing with sterile needle and needle cover, and aseptically insert 10-mL syringe in short microbore tubing.
15. Unclamp short microbore tubing. Aspirate (slowly and steadily) 5 to 10 mL blood. Remove syringe with blood and discard.
16. Aseptically insert syringe of correct size for needed blood specimen into short microbore tubing.
17. Open the slide clamp on short microbore tubing and slowly aspirate blood in the quantity needed.
18. Close slide clamp on short microbore tubing. Remove syringe and place sterile needle on syringe.
19. Quickly and aseptically insert the 10-mL syringe with normal saline into the short microbore tubing. Open slide clamp on short microbore tubing.
20. Gently irrigate catheter with 5 mL normal saline.
21. Close slide clamp on short microbore tubing; temporarily leave syringe with 5 mL normal saline in place.
22. Place blood into blood collection tubes as previously described.
23. Open slide clamp on short microbore tubing. Complete irrigation of

catheter with remaining 5 mL normal saline. Close slide clamp on short microbore tubing.

24. Aseptically reconnect IV tubing to short microbore tubing. Open clamp on IV tubing and slide clamp on short microbore tubing.

25. Determine that IV fluids are infusing properly at rate set by unit nurse. *Note:* If pump is being used, make certain pump is ON and alarm is ON. If the rate of IV flow appears altered, the nurse should be notified *immediately.*

Retape connection between short microbore tubing and IV tubing.

26. Make sure the patient is in a safe and comfortable position with the bed down, siderails up, and bedside table and call light accessible to patient. Place used equipment and supplies in appropriate discard containers. The needles should NOT be recapped before discarding.

27. Write the date, time, and initial labels on blood specimens and place tubes of blood with the correct lab requisitions. Dispatch to laboratory in usual manner.

28. Document completion of procedure and any problems in the patient's medical record.

Note: The uncapped used needles should NOT be placed on the patient's bed but rather in an appropriate container until they can be properly discarded.

Cannulas and Fistulas

A *cannula* is a tubular instrument that is used in kidney patients to gain access to venous blood for dialysis or blood drawing. Drawing blood from the cannula of a kidney patient should be performed only by specially trained personnel since it requires special techniques and experience.

A *fistula* is an artificial shunt in which the vein and artery have been fused together through surgery. It is a permanent connection tube located in the arm of kidney dialysis patients. The phlebotomist should use extreme caution when collecting a blood specimen from a kidney dialysis patient and avoid using the patient's arm with the fistula as the site for venipuncture. If no other location can be found for the venipuncture site, the patient's arm must be cleaned *thoroughly* prior to blood collection. If the venipuncture site in this arm becomes infected, the inflammation in the blood vessels of the arm may shut down all the veins, requiring surgery to place a new shunt in the kidney dialysis patient.

Donor Room Collections

Properly trained phlebotomists may be employed in a regional blood center or hospital blood donor center to screen and collect blood from donors. This section summarizes the procedure outlined by the American Association of Blood Banks (AABB).[9] Only an experienced, properly trained phlebotomist or technologist should be considered for this function. A physical, emotional, or traumatic experience may keep a donor from volunteering in the future.

Donor Interview and Selection.   Not everyone who wishes to donate his blood is eligible. It is up to the interviewer to determine the eligibility of the donor. Carefully determining donor eligibility helps prevent the spread of disease to blood product recipients and prevents untoward effects for the potential donor.

The following information should be kept on file on every donor for a minimum of 5 years and initially obtained on every prospective donor, regardless of ultimate acceptability.[9]

1. Date of donation
2. Name: last, first, and middle
3. Address
4. Telephone number
5. Gender
6. Age and date of birth (donors should be between the ages of 17 and 66 years). Minors may be accepted if written consent has been obtained in accordance with applicable law in the state
7. After the 66th birthday, donors may still be accepted at the discretion of the blood bank physician
8. Written consent form signed by the donor: (1) allowing the donor to defer from being a donor if he or she has risk factors for human immuno-deficiency virus (HIV), the causative agent of AIDS, or (2) authorizing the blood bank to take and use his or her blood
9. A record of reason for deferrals, if any
10. Social security numbers or driver's license numbers may also be used for additional identification but are not mandatory
11. The race of a donor is not mandatory, but this information can be useful in screening patients for a specific phenotype (chromosomal makeup)
12. Unique characteristics about a donor's blood can also be helpful; blood from donors that is negative for cytomegalovirus or that is Rh-negative group O blood is used for neonatal patients.

To help minimize the incidence of dizziness, fainting, or other reactions to blood loss, donors are encouraged to eat within 4 to 6 hours of donating blood. A light snack just before phlebotomy may help avoid these reactions, but a donor should not be required to eat if he or she does not wish to do so.

Blood bank records must be able to trace all components of a donor unit [red blood cells (RBCs), white blood cells (WBCs), platelets, etc.] to its disposition. If the donation is a "replacement for credit" for a particular patient, then the donor must supply the patient's name or the group name that is to be credited.

A brief physical examination is required to determine if the donor is in general good condition on the day he or she is to donate blood. The physical examination entails a few simple procedures easily mastered by the blood bank phlebotomist.

1. *Weight.* Donors must weigh at least 110 lb (50 kg); if the weight is less, the volume of blood donated must be carefully monitored and care taken that not too much blood is taken; also the anticoagulant in the bag must be modified for the lesser donation. Most blood banks will not routinely accept donors who weigh less than 110 lb.

2. *Temperature.* Oral temperature must not exceed 37.5°C (99.6°F).

3. *Pulse.* It should be a regular, strong pulse between 50 to 100 beats/minute. The pulse should be taken for at least 30 seconds.

4. *Blood pressure.* The systolic blood pressure should measure 90 to 180 mm Hg and the diastolic blood pressure should be between 50 and 100 mm Hg. People outside of these limits should be deferred as donors and referred to their physicians for evaluation of a possible health problem.

5. *Skin lesions.* Both arms should be examined for signs of drug abuse such as needle marks or sclerotic veins. The presence of mild skin disorders such as psoriasis, acne, or poison ivy rash does not necessarily prohibit an individual from donating unless there are lesions in the antecubital area or the rash is particularly extensive. Donors with purulent skin lesions, wounds, or severe skin infections should be deferred. The skin at the site of the venipuncture must be free of lesions.

6. *General appearance.* If the donor looks ill, excessively nervous, or under the influence of alcohol or drugs, he or she should be deferred.

7. *Hematocrit or hemoglobin.* The hematocrit must be no less than 38 percent for female donors and no less than 41 percent for male donors. The hemoglobin value must be no less than 12.5 g/dL for female donors and no less than 13.5 g/dL for male donors. A fingerstick is commonly used to determine these values. The phlebotomist may either collect a hematocrit tube for centrifuging and reading or use the copper sulfate method in which the hemoglobin is qualitatively determined. (For further details on the copper sulfate method, please refer to the AABB Technical Manual.[9])

An extensive medical history must be taken on all potential donors regardless of the number of previous donations on record. Most blood bank donor rooms have a simple card listing all the questions to be asked and "yes" or "no" columns to check the donor's responses. Refer to the protocol of the donor room at the institution's blood bank or the AABB Technical Manual, which sets guidelines for donor screening and acceptance.

Collection of Donor's Blood.   The phlebotomist in a donor room must operate under the supervision of a qualified, licensed physician. Blood should be collected using aseptic technique, a sterile, closed system, and a single venipuncture. If a second venipuncture is needed, an entirely new, sterile donor set is necessary; the first is discarded according to the contaminated material disposal protocol of the institution. A donor should never be left alone either during or immediately after collection of blood. The phlebotomist should be well versed in donor reactions, equipment safety precautions, first aid techniques, and location of first aid if it should be needed in the course of donation.

The phlebotomist should prepare the antecubital portion of the donor's arm in the same manner as for collection of a blood culture specimen. (Refer to the section Blood Cultures in this chapter.) The blood collecting bag should be placed conveniently and the tubing should be extended to make sure there are no kinks in the tube that would prevent a free flow. When the arm is properly prepped, the tourniquet should be replaced and the donor given instructions to open and close the hand during the course of phlebotomy. A 15-gauge "regular" or 17-gauge "thin-walled" needle is most often used. The 17-gauge thin-walled needle is preferable because it has the internal diameter of a 15-gauge needle and the outside diameter of a 17-gauge, that is, it has the large bore size of a 15-gauge needle, but the smaller total size of the 17-gauge needle. The sterile needle is uncapped and with a quick, sure motion, the needle is slipped under the skin and into the vein. As the draw begins, the needle and tubing should be taped in place and a dry, sterile gauze sponge laid on top. The phlebotomist should encourage the donor to continue to slowly open and close the hand and to report any discomfort or dizziness if it should occur.

The phlebotomist should make sure that the blood in the bag mixes with the anticoagulant during the collection, either manually or by placing it on a mechanical agitator. If the collection process takes more than 8 minutes to complete, it is possible that platelet concentrates or antihemophilic factor preparations may not be possible. However, as long as the flow is constant and the bag contents continue to be mixed well, no time constraints are necessary.

Once the proper amount of blood has been collected (405 to 495 mL), the phlebotomy should be stopped, the tubing clamped off with a hemostat or some other temporary clamp, the tourniquet or blood pressure cuff released, the needle removed, and pressure placed over the site for several minutes. It is advisable that the donor be instructed to raise his or her arm over the head while holding the gauze with pressure over the puncture site. This method minimizes bleeding into the site and surrounding tissues as well as helps restore the integrity of the vascular tissue. The donor should not be allowed to bend the arm until bleeding stops as this may cause the tissue to be further traumatized by bleeding into the area below the skin as well as encouraging the vascular tissue to overlap and form scar tissue on the site during the healing process. A pressure bandage may be placed over the site once bleeding has stopped. The blood in the bag and tubing should be mixed well, properly labeled, and stored in accordance with blood bank standards.

The donor should be encouraged to remain seated or prostrate for 10 to 15 minutes or longer if the donor complains of dizziness or other discomfort. If the donor appears to be well, he or she should be encouraged to drink more fluids than usual to replace the volume loss and to refrain from strenuous exercise or work until after a full meal. Refreshments should be offered to the donor as a courtesy as well as in an effort to restore some of the lost body fluids. Any adverse reactions experienced by the donor should be recorded on the donor card. If the donor leaves before staff members recommend, it should also be noted on the record.

Therapeutic Phlebotomy

Therapeutic phlebotomy is used in the treatment of some myeloproliferative diseases, such as polycythemia, or other conditions in which the removal of blood benefits the patient. Records in the Blood Bank should be kept indicating the patient's diagnosis, the physician's request for the phlebotomy, and the amount of blood to be taken. It is up to the medical director of the blood bank to decide if the patient is to be bled in the donor room or in a private section of the blood bank. Some patients are visibly ill and weak and may have some psychological effects on healthy donors present. When a patient is obviously ill, his or her physician or the medical director of the blood bank should be present during the phlebotomy. Generally, the patient should be bled more slowly than a healthy donor and the resting period should be extended.

The blood obtained through therapeutic bleeding may be used for homologous transfusion if the unit is deemed suitable by the director of the blood bank. If it is to be used, the recipient's physician must agree to using the blood for his or her patient and a record should be kept of the agreement. The unit is then labeled and processed in the usual manner. The label must indicate that the blood is the result of a therapeutic bleed and include the patient's diagnosis. If the unit is not suitable for transfusion, the entire unit is disposed of in the usual manner of contaminated waste.

Autologous Transfusion

A practice that is frequently used now is *autologous transfusions*. The patient donates his or her own blood before anticipated surgery. The reason for this type of transfusion is that the safest blood a recipient can receive his or her own blood. The autologous transfusion prevents transfusion transmitted infectious diseases (i.e., HIV, hepatitis) and also eliminates the formation of antibodies in the transfused patient.

THE EMERGENCY CENTER

The phlebotomist's role in an emergency center [emergency room (ER), etc.] may vary from state to state, city to city, and hospital to hospital. Local laws may prohibit unlicensed persons from starting an IV in one state whereas there may be no restrictions in a neighboring state. The limitations placed on an unlicensed person may vary considerably; therefore, a phlebotomist who is to be involved in the Emergency Center should become familiar with the limitations and expectations at the health institution.

The atmosphere in an emergency center is very different from any other area of the hospital. Most emergency rooms are chronically filled with people in pain, ranging from relatively minor injuries or illnesses to major, traumatic injuries. In addition to those who have come to the Emergency Center for immediate treatment of acute injuries or illness, there are those who have no regular physician and use the local emergency center for treatment of chronic illnesses such as coughs and colds. Family members often accompany the patients and may be highly emotional and vocal about their concern for loved ones.

This range of patients and families with varying needs, demanding attention from the limited staff, can create a highly charged atmosphere. Most Emergency Centers have a central reception area that prioritizes the patients as they come in. It is often referred to as a triage area. Those who need immediate attention are seen first and those whose conditions are more stable are seen later. However, even when the patients are prioritized according to their illnesses, the routine can be assaulted if a trauma patient arrives by ambulance and requires immediate life-saving measures. Although the triage desk may attempt to put order and stability in the Emergency Center workflow, medical emergencies and critically ill or injured patients are unavoidable and must be handled professionally. It is easy to see that the Emergency Center is an unpredictable setting. Although guidelines are placed on the flow of patients, the unexpected can occur at any moment.

Recognizing that the Emergency Center setting is a stressful one, the phlebotomist has two very important responsibilities. First, he or she must be completely familiar with all of the equipment and well-versed in all blood collecting procedures. If called upon to collect "STAT" blood specimens from a critically injured person about to go to surgery, the phlebotomist must respond quickly and successfully obtain the correct specimen in the right volume. There may not be enough time to re-collect the specimen if the first one is unsuitable. Only experienced phlebotomists should accept positions in the Emergency Center, where skills must be well mastered and automatic. The second responsibility is to follow directions quickly and correctly. In a critical situation, it is vital that the phlebotomist follow the orders exactly and not require extensive time-consuming directions. An experienced, confident, mature phlebotomist is best suited to the unpredictable emergency environment.

Another factor present in the Emergency Center, which may cause a great deal of stress in some persons, is the sight and sound of traumatically injured patients in pain. Profuse bleeding, disfigurement, moaning, and groaning are common occurrences in this setting. It is wise for phlebotomists to be aware of their reactions to critically injured patients. If they find it too stressful, they should opt for work on the general floors of the hospital or in a clinic setting where the sights and sounds are more predictable and controlled. The phlebotomist who works in an Emergency Center must learn to do his or her job with single-mindedness and ignore anything that may distract from obtaining high-quality samples with speed and accuracy.

Obviously in such a stress-charged atmosphere, tension runs high and minor personality conflicts occur more readily than in other more routine surroundings. The phlebotomist, like all Emergency Center personnel, must learn to resolve and quickly dismiss irritations and losses of temper that may otherwise interfere with the delivery of good emergency medical care. A mature, responsible person can best cope with the Emergency Center environment.

Emergency medicine is not for everyone; some can work in that environment for only a limited amount of time; others would work nowhere else. The excitement of being part of a team of professionals who routinely provide life-saving treatment to critically injured victims has an attraction that cannot be easily duplicated in any other area of patient care. Phlebotomists must choose the environment that is best suited to their temperament and where they can best deliver quality patient care.

KEY TERMS

aerobic bottle	fasting specimen	rapid methods for
anaerobic bottle	fistula	glucose testing
arterial blood gases	forensic specimens	sodium polyanethole
autologous	gastric analysis	sulfonate (SPS)
transfusion	glucagon tolerance	STAT specimen
bleeding time test	test	sweat chloride test
blood culture	glucose tolerance test	test collection
cannula	Hollander test	priorities
capillary blood gases	lactose tolerance test	therapeutic drug
central venous	Lee-White clotting	monitoring (TDM)
catheters (CVC)	time	therapeutic
chain-of-custody	nasopharyngeal	phlebotomy
xylose test	culture	throat culture
epinephrine tolerance	postprandial glucose	timed specimen
test	test	trace metals

STUDY QUESTIONS

1. Why should the thumb not be used for palpating arteries in an arterial puncture?
2. Describe the preparation for an arterial puncture.

3. Why is the Duke method for bleeding time no longer the method of choice?
4. Describe the technique for properly preparing a site for a blood culture sample.
5. What is the purpose of skin testing?
6. What instructions should be given to a patient who is about to undergo a glucose tolerance test?
7. What role can a phlebotomist play in epinephrine or glucagon tolerance tests?
8. What is the sweat chloride test used for?
9. List the parts of the physical examination for donor acceptability.
10. What is the proper amount of blood taken from a donor to make one unit of blood?
11. Explain the purpose of therapeutic phlebotomy.
12. Name three ways in which blood specimens are ordered that influence the sequence in which the phlebotomist collects blood from patients.
13. What are two important responsibilities that the phlebotomist has in an emergency room?

REFERENCES

1. National Committee for Clinical Laboratory Standards: Use of Devices for Collection of Skin Puncture Blood Specimens. H14–A. NCCLS, Vol 5, no 9, 1985.
2. Smith C: Surgicutt: A device for modified template bleeding times. *J Med Technol* 3(4): 1986.
3. Surgicutt: Package insert of procedure. International Technidyne Corporation, Edison, N.J.
4. Balows A (ed): *Manual of Clinical Microbiology*, 5th ed. American Society for Microbiology, Washington, D.C., 1991.
5. Woodard E: *Laboratory Liaison Technician Manual*. Division of Laboratory Medicine, M.D. Anderson Hospital and Tumor Institute, Houston, Tex., 1988.
6. Ayers M, Brown M, Burritt M: Reflectance meter glucose analysis by the phlebotomy team. *J Med Technol* 4(5):195, 1987.
7. Eason M: A lab program to do bedside glucoses. *Med Lab Observ* 18(1):69, 1986.
8. "Sweat Chloride by Iontophoresis," procedure used in Special Chemistry section of the Department of Pathology and Laboratory Medicine, Hermann Hospital, Houston, Tex. Method developed by Karen Kumor, M.D., 1981.
9. Walker RH (ed): *Technical Manual of the American Association of Blood Banks*, 10th ed. Arlington, Va., AABB, 1990.
10. Janknegt R, Lohman J, Hooymans PM, et al: Do evacuated blood collection tubes interfere with therapeutic drug monitoring? *Phar Weekbl (Sci)* 5:287–291, 1983.
11. Quattrocchi F, Karnes H, Robinson J, et al: Effect of serum separator blood collection tubes on drug concentration. *Ther Drug Monit* 5:359–362, 1983.

12. Meranger J, Hollebone B, Blanchette G: The effects of storage times, temperature and container types on the accuracy of atomic absorption determination of Cd, Cu, Hg, Pb and Zn in whole heparinized blood. *J Anal Toxicol* 5:33–41, 1981.
13. National Committee for Clinical Laboratory Standards: *Collection Containers for Specimens for Toxicological Analysis. Proposed Guidelines.* NCCLS Document H31–P. Villanova, Penn., NCCLS, 1986.
14. College of American Pathologists: *Clinical Laboratory Handbook for Patient Preparation and Specimen Handling: Fascicle IV—Therapeutic Drug Monitoring and Toxicology.* Skokie, Ill., College of American Pathologists Pub., 1985.
15. Bittikofer J: Toxicology (Chap 27). In Bishop M, Duben Engelkick J, Foely E (Eds): *Clinical Chemistry: Principles, Procedures, Correlations.* Philadelphia, Lippincott, 1992.
16. National Diabetes Data Group: Classification and diagnosis of diabetes mellitus and other categories of glucose intolerance. *Diabetes* 28:1039, 1979.
17. Isaacman DJ, Karasic RB: Lack of effect of changing needles on contamination of blood cultures. *Pediatric Infect Dis J* 9:274, 1990.
18. Krumholz HM, Cummings S, York M: Blood culture phlebotomy: Switching needles does not prevent contamination. *Ann Intern Med* 113:290, 1990.
19. Jones AW, Jönsson K-A, Korfeldt L: Differences between capillary and venous blood-alcohol concentrations as a function of time after drinking, with emphasis on sampling variations in left vs. right arm. *Clin Chem* 35:400, 1989.
20. National Committee for Clinical Laboratory Standards: *Blood Gas Preanalytical Considerations: Specimen Collection, Calibration, and Controls.* NCCLS Document C27–T. Villanova, Penn., NCCLS, 1989.

Infection Control and Equipment Safety in Health Care Facilities

6

Sterile Techniques for Phlebotomists
    Disinfectants and Antiseptics
Equipment and Safety in Patients' Rooms
Patient Safety Outside Patients' Rooms
Key Terms
Study Questions

INTRODUCTION TO INFECTION CONTROL

The condition in which the body is invaded with pathogenic bacteria, fungi, viruses, or parasites is called infection. *Nosocomial infections* are those that are acquired after admission to a health care facility, including hospitals, clinics, nursing homes, and psychiatric institutions. Approximately 5 percent of hospitalized patients in the United States acquire nosocomial infections.[1] These infections are often harmful to the patient and costly to both patients and insurers. Each year millions of dollars are spent on nosocomial infections. In an attempt to control them, "infection control programs" have been developed. Based on guidelines established by the Centers for Disease Control (CDC), the Joint Commission for Accreditation of Health Care Organizations (JCAHO), and state regulatory agencies, each health care institution is responsible for developing and implementing an *infection control* program. These programs usually address the issues of *surveillance,* reporting, *isolation procedures,* education, and the investigation of epidemics within the health care institution. An infection control nurse or practitioner usually works closely with or in the clinical microbiology laboratory and communicates with personnel on the hospital ward to make the necessary assessments.

Surveillance
In most health care institutions, the infection control program monitors and collects data on several specific populations such as (1) patients at a high risk of infection, (2) patients with already acquired infections, (3) personnel or patients accidentally exposed to communicable disease, contaminated equipment, or hazardous reagents, and (4) patients in certain areas of the hospital or in certain rooms. It is helpful to the phlebotomist to be aware of these special circumstances for two reasons. First, the phlebotomist can take the necessary precautions to avoid infecting him or herself or the patient. Second, the phlebotomist can mentally prepare him or herself to deal in a professional and humanistic manner with these special patients. Because each hospital has its own infection control program, policy manual, or both, it behooves the phlebotomist to read and be familiar with it.

Infection control surveillance also involves classification of infections according to prevalence rates. One example of a report depicting the prevalence of nosocomial infections is represented in Figure 6–1. Each of these infections

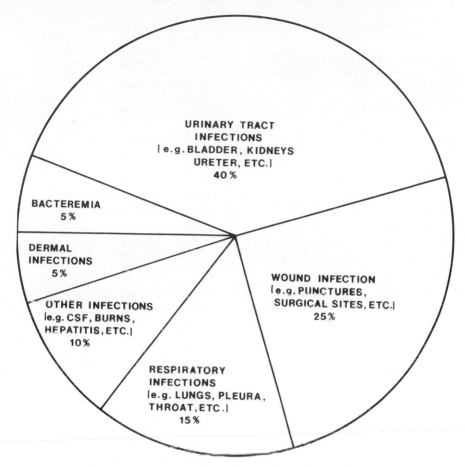

Figure 6–1. Prevalence of nosocomial infections. CSF, cerebrospinal fluid. *(From Castle M, Ajemian E: Hospital Infection Control. New York. John Wiley & Sons, 1987, New York, with permission.)*

can be transmitted in a variety of ways. The phlebotomist should realize that he or she can be a potential recipient or transmitter of infectious agents. Table 6–1 lists causative agents for nosocomial infections.

Infection control programs monitor employee health programs. A primary objective of both programs is to minimize the risk of infection or hazardous circumstances for employees and patients. Most employees are screened for the following diseases prior to working: measles, mumps, tuberculosis, hepatitis, diarrheal disease, syphilis, and skin diseases. Immunization for a variety of diseases is often made available initially and throughout employment, free of charge. Often, the hospital stipulates policies for employees with specific infections or who have been exposed to certain infections as in Table 6–2.

For the employee's protection, many types of warning labels are used.

TABLE 6–1. PATHOGENIC AGENTS CAUSING NOSOCOMIAL INFECTIONS

Body Areas or Hospital Areas	Commonly Identified Pathogenic Agents
Blood and cerebrospinal fluid	Any microorganisms
Burn unit	All gram-negative bacilli
	Gram-positive rods
	Fungi
Dialysis unit	Hepatitis and other viruses
	Bacteria
	Fungi
Ear	*Pseudomonas aeruginosa*
	Streptococcus pneumoniae
	Gram-negative bacilli
Eye	*Staphylococcus aureus*
	Neisseria gonorrheae
	Gram-negative bacilli
	Moraxella lacunata
	Hemophilus influenzae
	Streptococcus pneumoniae
	Pseudomonas aeruginosa
Gastrointestinal tract	*Salmonella* sp.
	Shigella sp.
	Yersenia enterocoliticus
	Enteropathogenic *Escherichia coli*
	Vibrio cholerae
	Campylobacter sp.
	Parasitic protozoans
	Candida albicans
	Some viruses
Genital tract	*Neisseria gonorrheae*
	Hemophilus vaginalis
	Candida albicans (yeast)
Intensive care or postoperative unit	Any microorganisms
Nursery unit	*Staphylococcus aureus*
	Group B *Streptococcus*
	Escherichia coli
	Streptococcus pneumoniae
	Other gram-negative bacilli
	Viruses
Respiratory tract	*Streptococcus pyogenes*
	Corynebacterium diphtheriae
	Bordatella pertussis
	Staphylococcus epidermidis
	Staphylococcus aureus
	Streptococcus pneumoniae
	Hemophilus influenzae
	Any gram-negative bacilli
	Fungi
	Certain viruses

(continued)

TABLE 6–1. *(Continued)*

Body Areas or Hospital Areas	Commonly Identified Pathogenic Agents
Skin	*Staphylococcus aureus*
	Streptococcus pyogenes
	Candida albicans
	Smallpox
	Herpes virus
	Enterovirus
	Measles
Urinary tract	Any microorganism in sufficient numbers
Wounds and abscesses	Any microorganisms

Among these are color-coded isolation signs and radiation hazard signs. Radiation signs may be posted on the hospital door of patients treated with radioactive isotopes. Generally speaking, a short period of contact with these patients would not be significant; however, the College of American Pathologists (CAP) recommends that pregnant employees avoid contact with these patients.[2]

Modes of Transmission

Nosocomial infections result when the *chain of infection* is complete. The three components that make up the chain are *source, modes of transmission,* and *susceptible host.*[1] In a normal environment, relatively few things are sterile; therefore, sources include a wide range of things. Inanimate objects, as well as people, are colonized with a variety of microorganisms, many of which help carry out normal bodily functions. Some of these microorganisms, however, are more pathogenic than others. For example, relatively few *Shigella* organisms need to be ingested for a diarrheal infection to occur. However, with *Salmonella,* large numbers of organisms need to be ingested before acquiring symptoms. On the other hand, numerous anaerobic and aerobic bacteria must be present in the gastrointestinal tract for normal metabolism to occur.

Regarding the sources of nosocomial infections, infection control practitioners must consider amount of contamination, viability of the infectious agent, virulence of the agent, length of time from contamination to contact, and how the agent was transmitted from the source. Sources of nosocomial infection can be hospital personnel, other patients, and visitors, and medical instruments, such as contaminated needles, intravenous catheters, Foley catheters, cardiac catheters, bronchoscopes, respiratory therapy equipment, and medical reagents (intravenous fluids and saline).

Human hands provide a warm moist environment for microorganisms. Therefore, a physician, phlebotomist, or nurse can transmit organisms from themselves or an infected patient to another potential host. Uniforms or other clothing, which have had contact with infectious agents and are then used with other patients, are potential sources of infection. Medical instruments that

TABLE 6–2. EMPLOYEE INFECTIONS OR SPECIAL CIRCUMSTANCES[a]

Disease	Work Status	Duration of Work or Work Limitations
AIDS	May work with restriction	Evaluated by Employee Health Physician
Draining abscess, boils, and so forth	Off	Until drainage stops, if employee has patient contact
Chickenpox (varicella)	Off	For 7 days after eruption first appears in normal host, provided lesions are dry and crusted when they return
Diarrhea Shigella Salmonella	Variable	Individual, depending on extent of symptoms, cultures, and evaluation by Personnel Health Service
Gonorrhea	May work	
Hepatitis A	Off	Must bring note from private physician upon return
Hepatitis B	Off	Must bring note from private physician upon return
Herpes simplex	May work	Evaluation by Personnel Health Service, depending on work area
Herpes zoster	No patient contact	If able to work, may do so
Influenza and URI	Variable	Evaluation by Personnel Health Service, depending on work area
Impetigo	Off	No patient contact until crusts are gone
German measles (rubella)	Off	Until rash is cleared (minimum of 5 days)
Measles	Off	Until rash is cleared (minimum of 4 days)
Mononucleosis	Off	At discretion of private physician
Positive PPD conversion	May work	Evaluation and follow-up by Personnel Health Service
Pregnancy (first or second trimester)	May work	Avoid patient contact with patients having viral or rickettsial infections or those being treated with radioactive material
Pregnancy (third trimester)	May work	Avoid contact with patients in any type of isolation
Active TB	Off	Until under treatment and smears are negative for 2 weeks
Scabies	Off until treated	
Strep throat (group A)	Off	May work 24 hours after being placed on appropriate antibiotic and symptom free

Abbreviations: PPD, Purified Protein Derivative; URI, upper respiratory infection; TB, tuberculosis.
[a]Sample guideline for employees with infections, their work status, and when they can return to work.
Adapted from Castle M, Ajemian E: Hospital Infection Control, New York, John Wiley & Sons, New York, 1987, with permission.

come into contact with open wounds, mucous membranes, or organs present a possible source of infection. For example, an instrument, such as a fiberoptic bronchoscope, may be used repeatedly only if thoroughly decontaminated between patient use. Otherwise, it may be implicated in transmitting bacterial pneumonia. Many other pieces of invasive equipment are potential transmitters unless adequately sterilized. Some equipment can become contaminated with bacteria, yet is less likely to cause infection. As an example, tourniquets come in contact with intact skin, but are less likely to be a source of infection.

The next step in the link involves transmission from the source to the next host. *Pathogenic agents* may be transmitted by direct contact, via air, by medical instruments or other objects, or other vectors. Direct contact involves close or intimate contact with an infected person. For example, some patients acquire staphylococcal infections, chicken pox, hepatitis, or diarrhea after touching other infected individuals. During contact, the infective microorganism is rubbed off one person onto another. Handwashing is the best means of preventing infections by this route.

Microscopic airborne droplets may carry infectious agents, such as the causative agent of tuberculosis and Legionnaire's disease. Droplets may become airborne in the following instances: when an individual coughs or sneezes, when linens are shaken, when dust is stirred by sweeping, or when ventilation is not adequate. Means of prevention are wearing a mask, isolating specific patients, and good ventilation.

Invasive medical instruments, as well as other inanimate objects, may expose a susceptible patient to pathogenic agents. Instruments such as tourniquets and catheters should be changed after use or decontaminated. Needles should be disposed of after each use. Other objects, such as toys in the pediatric areas, common toilets and sinks, linens, and water fountains are all potential modes of transmission. Preventing these transmission modes can be accomplished by isolation techniques, use of sterile technique for injections or venipuncture, wearing gloves during equipment handling, and restricting use of common toys or facilities.

Many insects (mosquitoes, ticks, fleas, mites) and rodents act as vectors in transmitting infectious diseases such as plague, rabies, and malaria. Patients may be exposed to them in unsanitary conditions or in areas where the diseases are prevalent.

The third area in the infectious chain is the susceptible host. Factors that affect host susceptibility are age, drugs, degree and nature of the illness, and status of the host immune system. The progress of the patient in the hospital greatly affects the chances of acquiring an infection. Underlying diseases, such as diabetes, acquired immune deficiency syndrome, cancer, and therapeutic measures (chemotherapy, radiation therapy, antibiotics), all change the status of the body making it a potential host for infection.

Infection control programs aim at breaking the infection chain at one or more spots, as shown in Figure 6–2. Handwashing procedures for *sterile tech-*

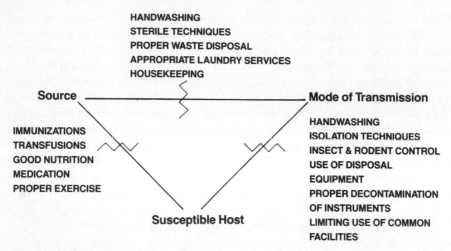

HANDWASHING
STERILE TECHNIQUES
PROPER WASTE DISPOSAL
APPROPRIATE LAUNDRY SERVICES
HOUSEKEEPING

Source ——————————————————— Mode of Transmission

IMMUNIZATIONS
TRANSFUSIONS
GOOD NUTRITION
MEDICATION
PROPER EXERCISE

HANDWASHING
ISOLATION TECHNIQUES
INSECT & RODENT CONTROL
USE OF DISPOSAL
EQUIPMENT
PROPER DECONTAMINATION
OF INSTRUMENTS
LIMITING USE OF COMMON
FACILITIES

Susceptible Host

Figure 6–2. The chain of nosocomial infection can be interrupted by infection control procedures.

niques, proper waste disposal, appropriate laundry services, and housekeeping are ways of controlling the sources. Isolation techniques, control of insects and rodents, and use of disposable equipment and supplies help interrupt the modes of transmission. Host susceptibility is controlled by speeding the patient's recovery. Immunization, transfusions, nutrition, medication, and exercise all help the patient to regain health.

ISOLATION PROCEDURES

Isolation procedures, methods of removing diseased individuals from society, date back to antiquity. Although the supplies and methods have been updated, the fear of being contaminated and the stigma associated with a patient in isolation are still present. The psychological effects of being a patient in isolation are profound. The phlebotomist should make an effort to reduce the anxiety of these patients by communicating in a calm, professional, and reassuring manner.

Isolation procedures are established in varying degrees. They range from sterile rooms or wards to isolation procedures for one disease only. However, in general, isolation techniques are divided into two types: procedures for patients with communicable diseases and procedures for patients who are extremely susceptible to infections.[1]

Most hospitals have special color-coded posters or signs on the patient's door indicating which type of isolation procedure is to be employed. The most common types and actual procedures are listed below and shown in Figure 6–3 and Table 6–3.

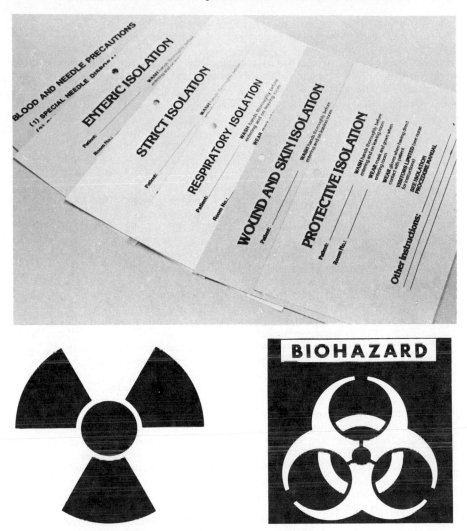

Figure 6–3. Isolation systems and warning signs.

Strict or Complete Isolation

Strict or complete isolation is required for patients with contagious diseases, that is, diseases that may be transmitted by direct contact and via the air. Examples include anthrax, rabies, smallpox, measles, chickenpox, plague, diphtheria, and streptococcal and staphylococcal pneumonia. The patients are housed in private rooms with doors closed and all articles in the room should be handled as if they were contaminated. Patients are usually restricted to their rooms. If they must be moved, they should be appropriately covered. Personnel entering these rooms must wear gowns, a mask, and gloves. Handwashing is

TABLE 6–3. ISOLATION TECHNIQUE FOR LABORATORY PERSONNEL

Principle:

Isolation techniques must be practiced by laboratory personnel when collecting specimens from infectious patients. This helps prevent the transmission of the disease to the laboratorian and to other patients via the technologist.

Procedure:

1. A sign posted on the door of an isolation room will tell the laboratorian the type of isolation and to what extent the isolation procedures must be followed. The types of isolation are as follows:
   a. *Complete:* anthrax, rabies, smallpox, measles, chickenpox
   b. *Respiratory:* tuberculosis, whooping cough, meningococcal meningitis, mumps, rubeola
   c. *Protective (reverse):* immune-suppressed or burn patients
   d. *Wound and skin:* postoperative
   e. *Enteric:* AIDS, hepatitis, salmonella, shigella, typhoid fever
      Should also have "Needle and Blood Precautions" sign on the door
2. Check with the nursing station to find out the diagnosis. Women who are pregnant or think they might be should avoid all patients isolated for viral or rickettsial infections. Pregnant women in their last trimester should not go into *any* isolation rooms.
3. Except for protective isolation, any equipment taken into the room must be left there. Make sure a Vacutainer adapter, tourniquet, and pen are in the room before entering. Protective isolation rooms should have an adapter and a tourniquet already in the room.
4. Isolation rooms will have either an anteroom in which isolation equipment is kept or a cart outside the door for the same purpose.
5. Place a mask over your nose and mouth. Tie both ties comfortably around your head.
6. Put on a sterile gown, touching only the insides. Make sure your back is completely covered and tie the belt. Pull the sleeves all the way down.
7. Put on disposable gloves, trying not to touch the palm with your hands. When entering a protective isolation room, wash your hands thoroughly before you put on *sterile* disposable gloves. Pull the gloves up over the sleeves of the gown.
8. Invert the isolation bag halfway inside out and leave near the door outside room. Take only the equipment you will need into the room. Leave the requisition on the cart outside of the room.
9. Check the patient's armband and draw your specimen. Label the specimen from the patient's armband, leaving pen in the room.
10. Dispose of the Vacutainer needle in the dirty needle box in the room. Throw the cotton swab and any gauze flats in the trash.
11. Before placing the tube in the isolation bag, wipe the outside of the tubes with a paper towel moistened with cold water to remove any blood that may be on the outside of the tube. Touching only the inside of the biohazard bag, place the tubes inside the bag, standing in the doorway of the room. Touch only the inside of the bag; avoid touching other items or areas outside the room with gloved hands.
12. Wash your gloved hands in the patient's room. Dry your hands and turn off the faucet with a paper towel.
13. Remove your gown by breaking the paper tie and touching only the inside. Fold it with the contaminated side on the inside and discard it.
14. Remove first glove.
15. Remove your last glove by sliding the pointer finger of the opposite hand between the glove and your hand. Discard the gloves.

(*continued*)

TABLE 6-3. (Continued)

16. Wash your hands again, using a paper towel to turn off the faucet.
17. Leave unit: Place clean paper towel over door knob and open door. Hold door open with feet and discard paper towel in wastebasket beside door. Place tubes of blood in isolation container for return to lab.
18. Check labeled tubes against requisition slip to be sure that the patient collected *was* the patient with tests ordered.
19. Wash your hands at the nursing station before going to the next patient's room.
Quality Control:
The only means of quality control is strict adherence to the procedure.

From Hermann Hospital Clinical Laboratories, Houston, Tex., with permission.

critically important. All items taken into the room must be left there in the appropriate location (see Table 6–3).

Respiratory Isolation

Respiratory isolation is required for patients with infections that may be transmitted through the air. Examples include tuberculosis, whooping cough, meningococcal meningitis, mumps, and measles. Patients are housed in private rooms with doors closed. Anyone entering the room must wear a mask, as should the patient if he or she is moved. All contaminated supplies should be disposed of in the patient's room.

Enteric Isolation

Enteric isolation is required for patients with infections that are transmitted by ingestion of the pathogen. Examples include diarrheal diseases, such as *Salmonella, Shigella, Escherichia coli, Yersinia, Staphylococcus, Campylobacter, Vibrio,* amebic dysentery, and other parasitic infections. Ideally, patients should be housed in private rooms. Their bathroom facilities should *not* be used by hospital personnel, other patients, or visitors. People entering these rooms should wear gowns and gloves. All contaminated materials should be disposed of in the patient's room.

Wound and Skin Isolation

Wound and skin isolation may be required after surgery or if a patient is admitted with a skin infection. Postoperative wounds, catheters, and intravenous apparatus may become infected and microorganisms can be transmitted to other patients by direct or indirect contact. Patients are generally restricted to their rooms and all entering people should wear gowns and gloves. When these patients are moved, procedures to prevent transmission should be used, for example, covering the infected site.

Universal Precautions for Hepatitis and Human Immunodeficiency Virus (HIV)

Patients who are infected with blood-borne pathogens such as hepatitis or human immunodeficiency virus (HIV) cannot always be readily detected. Therefore, the CDC states that "under universal precautions, all patients should be assumed to be infectious for HIV and other blood-borne pathogens."[3] *Universal precautions* eliminate the need for a separate isolation category of "blood and body-fluid precautions." Other categories of isolation precautions should still be retained if conditions are appropriate. The following summary indicates the necessary precautions for prevention of blood-borne pathogens:[3,4]

1. All health care workers should routinely use appropriate barrier precautions to prevent skin and mucous membrane exposure when contact with blood or other body fluids of any patient is anticipated. Gloves should be worn for touching blood and body fluids, mucous membranes, or nonintact skin of all patients, for handling items or surfaces soiled with blood or body fluids, and for performing venipuncture and other vascular access procedures. Gloves should be changed after contact with each patient. Masks and protective eyewear or face shields should be worn during procedures that are likely to generate droplets of blood or other body fluids to prevent exposure of mucous membranes of the mouth, nose, and eyes. Gowns or aprons should be worn during procedures that are likely to generate splashes of blood or other body fluids. A personal respirator should be used if risk of aerosolized *M. tuberculosis* is present.

2. Hands and other skin surfaces should be washed immediately and thoroughly if contaminated with blood or other body fluids. Hands should be washed immediately after gloves are removed.

3. All health care workers should take precautions to prevent injuries caused by needles, scalpels, and other sharp instruments or devices during procedures; when cleaning used instruments; during disposal of used needles; and when handling sharp instruments after procedures. To prevent needlestick injuries, needles should not be recapped, purposely bent or broken by hand, removed from disposable syringes, or otherwise manipulated by hand. After they are used, disposable syringes and needles, scalpel blades, and other sharp items should be placed in puncture-resistant containers for transport to the reprocessing area.

4. Although saliva has not been implicated in HIV transmission, to minimize the need for emergency mouth-to-mouth resuscitation, mouthpieces, resuscitation bags, or other ventilation devices should be available for use in areas in which the need for resuscitation is predictable.

5. Health care workers who have exudation lesions or weeping dermatitis

should refrain from all direct patient care and from handling patient-care equipment until the condition resolves.

6. Pregnant health care workers are not known to be at greater risk of contracting HIV infection than health care workers who are not pregnant; however, if a health care worker develops HIV infection during pregnancy, the infant is at risk of infection resulting from perinatal transmission. Because of this risk, pregnant health care workers should be especially familiar with and strictly adhere to precautions to minimize the risk of HIV transmission.

Furthermore, the CDC and NCCLS recommend that all health care facilities should be responsible for continuing education and training, monitoring, and providing necessary supplies for compliance with the listed procedures.[3,4]

Isolation for Hospital Outbreaks

Occasionally, outbreaks of particular infections occur in one or more hospital areas. For example, infection control surveillance may reveal that the nursery unit is having many cases of staphylococcal infection. The infection control staff may dictate the need for special precautions, isolation procedures, or screening employees for staphylococcal carriers in order to control the outbreak. Anyone entering or exiting these areas, including phlebotomists, should be made aware of special circumstances.

Protective or Reverse Isolation

Many patients are put in isolation because they are highly susceptible to infection and need to be protected from the external environment. Therefore, it is referred to as *protective or reverse isolation*. The patient does not necessarily have an infection but has a lowered resistance. In general, a private room and good handwashing techniques are sufficient but more serious precautions such as gowns, gloves, and masks may be used. Articles may be removed from the room and do not need to be double-bagged since these patients do not have infections. However, articles entering the room must be sterile or carefully decontaminated.

A few hospitals in the United States have large protective isolation facilities. Patients with combined immunodeficiencies need to live in environments that are completely sterile. All food and articles are sterilized prior to entering the patient's room. Some patients must live their entire lives in this protected environment.

Other areas where patients are at a high risk of infection are the nursery, burn units, postoperative or intensive care units (ICUs), and dialysis units.

Infection Control Procedures in a Nursery Unit

Newborn infants are easy candidates for infections of all sorts because their immune systems are not fully developed at birth. They may pick up pathogens from their mothers, other babies, or hospital personnel. The best way to minimize infection is to use gloves and an antiseptic for handwashing. Special clothing changed daily may be worn by nursery personnel and limited to that unit. It has been recommended that bibs be used and discarded after contact with each baby. Often a baby is assigned only one nurse so as to limit the possibility of transmitting infection. Babies whose mothers have genital herpes must be isolated from other infants. Mothers with genital herpes must also be isolated. All individuals having contact with either the mothers or children must be gowned and gloved, and double-bagging procedures must be employed for disposal of contaminated articles in the patient's room.

Infection Control in a Burn Unit

Patients with burns are also highly susceptible to infection. In some institutions, infection rates are lower because of the availability of a completely isolated environment for each patient. Each bed is surrounded by a plastic curtain containing sleeves. Hospital personnel use these sleeves when contacting the patient. All supplies and equipment are kept outside of the curtain.[1]

In hospitals lacking these facilities, burn patients are housed in private rooms. Gowning, gloving, double-bagging (as described in Specific Isolation Techniques, below), and strict handwashing procedures should be used. All articles in the room, as well as the room itself, should be disinfected or sterilized frequently.

Infection Control in an Intensive Care or Postoperative Unit

Patients in ICUs are more critically ill and, by the nature of being there, are more susceptible to infections. In most hospitals, ICUs are open areas with numerous patients in one large room so as to be more easily monitored. Patients with known infections should be isolated according to the type of infection they have, and strict handwashing and gloving policies are necessary in all ICUs.

Postoperative patients are susceptible to infection because surgical wounds or drains enable bacteria to gain easy access to deeper tissues. Here again, patients should be isolated and dealt with according to the type of infection acquired.

Infection Control in a Dialysis Unit

Patients needing dialysis are most often immunosuppressed, making them a high-risk group for contracting infection, especially hepatitis. Protective gowns and gloves may be worn on the unit, and strict handwashing and gloving techniques should be employed.

Infection Control in the Clinical Laboratory

The clinical laboratory contributes to infection control programs in the following manner:

1. Maintenance of laboratory records for surveillance purposes
2. Reporting of infectious agents, drug-resistant microorganisms, and outbreaks
3. Evaluating the effectiveness of sterilization or decontamination procedures

Laboratory personnel must be cautious because they often handle specimens with infectious agents. Laboratorians have higher incidence of hepatitis antigen, tuberculosis, tularemia, and Rocky Mountain spotted fever than other hospital personnel.[1] Many of these infections are acquired by aerosols, needlesticks, spills, mouth pipetting, and eating, drinking, or smoking in the laboratory. These can be easily avoided or minimized by adhering to policies that prohibit mouth pipetting, eating, drinking, and smoking in the laboratory. Handwashing, gloving, protective clothing such as lab coats and face shields if appropriate, surface decontamination, and careful disposal of needles are also useful procedures.

Phlebotomists are usually headquartered in the clinical laboratory. It should be remembered that quality of laboratory results is only as good as the specimen collected. If the specimen is contaminated or improperly collected, laboratory results reflect this and may be misleading. If sloppy techniques are used, the potential for mistakes and infection is greater.

Phlebotomists are partially, if not fully, responsible for the specimen collected. This includes proper collection procedures and adherence to policies. Infection control policies are often time consuming and cumbersome; however, failure to follow the policies results in more severe consequences. Because phlebotomists perform skin and venipunctures on numerous patients daily, their direct patient contact is considerable. In one day, a phlebotomist may collect specimens from 50 or so patients. Imagine the potential of that single phlebotomist to spread infections to all those patients if inappropriate procedures are followed. Phlebotomists are also fairly mobile individuals, that is, they often have to collect specimens on several floors or in various parts of the health care facility. This increases the likelihood of spreading infections to these areas if infection control policies are not followed. Table 6–4 details the responsibilities of the phlebotomist with regard to infection control policies.

SPECIFIC ISOLATION TECHNIQUES

In most hospitals, all supplies required for isolation procedures are located in an area or cart just outside the patient's room. After washing hands, the appropriate garb may be put on just prior to entering the room (Fig. 6–4).

Handwashing
Handwashing is the most important procedure in the prevention of disease transmission in hospitals. It should be the first and last step of any isolation

TABLE 6–4. INFECTION CONTROL RESPONSIBILITIES OF THE PHLEBOTOMIST

1. Maintaining good personal hygiene including wearing clean clothes, keeping hair clean and tied back if necessary, keeping nails clean, and washing hands frequently.
2. Maintaining good health by eating balanced meals in the designated areas, getting enough sleep and exercise.
3. Reporting personal illnesses to supervisors.
4. Become familiar with and *observe all isolation policies.*
5. Learn about the job-related aspects of infection control and share this information with others.
6. Caution all personnel working with known hazardous material. This can be done with proper warning labels.
7. Report violations of the policies.
8. Report potential candidates for infection control, for example, patients who are jaundiced.

procedure. Scrubbing for surgery requires a different procedure than washing hands for general patient care. For general purposes, handwashing usually removes potential pathogens, but not necessarily sterilizes the hands. Good technique involves soap, warm running water, and friction.[1] Soap removes oils that may hold bacteria to the skin. Many varieties of soap are available for general purposes. However, it is recommended that health care facilities choose those that are mild, easy to use, and form a good lather. Warm running water washes away loosened debris and lathers the soap. Friction from rubbing one's hands together loosens and removes dead skin, oil, and microorganisms. One should thoroughly rub both sides of each hand and in between each finger. Hands should be rinsed in a downward position. After rinsing, the faucet should be turned off using paper towels so as to avoid reinoculation of microorganisms onto hands.

Masking
After washing hands, a mask (if necessary) may be put over the nose and mouth. Often a small metal band on the mask can be shaped to fit one's nose. Two ties are usually made, first one around the upper portion of the head, and second, around the upper portion of the neck. Most masks become ineffective after prolonged use (20 minutes).[1]

Gowning
A sterile gown should be put on by touching only the inside surface of it. It should have long sleeves and be large and long enough to cover all clothing. They are generally made of cloth or paper. The back must be completely covered, the belt tied, and the sleeves pulled all the way to the wrists.

Gloving
Clean disposable gloves may be used for most isolation procedures. The exception is with protective isolation where sterile disposable gloves should be used.

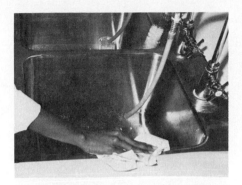

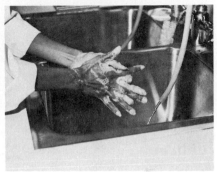

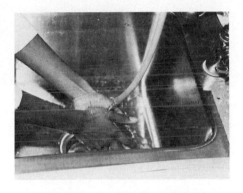

A. Good handwashing involves soap, warm running water, and thorough rubbing.

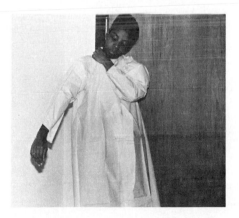

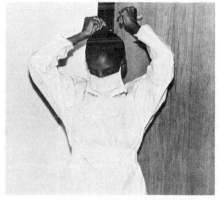

B. Gowns should be large enough to cover all clothing. Sleeves should be pulled down and back should be covered.

C. Masks should be tied in two places and fit comfortably.

Figure 6–4. Specific isolation techniques: handwashing, gowning, masking, gloving, and double-bagging.

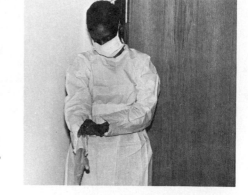

D. Gloves should be pulled over ends of gown sleeves. After specimen collection, removal of the gown should be from inside out.

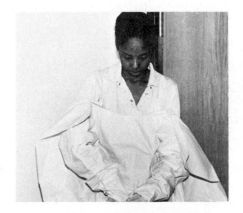

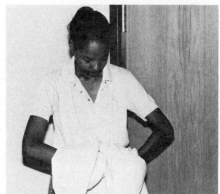

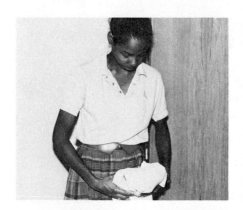

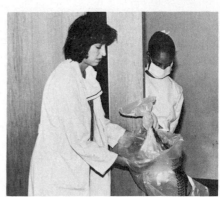

E. Double-bagging involves two individuals, one inside the room and one outside.

Figure 6–4. (Continued)

Gloves should be pulled over the ends of the gown sleeve. It is recommended that rings or other jewelry not be worn as they may puncture the glove during patient contact.

Entering and Exiting the Room

Isolation bags for transporting specimens are often available. The bag may be turned halfway inside out and left near the door outside the room, or someone may be available to hold the bag outside the door. Only the needed supplies should be taken into the room. Phlebotomy requisitions may be left outside the room on the isolation cart. If drawing a blood specimen, the phlebotomist may use a tourniquet in the room, or leave the one brought in. The specimen should be labeled at the bedside and the pen left in the room. Used needles, swabs, and so on should be put in appropriate containers inside the room. Any blood on the outside of the specimen container should be removed with a paper towel. While standing in the doorway, and touching only the inside of the isolation bag, the specimen should be placed inside the bag. Gloved hands should be washed in the room. The faucet may be turned off with a paper towel.

The mask, if used, can be removed by carefully untying the lower tie first, then the upper one. Only the ends of the ties should be held. It should then be properly disposed of inside the room. In some cases, a special container for masks is placed just outside the room to avoid exposure of hospital personnel to airborne diseases while inside.

The gown is removed first by breaking the paper tie or untying the sash. It should be removed and folded with the contaminated side turned inside and with care not to touch one's uniform. One glove may be removed, and the second one can be slipped off by sliding the index finger of the ungloved hand between the glove and the hand.

Just before leaving the room, however, hands must be washed again, using a paper towel to turn off the faucet. A clean paper towel should be used to open the door. The door should be held open with one's feet and used paper towels discarded in the waste basket directly inside the patient's room. Once outside the room, the requisition forms may be checked again, placed carefully in the isolation bag and sealed. Care must be taken to avoid touching the inside of the bag holding the specimen. Personnel should wash hands again before proceeding with other duties.[5]

Double-bagging

Trash, linens, and other articles in an isolation room must be removed by using the double-bagging procedure. *Double-bagging* involves putting contaminated material in one bag and sealing it inside the room. A different person should stand outside the doorway with another opened, clean, impermeable bag. The person standing outside the room should have the ends of the bag folded over the hands to shield them from possible contamination. The sealed bag from the room may then be placed inside the clean bag. The person outside the room can then fold over the edges, expel the air, and seal the outer bag. It should then be labeled with appropriate warnings.

PREVENTION OF LABORATORY-ACQUIRED INFECTIONS

As previously mentioned, the phlebotomist must be extremely cautious with biohazardous specimens. Policies and procedures for handling such specimens should be defined in the laboratory policy manual and should be reviewed periodically by the phlebotomist. Infections from these specimens may be spread in collection and handling by several routes. The actual occurrence of an infection from a biohazardous specimen depends upon the virulence of the infecting agent and the susceptibility of the host. The following are possible routes of infection from collected specimens and, therefore, should be considered when collecting or processing specimens for laboratory assays:

1. *Skin contact.* Virulent organisms can enter through skin abrasions and cuts or through conjunctiva of the eye. Thus, scratches from needles and broken glass must be avoided. If the phlebotomist has a cut or abrasion, he or she should always wear a lab coat, gloves and protective adhesive tape to prevent possible inoculation from infectious specimens. The phlebotomist must avoid rubbing his or her eyes in order to prevent possible transmission of an infection from a biohazardous specimen.

2. *Ingestion.* Failure to wash contaminated hands and subsequent handling of cigarettes, gum, food, or drinks can result in an infection from a biohazardous specimen. The phlebotomist must comply with the safety rules of the laboratory to prevent transmission of infections.

3. *Airborne.* As discussed in other sections, aerosols created from patients' specimens by careless splashing or centrifugation must be prevented by the phlebotomist and other laboratory personnel. The phlebotomist should be aware that dangerous, infectious aerosols can be caused from popping stoppers off of the blood specimen vacuum tubes and centrifugation of the blood specimens. To protect against blood exposure during this hazardous step, different types of items have been recently developed by manufacturers (see Chapter 3, Syringes, Needles and Safety Devices). Vacuum tubes should be inspected for cracks prior to centrifugation. Tubes with wet rims should be wiped dry prior to centrifugation. The centrifuge brake should not be applied to save time because braking can cause infectious aerosol formation. Centrifuged infectious specimens must not be poured because of the potential hazards from aerosol formation. Instead, the contents should be transferred using a disposable pipet with rubber bulb or equivalent

and gently transferring the contents down the wall of the aliquot tube(s).

STERILE TECHNIQUES FOR PHLEBOTOMISTS

All hospital personnel should realize that bacteria and other microorganisms can be found everywhere. For example, human skin is covered with bacteria. Because of this fact, all hospital personnel should be responsible for cleanliness and maintaining sterility when handling instruments, catheters, IV supplies, or other devices that contact patients.

The phlebotomist has the responsibility of using sterile supplies for skin and venipuncture and antiseptics for patient preparation. Alcohol pads are often used to cleanse skin sites for venipuncture. Although rubbing with alcohol pads destroys most of the bacteria, it does not destroy all microorganisms. A special decontamination procedure is required to obtain a sterile site. Venipuncture for blood cultures requires this type of preparation, as discussed thoroughly in Chapter 5. It involves cleansing the site with surgical green soap for 2 minutes, removing the soap using a sterile alcohol pad, and applying an iodine solution in concentric circles beginning at the site and working outward. The iodine solution should be allowed to dry. In some hospitals, it is recommended that the tops of the blood culture bottles or tubes and the phlebotomist's gloved finger used for palpation be sterilized in the same manner. (See Chapter 5 for further details of the procedure.) Failure to use the proper technique may result in false-positive blood cultures that are due to skin or needle contaminants.

New needles and most blood collection tubes are sterilized by the manufacturers. Once the covering of a needle or lancet has been removed, it should not touch anything until it punctures the skin. If it accidentally touches *anything* prior to the skin site, it must be appropriately discarded and replaced with a new one. If a needle is used for an unsuccessful venipuncture, it *must* be discarded and replaced with a new one before attempting another puncture.

Sterile techniques and isolation procedures may require sterile gloves. If such is the case, the phlebotomist must make sure that the package of gloves indicates that they are sterile. Some manufacturers produce gloves that are chemically clean but not necessarily sterile. Most sterile gloves come in various hand sizes. If gloves do not fit properly, they may interfere with the procedure.

Disinfectants and Antiseptics

Disinfectants are chemical compounds used to remove or kill pathogenic microorganisms. Chemical disinfectants are regulated by the Environmental Protection Agency. *Antiseptics* are chemicals used to inhibit the growth and development of microorganisms but not necessarily kill them. Antiseptics may be used on human skin. Disinfectants are generally used on surfaces and instru-

TABLE 6–5. COMMON HOSPITAL ANTISEPTICS AND DISINFECTANTS

Compound	Uses and Restrictions
Alcohols	
Ethyl	Antiseptic for skin
Isopropyl	Antiseptic for skin
Chlorine	
Chloramine	Disinfectant for wounds
Hypochlorite solutions	Disinfectant
Ethylene oxide	Disinfectant (toxic)
Formaldehyde	Disinfectant (noxious fumes)
Glutaraldehyde	Disinfectant (toxic)
Hydrogen peroxide	Antiseptic for skin
Iodine	
Tincture	Antiseptic for skin (can be irritating)
Iodophors	Antiseptic for skin (less stable)
Mercury compounds	Antiseptic for skin
Phenolic compounds	
1%–2% Phenols	Disinfectant
Chlorophenol	Disinfectant (toxic)
Hexachlorophene	Antiseptic for skin (used in surgery)
Chlorohexidine	Antiseptic for skin
Hexylresorcinol	Antiseptic for skin
Quarternary ammonium compounds	Antiseptic for skin (ingredient in many soaps)

ments because they are too corrosive for direct use on skin. Intermediate-level disinfectants having a product label claim for HIV-cidal or tuberculocidal or containing 500 ppm of free chloride should be used to disinfect tourniquets and items contaminated with blood or other body fluids.[6] Table 6–5 lists some of the more common hospital disinfectants and antiseptics used.

EQUIPMENT AND SAFETY IN PATIENTS' ROOMS

As a member of the health care team, the phlebotomist is responsible for the safety of the patient. All health care professionals are responsible for patient safety from the time the patient enters the health care setting until departure. As a matter of general patient safety, the phlebotomist should be aware of the following precautions in the patient's room:

1. Make certain that all specimen collection supplies, needles, and equipment are either properly disposed of or returned to the specimen collection tray after collection.
2. Check to see if the bedrails are up or down. Always place bedrails up before leaving the patient if they were up when you entered the room.
3. Unusual odors should be reported to the nursing station because a pipe may be broken and leak gas or liquid.

4. Check for food or liquid spilled on the floor, urine spills, or IV leakage. Areas on which the patient and health care professionals walk must be dry. They should be free of obstacles and slipping hazards. Thus, in case of spills, make certain that the area is cleaned and dried for the safety of the patient and hospital personnel.

5. During blood collection, be very cautious not to touch any electrical instrument located adjacent to the patient's bed. If the instrument should malfunction, then the phlebotomist may ground the patient and as a result, a microshock would pass through the phlebotomist into the patient. A serious problem could result from this shock to a patient with an electrolyte imbalance or one who is wet with perspiration or other fluid. The needle inserted in the patient's arm could produce ventricular fibrillation and death if the patient has a pacemaker or an unstable heart ailment.

6. If the patient has an IV and the site is swollen and red in appearance, the IV needle is probably no longer in the vein and the IV solution is infiltrating into the surrounding tissues. Report this problem immediately to the nursing station because some chemicals in IV solutions are toxic to body tissue, and gangrene could result due to infiltration. Also, if blood is backing up the IV line from the needle insertion to the IV drip container, the IV solution container is empty. Report this problem immediately.

7. If the patient's alarm for the IV drip is sounding, report this problem to the nursing station immediately.

8. If the patient is in unusual pain or is unresponsive, notify the nursing station immediately.

PATIENT SAFETY OUTSIDE PATIENTS' ROOMS

The phlebotomist should be aware of possible hazards to patients outside the patients' rooms. As a matter of general safety practice, the phlebotomist should follow the following guidelines:

1. Because trays, carts, and ladders may be placed around a hallway corner, the phlebotomist should be careful about traveling too quickly from one room to another and around corners.

2. Items lying on the floor, such as flower petals, may cause someone to slip and should be reported for cleaning.

3. Avoid running in a hospital because patients and visitors may become alarmed and begin to run as well. Also, someone may be hurt if the phlebotomist runs into him or her (for example, a cardiac patient walking in hall with inserted IV stand, another phlebotomist carrying specimen collection tray, and so forth).

KEY TERMS

antiseptics	isolation procedures	respiratory isolation
chain of infection	masking	source
disinfectants	mode of transmission	sterile techniques
double-bagging	nosocomial infections	susceptible host
enteric isolation	pathogenic agents	surveillance
infection control	protective or reverse	universal precautions
isolation	isolation	wound isolation

STUDY QUESTIONS

The following questions may have one or more answers:

1. Which of the following nosocomial infections is most prevalent?

   a. dermal infections   c. respiratory tract infections
   b. wound infections   d. urinary tract infections

2. Name the links in the infection control chain.

   a. poor isolation technique   c. source
   b. susceptible host   d. mode of transmission

3. What is (are) the primary function(s) of isolation procedures?

   a. Keep the hospital clean.
   b. Prevent transmission of communicable diseases.
   c. Protect the general public from disease.
   d. Provide protective environments.

4. Phlebotomists are responsible for knowing procedures of which type(s) of isolation?

   a. strict   d. protective/reverse
   b. wound and skin   e. respiratory
   c. enteric   f. universal precautions

5. Which of the following precautions to avoid infectious aerosols is (are) true?

   a. To open a vacuum collection tube, pop the cap rather than twist it.
   b. Vacuum tubes should be inspected for cracks prior to centrifugation.
   c. The centrifuge brake can be applied to save time when centrifuging these specimens.
   d. It is best to pour the specimens into the required aliquots to avoid infectious aerosols.

6. Which of the following safety rules should be maintained in patient rooms?

  a. Full ashtrays should be emptied into the trash can to avoid a fire hazard.
  b. Unusual odors in the patient's room should be reported to the nursing station.
  c. Phlebotomists should not touch electrical instruments located adjacent to the patient's bed.
  d. If the patient has an IV and the site is swollen and reddish, this problem should be reported to the nursing station.

REFERENCES

1. Castle M, Ajemian E: *Hospital Infection Control.* New York: John Wiley & Sons, 1987.
2. College of American Pathologists: *So You're Going to Collect a Blood Specimen* (4th ed). Northfield, Ill., College of American Pathologists, 1989.
3. Guidelines for Prevention of Transmission of Human Immunodeficiency Virus and Hepatitis B Virus to Health-Care and Public-Safety Workers. *MMWR,* 38 (no. S-6), 1989.
4. National Committee for Clinical Laboratory Standards: Protection of laboratory workers from infectious disease transmitted by blood, body fluids, and tissue; Tentative guideline. NCCLS Document M29-T2. Villanova, Penn., NCCLS, 1991.
5. Hermann Hospital: Procedure Manual: Isolation Technique for Laboratory Personnel. Houston, Tex., Hermann Hospital, 1991.
6. Luebbert P: Choosing the appropriate disinfectant. *Lab Med* 23(2): 126, 1992.

Specimen Requisitions, Transportation, and Reporting Results

7

CHAPTER OUTLINE

Verbal Reports
Computerized Reports
Interim Reports and Cumulative Summaries
Distribution of Results
Medical Records and Charts

Key Terms
Study Questions

PHYSICIAN–PATIENT–LABORATORY NETWORK

The major purpose of a clinical laboratory is the acquisition and determination of valid data by analytic procedures performed on patient specimens and the timely communication of those data to the physician. It is essential that a physician–patient–laboratory communication cycle be established to achieve this end. The number of persons and steps involved in this cycle varies greatly depending on the size of the institution and type of laboratory involved. With each additional step or person involved, however, another potential source of error or delay is introduced into the system. Therefore, it is the responsibility of the clinical laboratory to concern itself with all parts of the cycle rather than limit its attention solely to data acquisition. The phlebotomist is a vital link in this cycle and can serve to enhance communication among the patient, the laboratory, and the physician.

Various illustrations conceptualize this cycle pattern, ranging from a simplified version, as in Figure 7–1, to more complex representations as in Figure 7–2. Although these illustrations are quite different, they show that the clinical laboratory is intimately involved in extralaboratory activities in its effort to deliver effective services, and also that there is a constant overlapping or interaction between internal and external functions of the laboratory. This chapter addresses the importance of this network, both inside and outside the laboratory, as well as the various nonanalytic communication components of laboratory test request specifications, test requisitioning, patient and specimen identification, specimen transport, reporting of results, and distribution of results.

The College of American Pathologists (CAP), *Standards for Accreditation of Medical Laboratories,* states that, "channels of communication within the laboratory as well as with all other closely affiliated sections of services in the hospital and the medical staff shall be appropriate to the size and complexity of the organization."[1] In a relatively small laboratory, as in the case of a physician's office laboratory, the communication processes, both within the laboratory (intralaboratory) and with all others outside the laboratory (extralaboratory), are essentially the same. As the size of the institution increases, however, the requirements for effective and efficient intralaboratory and extralaboratory communications are greatly expanded.

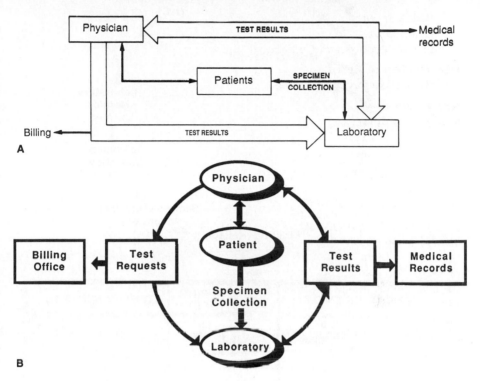

Figure 7–1A. The patient–physician–laboratory network can be depicted very simply.
B. The network can be considered a cyclical one.

INTRALABORATORY COMMUNICATIONS NETWORK

Policy Manual

Usually, each clinical laboratory has an administrative or personnel policy manual that can be consulted by all workers. The manual contains policies that are consistent with those of the larger organization (i.e., hospital, clinic). They are general in scope and particularly concerned with, but not limited to, such subjects as management authorizations, tables of organization, responsibilities, personnel practices, e.g., attendance and punctuality policies, dress codes, and rules about coffee breaks, and professional protocol. As points of reference, written policies for the laboratory ensure consistency of intent and save considerable time by removing the need to remake decisions. They are written in consultation with the clinical laboratory employees involved and reviewed for consistency with the institutional policies. The policies are generally approved and signed by the laboratory director. Because many changes occur in the clinical laboratory, the policies must be reviewed by the supervisory staff and

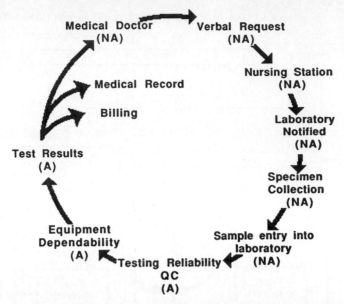

A

PATIENT ORIENTED	OVERLAPPING FUNCTIONS	TEST ORIENTED
Patient Medical Records ▶	Compiled Recorded	Medical Doctor reviews/ assesses
Medical Doctor requests tests ▶	Divided	Laboratory Record
Mechanism for test request ▶	Sorted Checked	Reporting
Phlebotomist receives orders ▶	Batched	Calculations Evaluations
Process of specimen collection ▶	Delivered Collated	Analysis
Venipuncture ▶		▶ Sample Collection

B

Figure 7–2A. The patient–physician–laboratory network can be depicted in an "analytical" (A) phase and a "nonanalytical" phase (NA). **B.** The network can also be shown as "patient oriented" and "test oriented" functions.

updated at least annually with a signature and a date to document the review. A staff technologist, technician, or phlebotomist who accepts a position in a clinical laboratory section should become acquainted with the laboratory policies.[2]

Procedure Manuals

Written procedures that provide information relevant to a given situation, event, or problem or protocol to be followed are usually made available to the clinical laboratory employees. Various types of written procedural manuals include the following.[2]

Technical Procedures.   Technical procedures describe in detail the steps to be followed in the performance of specimen collection and each laboratory test. Technical procedures are approved and signed by the supervisor, the medical director, or both individuals from the section responsible for the performance of the particular laboratory test. The CAP requires technical procedures to be made available, on site at all times, to technical personnel who perform specimen collection and laboratory assays. The technical procedure format includes name and title of procedure, a description of the method, specimen requirements, procedural steps, reagents and preparation, *reference ranges,* clinical significance of results, quality control instructions, calculations, reporting requirements, approval signatures, dates, and references.[3]

Laboratory Administrative Procedures.   Laboratory administrative procedures pertain to administrative concerns. They are distributed to laboratory management and made available to all other relevant personnel. The following information is generally found in an administrative procedure manual:

- Technical procedure format
- Assignment of test code numbers to laboratory procedures
- Communication with physicians and other health care professionals
- Time cards
- Attendance records
- Laboratory equipment identification and centralization of specification files
- Handling of samples for reference laboratory work
- Acceptable symbols, abbreviations, and units of measure
- Handling of laboratory charge tickets
- Purchase and repair requisitions
- Performance evaluation procedure
- Employee folders, color blindness records, certification records
- Distribution of laboratory documents
- Quality assurance procedures
- Quality control procedures

- Safety procedures, including fire, chemical, radiation safety, and a disaster plan
- Loan of laboratory equipment
- Compensatory time off, annual leave, and overtime policies
- Employee accidents
- Laboratory libraries
- Inventory of capital equipment
- Consent to donate blood and urine specimens
- In-service records
- Clinical laboratory samples referred from outside sources
- Formal disciplinary action
- Hepatitis testing of laboratory personnel
- Dress code

Safety Procedures.   Safety procedures should be distributed to all management and made known to all personnel. One book of safety procedures should be available in each laboratory section, including the specimen collection area. Safety manuals should include fire safety, internal/external disaster plans, radiation safety, biologic hazards, *Hazard Communication Manual,* and Infection Control Manuals.

Hazard Communication Manual.   The *Occupational Safety and Health Administration* (*OSHA*) Hazard Communication Standard enacted in 1986 requires that employers maintain documentation related to any hazardous substances. This act is known as the *Right to Know Act.* Employers must have a written communication program, training for employees, sophisticated tracking and documentation of hazardous substances, and *material safety data sheets* (*MSDS*). The manual must include copies of the federal act as well as any state laws and regulations. All employees must be trained to read and understand MSDS sheets, biohazardous labels, and appropriate ways to react to accidents in the laboratory.

Quality Control Procedures.   *Quality control procedures* pertain to the conduct of diagnostic laboratory testing. Quality control procedures should be available in each laboratory section, including the specimen collection area, or can be indicated in each technical procedure.

QC records include information about hazards, proper use, storage, handling, stability, expiration dates, and indications for measuring precision and accuracy of analytic processes.

Infection Control (IC) Policy or Manual.   The Infection Control Manual usually includes procedures for handling specimens, isolation procedures, handling precautions, disposal policies, decontamination procedures, and handwashing procedures.

Other manuals or procedures that might be used in the clinical laboratory are instrument and equipment maintenance procedures.

Using well-written procedures in the clinical laboratory enhances the communication network by assuring continuity of methods; avoiding short-cuts; minimizing the chances of errors, specimen re-collections, and reruns; preventing expensive substitutions of reagents; and enhancing quality control, teaching, and safety. Overall, the procedures lead to more efficient data collection.

Continuing Education

In addition to procedure manuals, ongoing laboratory in-service education programs help increase communication and efficiency in patient care. With the increasing complexity of laboratory medicine services, it is essential for phlebotomists to attend in-service education sessions. Phlebotomists are also encouraged to attend other appropriate educational programs within the institution and elsewhere. (See Chapter 12 for information on planning educational programs.)

Staff Meetings

Intralaboratory communications are improved when regularly scheduled staff meetings are held within each laboratory section, such as the specimen collection area. They are useful for discussing problems, new policies, and procedures and for planning. Decisions made in such meetings are usually conferred to all members of the laboratory by written memoranda, by minutes of meetings, or by telephone contact in some cases. Minutes of these meetings should be reviewed by employees who were absent from the meeting. Employees in remote locations off-site can participate using conference calls. This saves the time and travel expense of leaving a worksite to come to "headquarters" for meetings.

Memoranda

Effective communication through *memoranda* requires a concise, clear message written about one subject. This form of written communication should be written in a positive, courteous, and constructive manner. Memoranda provide a method for documenting conversations, decisions, agreements, and policies. They can be filed for future reference and reviewed before meetings. To avoid overstepping boundaries of authority, the phlebotomist should follow the hierarchical structure of the organization if he or she wishes to send memoranda or other written communications.[2]

Other Modes of Intralaboratory Communications

Bulletin boards, posters, checklists, and clipboards are noncomputerized suggestions for disseminating current information. One person from each laboratory should be responsible for periodically checking and changing poster information. Computer software and hardware are also available for networking within the laboratory. Electronic mail (*E-mail*), electronic bulletin boards, product recall notices, and FAXes are all effective ways of communication. Sometimes off-site lab facilities also have a "speed dialing" telephone exchange.

EXTRALABORATORY COMMUNICATIONS NETWORK

Providing Information

Communication with other health care professionals working outside the laboratory is enhanced in a variety of ways. An information bulletin or "floor book" of laboratory services, made available at least in every patient unit, both inpatient and outpatient, is a handy reference. It contains a directory of the laboratory sections with listings of the key staff members, the location of the laboratory, telephone numbers, operating hours, reference ranges, instructions, and pertinent standard procedures of the laboratory. The methods used for collection of all specimens, and the proper identification, storage, preservation, and transportation mechanisms to be used are clearly specified. In addition, an alphabetical listing of all laboratory determinations, specimen requirements, special instructions, and normal values for each measurement are included (Figs. 7–3 and 7–4). The phlebotomist should be familiar with the floor book in order to answer questions related to the clinical laboratory specimen collections and procedures. In some hospitals, this information can be reproduced as a pocket-sized resource. This is particularly helpful to medical students, residents, fellows, and new trainees.

Periodic hospital and departmental newsletters or bulletins, circulated to all departments and medical staff, are another method of communicating information about new institutional and departmental services or policies. The phlebotomist should read these bulletins in order to learn more about the health care institution and laboratory in which he or she works.

Use of the Telephone

The telephone is the most frequently used method of two-way communication in any setting. Phlebotomists should be aware of the following procedures for operating it: how to transfer calls, putting someone on "hold," use of an intercom system, use of conference call and speaker phone functions, and writing legible messages. In addition, conversational techniques and manners should be reviewed. The following suggestions may help the phlebotomist communicate effectively and politely on the telephone.[3] Additional suggestions for communication techniques are covered in Chapter 8.

1. When answering the phone, the department's name should be stated. This saves time for both parties on the phone in case of a wrong number. In addition, some hospitals require that the employee state his

or her name. To establish a cooperative relationship, he or she can offer statements such as "May I help you?" and "Thank you" at the end of the conversation.

2. The tone of voice is important in conveying a message and attitude about one's work. Because the phlebotomist represents the entire clinical laboratory, it is recommended that he or she be conscious of mood when answering the telephone. For example, just because a phlebotomist has had a difficult day at work does not mean that a negative attitude should be communicated to an innocent individual at the other end of the phone line.

3. Language in a hospital setting is very specialized and words are often difficult to pronounce. To avoid problems, the communicator should use appropriate terminology for the receiving individual. The phlebotomist should use words that are concise, direct, and uncomplicated. A simple explanation or definition may clarify or prevent a misunderstanding. Spelling a term may help the receiver understand or recognize what is being said.

4. Good listening habits also function in effective communications by gaining additional information about a problem, checking word meaning, conveying a cooperative attitude, and bringing the exact message into focus. Listening techniques which may help are as follows:

   a. Restating a sentence tells the communicator that one is actually hearing the correct message.

   b. Clarifying word usage also reassures the communicator that the correct message is being transmitted.

   c. Remaining neutral in a controversy helps maintain objectivity. If one gets angry, the emotion may confuse or alter what is really being said.

   d. Reflecting on the message for a moment rather than thinking about immediate response will reinforce it. However, too much silence may indicate lack of interest.

   e. Summarizing the message back to the communicator assures that it is correct and that both parties have fully understood and are in agreement about what was transmitted.

5. Asking pertinent questions and the ability to say "I do not know," are part of effective feedback. The communicator must realize that all individuals they speak to are not experts. The key to effective two-way communication is understanding each other and being cooperative. If it is impossible for one party to help or understand the other, then a statement such as this one will suffice: "I am sorry, but I simply cannot help you."

The importance of the role of the phlebotomist in public relations cannot be overlooked. Open communication and mutual respect should be maintained in the daily contacts between phlebotomists, other laboratory person-

TEST #	PROCEDURE	SPECIMEN	AVERAGE TURNAROUND TIME	REQUEST FORM	COLLECTED BY	INSTRUCTIONS
517	Herpes simplex, Virus culture	Must specify source	2 weeks	Special Test	Physician/Nurse	Contact Serology Laboratory (Ext. 3515). Performed by Reference Laboratory.
550	Heterophile Antibody (Monospot)	Blood 7cc-R.T.	24 hours	Serology	Laboratory	
586	HI Titer-St. Louis Encephalitis	Blood 7cc-R.T.	2 weeks	Special Test	Laboratory	Performed by Reference Laboratory.
861	Histamine	Blood 10cc-G.T.	5 days	Special Test	Laboratory	Collect on ice. Do not spin. Performed by Reference Lab.
526	Histoplasmosis, Complement Fixation (Fungal Serology)	Blood 10cc-R.T.	2 weeks	Serology	Laboratory	Performed by Reference Laboratory.

				Special Test	Laboratory	
3	HLA Typing (Microcytotoxicity)	Blood 10cc-G.T.				DO NOT refrigerate or freeze.
707	Homovanillic Acid (HVA)	Urine 24-hr	6 days	Chem Urine II	Nurse	72-hr diet restrictions; coffee, tea, vanilla ice cream, hypertensive drugs. Obtain specimen container with 25ml 6N HCl from Room C3.007. Performed by Ref. Lab.
761	Human Chorion c Gonadotrophin (HCG) (Immunoassay—beta)	Blood 10cc-R.G.T.	24 hours	Chemistry III	Laboratory	Available Mon–Fri only.
762	Human Chorinic Gonadotrophin (HCG)	Urine 24-hr	6 days	Chem Urine II	Nurse	Performed by Reference Lab.

Figure 7–3. Sample of a floor book of laboratory information listing pertinent requirements regarding laboratory determinations.

EXAMPLE OF REFERENCE RANGES IN HEMATOLOGY

TEST NAME	REFERENCE RANGES
Antithrombin III (AT III)	80%–120% normal activity
Bleeding Time	2.5–8.0 minutes
Differential Count	
Bands	3%–5%
Neutrophils (Polys)	42%–68%
Lymphocytes	24%–44%
Monocytes	2%–7%
Eosinophils	1%–3%
Basophils	0%–1%
Absolute Granulocyte Count	4300 ± 1520/µL
Eosinophil Count	Average of 200/µL
Erythrocyte Fragility	Initial hemolysis: 0.45%–0.39%
	Complete hemolysis: 0.33%–0.30%
Fibrin Degradation/Split Products (FSP)	<10 µg/mL
Fibrinogen	200–400 mg/100 mL
Fibrinopeptide A (FpA)	0–3.7 mg/mL
Hematocrit	40.0%–54.0% (male)
	37.0%–47.0% (female)
Hemoglobin	14.0%–18.0 g/dL (male)
	12.0%–16.0 g/dL (female)
Indices	
MCV	82–98 fl
MCH	27.0–31.0 pg
MCHC	31.0%–36.0%
LE Cell Prep	Negative—No LE cells present
Leukocyte Alkaline Phosphatase (Total Score)	25–139
Partial Thromboplastin Time (PTT)	24.3–36.3 seconds
Platelet Count	140–440 K/µL
Prothrombin Consumption Time	>20 seconds
Prothrombin Time (PT)	10.5–12.9 seconds
Red Blood Cell Count (RBC)	4.50–6.00 M/µL (male)
	4.00–5.50 M/µL (female)
Reticulocyte	0.5%–1.5%
Reticulocyte Count (Absolute)	20,000–90,000/µL
Reptilase Time	14.6–19.8 seconds
Sedimentation Rate (Erythrocyte)	0–9 mm/hr (male)
	0–20 mm/hr (female)
Sickle Cell Test	Negative—no sickling detected
Spinal Fluid Cell Count	Up to 10 lymphocytes/µL
Sucrose Presumptive Test for PNH	Negative
Thrombin Time	11.4–16.6 seconds
White Blood Cell Count (WBC)	4.0–11.0 K/µL

Figure 7–4. Sample listing of reference ranges determined for the routine hematology tests performed in the laboratory.

nel, patients, nursing, housekeeping, dietary, maintenance, purchasing, and other hospital personnel, sales representatives, and nonhospital personnel.

Confidentiality

Each state has statutes related to privileges between physicians and patients. However, communications between a physician and a patient are generally considered privileged and must not be shared with other people without written consent of the patient. Verbal and nonverbal communications must be kept confidential. Nonverbal matters include results of testing, e.g., laboratory and radiology, and monitoring. Exceptions to this are matters for legal consultation. Phlebotomists who have access to patient information must be careful not to disclose results or other patient information in a casual, unnecessary fashion. Discussion that does not directly relate to the phlebotomist's role in caring for the patient should be avoided. There is no need to discuss patients' medical status unless it affects the phlebotomist's ability to do his or her job. Disclosure of confidential information can lead to a breach of the patient's rights and an invasion of privacy, both of which can lead to litigation.

Electronic Transmission (Facsimile) of Printed Materials

Each laboratory or health care institution should have clear policies related to the use of test requests or patient information that has been FAXed. Most laboratories find the use of a *FAX machine* efficient, timely, and cost effective, especially when off-site services are offered. However, precautionary measures should be detailed in procedure manuals that relate to receiving an "official" laboratory order from the requesting physician. In addition, some FAX copies have been known to fade over time. Therefore one must reproduce (photocopy) the FAXed version onto a more permanent version.

COMPUTERIZED COMMUNICATIONS

Personal, mini, and mainframe computers have become essential instruments in the clinical laboratory and health care setting, and, thus, the phlebotomist needs to become acquainted with information systems. For example, in the clinical laboratory, the functions of a laboratory computer system include (1) entering lists of test requisitions for a patient, (2) printing patients' labels, specimen collection lists, and schedules, (3) updating the laboratory specimen accession records, (4) printing lists that identify what test procedures need to be performed on patients' specimens, (5) entering test results into the computer manually or through clinical laboratory instrumentation, (6) storing test results, (7) sending laboratory results to the nursing stations, and (8) sending patient charges to the accounting office.

Computers are composed of the same basic units that can transmit information, store information, and perform various types of calculations. The computer system has three main components: (1) CPU (central processing unit), (2) main memory, and (3) peripheral devices.

The *CPU* is the heart of the computer system. It performs the arithmetic operations and regulates the functions and sequence of events in the system. The main memory is the means by which the CPU stores data and programs for immediate use.[4]

Two types of memories frequently referred to are "read-only memory" (ROM) and "random access memory" (RAM). *ROM* is designed so that the memory is prewritten prior to being permanently placed in the computer. The memorized data are then read as needed by the computer. When the electrical power is switched off, ROM continues to store data. *RAM* is the memory that can be read and written by the computer as it operates. This type of memory is volatile in that the data and information are lost when the power is turned off.

Peripheral devices are devices that the computer uses for input, output, and secondary storage. Some peripherals that are used in computer systems include $3^1/_2''$ or $5^1/_4''$ diskettes, CDROM, optical disc drives, scanners, recording devices, modems, printers, and video terminals sometimes referred to as the *CRT* (cathode ray tube).

With major advances in computer technology, the phlebotomist sooner or later will become initiated to information processing by computerization. Thus, he or she should become thoroughly acquainted with computer terminology to provide quality health care services through effective communication networks. Some examples of computerization in the laboratory are given later in this chapter.

REQUISITION FORMS

The process of networking with which a phlebotomist becomes involved begins the moment the laboratory is notified of a requested test. This notification is done via the laboratory *requisition form* or via a computer-generated order. Therefore, the information or instructions must be explicit and the design and format of the request forms or computer screens to be used must be carefully considered in order to minimize handwriting, permit convenient handling, generate inexpensive and legible copies, and obtain all necessary information for laboratory testing.

Multiple-part forms, which serve as both request and report forms, represent one of the most widely used traditional formats for a manual hospital laboratory system. The forms are usually of a convenient size to be easily attached to $8^1/_2 \times 11$-in. paper as is customarily used for patients' medical records. Also, these forms are easy to transport, handle, sort, and store, as well as being cost effective. For example, the manual requisition forms designed for use at the University of Texas System Cancer Center, M.D. Anderson Hospital Cancer Center, Houston, Tex., are $3^1/_4$ in. in width by $7^3/_8$ in. in length and are

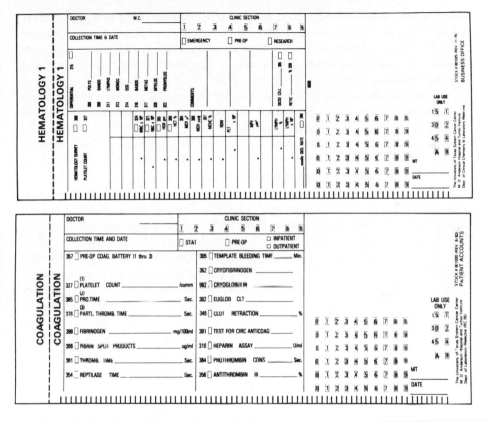

Figure 7–5. Multiple-part request forms that also serve as report forms. These forms are used with a computerized reporting system, but are designed to serve as temporary report forms on a backup basis. *(Courtesy of the University of Texas M.D. Anderson Hospital, Department of Laboratory Medicine, Houston, Tex., with permission.)*

usually positioned horizontally as seen on the Hematology and Coagulation request forms in Figure 7–5. Each form is divided into sections, one side for request information and the other for results. The information on the request side (physician's name, collection time, date, clinic section) is arranged so that it always appears in the same order. This consistency allows standardization between departments and facilitates correct usage. The request information must designate time specifications, or the promptness with which the test results are needed—"STAT," "routine," and so on; patient condition specifications or the circumstances at the time of specimen collection—"pre-op," "admission"; as well as patient category specifications such as "inpatient" or "outpatient." The request side also allows room for all patient identification information, whether done by means of an addressograph machine or handwritten. Each form is identified by name (i.e., Hematology 1, Coagulation, Chemistry 1) and is divided into test categories usually coinciding with the different sections of the laboratory. They are manufactured to provide clear copies and easy detachment (perforated edges). Color coding can be used for different request forms for ease of identification, both in the ordering of tests and in the charting of results. The name of the institution is usually included on each request form.

Certain additional specifications may be included on request slips that are to be used with a laboratory computer system or with instrumentation that generates printed results. Some request forms are used with a computerized reporting system, but are designed to serve also as a temporary report form on a backup basis. Exact spacing specifications must be met when the request form is to be used as a printout report for certain test results.

Other variations of computerized requisitions may also be used, such as those with barcoded identification numbers. Use of barcoding on patients' samples is becoming more commonplace to reduce transcription errors and speed up sample processing.

Barcodes represent a series of light and dark bands of varying widths. The configuration of these bands relate to specific alphanumeric symbols, i.e., numbers and letters. In other words, each letter of the alphabet and each number has a specific code (black and white bars of varying widths). When these bands are placed together in a series, they can correspond to a name (patient or test) or number (identification or test code). By scanning the bar with a sensitive light, or laser scanner, the series of numbers/letters are read into a computer in a very precise manner. This technology has been shown to be very accurate and fast. It saves time and personnel from entering or typing information, and it

Figure 7–6. Barcoded labels.

reduces clerical errors substantially. Barcodes not only represent patients' names and identification numbers, but the test codes, billing codes, inventory records, as well. Many instruments used in the clinical laboratory are functioning with automatic scanners to read a label directly from the patient's sample tube as it is run through the analyzer. In addition, many laboratory supplies are packaged with barcoded inventory labels (Fig. 7–6).

TRANSMITTING THE TEST REQUEST TO THE LABORATORY

The request mechanism formally initiates the cyclic procedure of the physician–patient–laboratory communication network. Two systems are commonly used for this activity. Orders for test requests can be transmitted directly to the clinical laboratory from the requesting authority via an on-line interactive computer system. In many institutions, however, manual requesting systems are still in use, sometimes using barcodes, which are then entered into the computer, or by a totally manual request system in which the request form also serves a dual purpose as the final report.

On-line computer input of request information is the most error free means of making requests. Because a computer system has the capability of performing automatic checks on the input, it does not accept a request for any test that is not in its test-information data base. Likewise, it does not accept a sample of plasma or urine for a test restricted to serum. It also allows the person entering the test request to obtain accurate and up-to-date information about specific determinations, such as revised specimen collection requirements, delivery instructions, assay techniques, reference ranges, and even charge fees.

In a manual system, the multipart request forms are commonly completed at each patient unit or nursing station by a nurse or ward clerk and delivered to the laboratory. This type of system is more subject to human error. The requisitions could be lost by the nursing service or ward clerk prior to arriving in the clinical laboratory or by the laboratory personnel after they reach the laboratory. Another common source of error comes from requests that are prepared in duplicate or not at all due to lack of communication on the nursing unit. These problems can be minimized by instituting a few organizational procedures. Providing a central location in the laboratory where all requisitions are to be delivered or scheduling laboratory personnel to make designated pickups of all request slips usually alleviates the problem of misplaced or lost forms. A sorting system is maintained once the requisitions reach the laboratory. The problem of whether or not a request slip has been made can be solved by removing one copy of the multi-part form that can be kept on the patient unit as a record of the test requested. A blood collection log sheet at the nurses' station can also be used for this purpose. The request slips are kept with the blood collection log and compared by the phlebotomist when the blood is drawn. This system also provides the added advantage of allowing the phlebotomist to make comments on the log sheet regarding problems in obtaining the blood specimens and provides a means of communicating this to the nursing personnel.

One system that works extremely well at University of Texas M.D. Anderson Cancer Center and alleviates errors in test requesting involves personnel that are trained and employed by the hospital clinical laboratory but stationed at the various nursing units in a phlebotomy/liaison capacity. The formal name of the program is the Laboratory Liaison Technician (LLT) program. It was designed to maintain open and accurate communications pertaining to laboratory services with physicians, nursing service, ward clerks, patients, and family members. The LLTs are mainly responsible for the collection of all blood work requested on their assigned unit after the 7:00 AM morning draw, and for delivery of these specimens to the laboratory, as well as all other specimens. They maintain a log of all specimens collected (Fig. 7–7) and review patient charts to ensure that the laboratory tests have been accurately transcribed to the request slips. It is easy to see how the intervention of personnel such as an LLT could alleviate problems encountered in request transcription, request delivery, specimen collection, and so forth. Other important functions served by these specialized phlebotomists are incorporated in Figure 7–8. Specific instructions for requesting laboratory work or ordering blood products may

LLT DAILY WORK SHEET

UNIT _____ DATE _____ LLT _____

TOTAL PATIENT SERVICES _____ TOTAL STAT SAMPLES _____   7:00-4:00 _____
(# OF VENIPUNCTURES)

                                                                                           3:00-11:00 _____

TOTAL TIMED SAMPLES _____

ROOM #	PATIENT'S NAME	PATIENT #	TESTS TO BE DONE OR SPECIMENS DELIVERED	LOGGED BY	TIME TO BE COLLECTED	TIME COLLECTED	OBTAINED BY	SPECIMEN	COMMENT

Figure 7–7. Daily log sheet documenting all specimens collected and delivery by the specialized phlebotomy personnel, Laboratory Liaison Technicians (LLTs): *(Courtesy of the University of Texas M.D. Anderson Hospital, Department of Laboratory Medicine, Houston, Tex., with permission.)*

DUTIES OF LABORATORY LIAISON TECHNICIANS
1. Blood collection—within laboratory guidelines.
2. Supervise and assist AM collection.
3. Deliver all Laboratory Medicine specimens to laboratories.
4. Deliver reports to assigned nursing units.
5. Maintain a daily log of all specimens collected.
6. Review patient charts as pertains to laboratory orders.
7. Review ward clerk's Kardex for laboratory orders.
8. Assist IV Team with collection of laboratory specimens. All LLTs who have been authorized to draw from CVC, IVH (except surgery IVH), and heparin locks may draw from these lines as time permits.
9. Advise nursing personnel on special collection techniques.
10. Serve as an information source regarding status of tests and retrieval of data from computer terminals.
11. Advise nursing staff on laboratory procedures and laboratory policy changes that will affect nursing.
12. Advise laboratory on laboratory needs of nursing and medical staff.
13. Work with Unit Managers in the orientation of Ward Clerks to laboratory procedures.
14. Review nurses' Kardex as pertaining to test ordered.
15. Secure printouts of reports as they are needed.
16. Coordinate laboratory collections to decrease the number of venipunctures.
17. Keep floors stocked with blood collecting supplies.
18. Maintain communications with patients and patient's family as pertaining to laboratory work.
LLTs with adequate training and in the presence of a RN or doctor may insert angicocaths, scalp vein needles, or butterflies to start an IV.

Figure 7–8. Listing of specific duties delegated to the specialized phlebotomy personnel: *(Courtesy of the University of Texas M.D. Anderson Hospital, Department of Laboratory Medicine, Houston, Tex., with permission.)*

be included in both a laboratory Bulletin of Information issued to each nursing unit and in an Administrative Services Manual issued to unit clerks. This is a good way of ensuring the proper handling of specimens and requisitions.

Verbal test requests are occasionally used in cases of emergency. The request should be documented on a standardized form in the laboratory prior to the collection of the blood specimen (Fig. 7–9). After the blood has been collected, the formal laboratory request slip can be filled out and accompany the specimen to the laboratory in the routine manner.

SPECIMEN LABELS

Clear and accurate specimen identification is essential and must begin immediately upon collection and continue through disposal of the specimen. Identification methods vary from manually copying all patient identification onto the

---

STAT REQUESTS

Nurse:

Requesting Physician:

Location: ICU_____ER_____Other_____
             Room:_____

Patient: Patient ID No._____

Pick up orders on unit:_____

Tests Ordered:_____
_____
_____
_____
_____

Requested by:_____

Order taken by:_____
Date_____   Time_____   AM_____PM_____

Figure 7–9. Sample of a documentation form used by the laboratory in cases of verbal test requests. *(Adapted from a form used at the University of Texas M.D. Anderson Cancer Center, Houston, Tex., with permission.)*

container to using prenumbered barcoded labels. Manually labeling specimens can be time consuming and is prone to transcription errors. This can be avoided by using preprinted labels, which are available from many commercial sources. Some labels are gummed hospital labels that can be attached to specimens. Other systems include those that can imprint a patient identification card or electronically print patient identification information onto the specimen label.

Among the most sophisticated, accurate, and efficient labels are those generated by a hospital computer system. Requisition slips for the morning draw can be sent to the laboratory in the afternoon of the previous day, or entered into the computer at any time. Based on the laboratory orders, the computer can generate enough labels containing all the appropriate patient identification criteria for each tube required to be drawn. The labels also contain the specific tests requested, the specimen collection tubes required for the requested tests, and unique accession numbers or sample numbers to be used for that particular collection time. Barcodes can also be used for any alphanumeric symbols. Smaller transfer labels may also be printed to label special aliquots, tubes, cuvettes, and microscope slides. This type of system eliminates the manually written entry log used by many hospitals to record the tests and accession number requested on each patient. Additional tests ordered later in the day are entered into the computer, which assigns a specific time to the tests, so they can be easily separated from the morning draw. Labels for later collection can be computer-printed or made with an addressograph machine. Blood drawing lists are also printed by the computer to provide a list of patients on each floor requiring blood work for the morning draw and the tests ordered, and to identify the assigned sample accession number. The phlebotomist initials this list after the patient's blood has been drawn, and a copy is left at the nursing unit so that caregivers attending the patient can see what tests have already been collected. Any additional specimens collected later in the day are written into the log book on the floor (see Fig. 7–7). In this way, the personnel on the nursing unit have a complete list of the tests collected on each patient throughout the day.

Computerization of the collection process can significantly decrease errors. Without a computer, collection and specimen information must pass through several people before the sample is actually processed in the laboratory. With a computer, data are continually being checked against the computer files, and authorized individuals can add to and receive information from the accumulated data.

SPECIMEN TRANSPORTATION AND DELIVERY

Both the communication network and the quality of laboratory test results are dependent upon the time that specimens are received for processing. Phlebotomists should assure that blood and other specimens are delivered expeditiously. However, specimen transportation procedures may vary considerably between institutions.

Hand Delivery

Many systems for specimen delivery involve hand-carried specimens and require standards for assuring promptness. The laboratory is most often the department responsible for the collection and delivery of blood specimens. The laboratory may also be responsible for the delivery of all other patient specimens as well. Phlebotomists, especially those permanently assigned to specific floors, as in the previously mentioned LLT system, can make scheduled pickups as well as delivery of "STAT" specimens. The specimens should be placed in an assigned area on each nursing unit after being written into the log book. The patient's name, hospital number, room number, specimens delivered, time, and initials of the person transporting the specimen should be included on the log sheet as specified in Figure 7–7. Specimen transportation can be more easily monitored when all personnel involved use the appropriate documentation procedures and communicate openly with one another.

Most phlebotomists organize their blood collection trays or carts to accommodate patient specimens that need to be taken to the laboratory. A test tube rack, slide rack, plastic holder, or cup are sufficient to hold the collected specimens. Some specimens require ice for transport, and so it is wise to carry a small container with ice that will not leak and will fit conveniently on the tray.

Transportation Department

Specimen delivery may also be performed by a transportation department within the hospital. Typically the transportation escort or orderlies are responsible for moving patients from their nursing units to service areas such as diagnostic radiology, physical therapy, etc. When a specimen and requisition form are to be delivered to the laboratory by the transportation department, the following information is usually required: type of specimen, name and hospital identification number of the patient, date and time of specimen collection, and destination of the specimen. After obtaining this information, the escort takes the specimen to the laboratory and logs it in on a log sheet as shown in Figure 7–10. The test request slip accompanying the specimen can also be "clocked-in" at this time so that actual delivery time can always be obtained. If any complications arise with the specimen, the escort notifies the nursing unit. Occasionally, specimens, especially "STAT" or timed requests, may be collected and delivered to the laboratory by a nurse or physician. Again, the requisition should be clocked-in.

Pneumatic Tube Systems

Some hospitals use *pneumatic tube* systems to transport patient records, messages, letters, bills, medications, x-rays, and laboratory results. However, reports from health care institutions differ as to the effectiveness of using tube systems for transporting blood specimens. Some reports indicate that certain test values are affected as a result of transporting specimens in pneumatic systems. Others report that with careful evaluation and use of the system, it can be a time-saving and cost-effective process.[5] The Mayo Clinic reports evaluating several aspects of a pneumatic system before employing it for transporting laboratory specimens. Among these are mechanical reliability, distance of transport, speed of carrier, control mechanisms, a soft landing mechanism, radius of loops and bends, shock absorbancy and sizes of carriers, and laboratory assessment of chemical and cellular components in transported specimens versus hand-carried specimens.[5] It is generally recommended that blood collection tubes be placed in the pneumatic tube with shock absorbent inserts padding the sides and separated from each other to avoid spillage or breakage. Plastic clear liners are also commercially available so that if leaks do occur,

SPECIMEN DELIVERY

Patient Name	Location	Specimens						Date	Time	Escort Name
		CSF	Blood	Urine	Sputum	Other	Test Ordered			

Figure 7–10. Sample of a log sheet used by the laboratory to document delivery of patient specimens by the institutional transport service.

they are visible and are contained to avoid contamination of the tube system, the carrier, and the personnel handling the specimens.

Transportation by Vehicle
Some manufacturers provide transport systems that are automated, motorized, or computerized. Delivery of specimens can be via a small container car attached to a network of track that is routed to appropriate sites in the laboratory, on the nursing stations, or in other specimen collection areas. Again, a thorough evaluation of such automated delivery systems needs to include mechanical reliability, transportation distances, speed of the carriers, control mechanisms, soft-landing provisions, radius of loops and bends, shock absorbency, size of carriers, method of cleaning containers, and overall time- and cost-effectiveness. When planning to renovate a laboratory area that includes this type of transport system, extra space above the ceiling tiles should be considered, as the transport vehicles require a sizable right-of-way.

Other Transport Equipment
Phlebotomists may also be required to order and use special transport containers. All should be evaluated for cost, protective ability, temperature con-

trol, sterilizing potential, appearance, labeling system, breakage, leakage, and tamper proofing.

Some hospitals send specimens to reference laboratories for special analysis. When packaging or receiving one of the specimens in a special transport container, care must be taken to pay attention to the following details:

1. Specimens such as human or animal feces, blood, body fluids, or tissue should be properly labeled and in containers that protect individuals from contamination.
2. Specimens containing viable microorganisms must be specially packaged so they can withstand leakage of contents, pressure and temperature changes, and rough handling. It is recommended that the specimen be placed in a "primary container" surrounded by absorbent packing material. If the contents were released, they would be maintained in the "primary container." It should be labeled with pertinent information and instructions about the specimen contents. It can then be placed in a secondary container. Biohazardous and mailing labels should be affixed to the outside container.[4]
3. Specimen requisition forms or special instructions should accompany the specimen.
4. Containers holding dry ice should be labeled, for example, "DRY ICE, FROZEN MEDICAL SPECIMEN."
5. It is recommended that, when shipping biohazardous material, the address and phone number of the Centers for Disease Control, Atlanta, Ga., be affixed to the container in the event of damage or leakage. Individuals outside the health professions may need advice on how to dispose of or clean up a biohazardous spill.
6. After receiving an intact specimen from an outside source, the container must be identified by name, number, and source. It should match the accompanying requisition and can then be processed accordingly.
7. If a leaky or broken specimen is received, it should be handled cautiously and according to safety procedures.

REPORTING MECHANISMS

Written Reports

The laboratory report is a feedback mechanism for transmitting vital data from the laboratory to the physician requesting the information. Both the Joint Commission of Accreditation of Health Care Organizations (JCAHO) and the CAP state that the results should be confirmed, dated, and accompanied by permanent report copies that are kept in the laboratory as well as sent to the patient's chart. The CAP also states that each report should contain adequate patient identification, be stamped to record the date and hour the procedures were completed, and be signed and initialed by the laboratory personnel performing the procedure. When computer-generated report forms are used, laboratory documentation on worksheets of those performing the procedures is sufficient. The CAP has suggested the following considerations when designing a report form:

1. Identification of patient, patient location, and physician
2. Date and time of specimen collection
3. Description, source of specimen, and labeled precautions
4. Compactness and ease of preparing the package for shipment
5. Consistency in format
6. Clear understandability of instructions or orders
7. Logical location in patient's chart for reference lab reports
8. Sequential order of multiple results on single specimens
9. Listing of normal ranges or normal and abnormal values
10. Assurance of accuracy of transcription of request
11. Administrative and record-keeping value[1]

Any unique institutional requirements needed for an acceptable report should be stated in the laboratory procedure manual and may include such criteria as quality control limits, absolute limits, and delta checks.[6] If these criteria cannot be met on the report form, a written policy including these requirements should be available when needed.

Results can be documented in one of the following three ways: manual recording of test results, laboratory instrument printed reports, and computer-generated reports. As previously mentioned, in most manual systems, combination test requisitioning/report forms are used. These contain multiple copies as depicted in Figure 7–5. Microprocessors are in wide use today in some laboratory instruments that can generate digital outputs and printed reports.

Verbal Reports

The use of verbal and telephone reports has declined in recent years because computer access to laboratory data is prevalent in most health care environments. If laboratory personnel take an active role in educating clerical, nursing, and physician staff on the acquisition of computerized data, the number of phone orders will decrease.

Verbal reports, although useful for reporting "STAT" results and "panic" values, may become a problem in laboratories. The possibility of error is so great that at the very minimum, a laboratory should always require proper identification of the patient and the name of the person receiving the report. Written documentation of verbally issued reports is recommended and should include the following information: patient name and hospital number, person receiving the information, date, information given, and person issuing the report (Fig. 7–11).

CULTURE RESULTS—TELEPHONE REQUEST

PATIENT NAME:_____

PATIENT ID NUMBER:_____

PHYSICIAN:_____

PERSON REQUESTING INFORMATION:_____

DATE	SOURCE	CULTURE #	INFO GIVEN

TIME OF INQUIRY:_____

DATE OF INQUIRY:_____

TECHNOLOGIST:_____

Figure 7–11. Sample form used by a microbiology laboratory to issue verbal results.

Computerized Reports

Various computer transmission devices can provide a rapid on-line report system, and are, in general, more reliable than verbal reports, as well as being faster than waiting for the written report. A hospital with an on-line laboratory computer system can have terminals located at each patient unit. After the tests have been completed and verified in the laboratory, the results can be immediately displayed on each patient unit. A printer can be attached to each terminal to generate a temporary hard-copy report. Another transmission method electronically transmits a handwritten report, which is generated in a similar form at the receiving end. A third transmission device transmits facsimile results, similar to a photocopy of the report, to an output device. All of these methods can provide a written report that is usually accurate, dependable, and consistent.

Interim Reports and Cumulative Summaries

Interim laboratory reports are typically sent to nursing units at specified times during the day, e.g., 11:00 AM and 2:00 PM. These reports may include test results completed, or "in progress." This type of reporting system is often used in facilities that are only partially computerized or as a backup process if the hospital computer system is malfunctioning or "down."

Cumulative summaries are a compilation of laboratory reports on one patient over a designated period of time, or after a certain number of tests have been performed on the patient. They are printed at designated times during the week and facilitate the medical record–charting process. They are helpful to nurses and physicians because groups of similar tests are reported together. Trends that reveal laboratory and physiological changes can be detected more easily than if each lab value was reported separately and charted in the medical record at random.

DISTRIBUTION OF RESULTS

The final communication involved in the physician–patient–laboratory network is the distribution of test results. Those who receive the laboratory data include nursing, clerical, and medical record personnel (chart attachment), the hospital business office (patient billing), and the laboratory (department record).

Medical Records and Charts

Manual Methods.   In order to provide a chronological type of reporting system in the patient's chart, the laboratory reports have traditionally been shingled one upon another. Color coding by the laboratory originating the results aids in coordinating them on a carrier page. The laboratory may also key chronological reports by having a master card prepared in the laboratory for each patient, beginning with the admitting laboratory results. The results of each day are added to the card, which can be photocopied and sent to the physician. This also allows the laboratory without a computer system to perform delta checks on the results before releasing them.[6]

Computerized Medical Records.   A hospital computer system can easily provide daily printed reports and cumulative reports for the patient's chart. All reports should be printed and delivered at times convenient for mounting on the chart and should also be suited to the schedule of the medical staff. Some hospitals send a second set of results directly to the physician in case errors or delays in chart attachments occur. This helps to ensure that the data are available to the physicians before making patient rounds.

The business office of the hospital also receives laboratory results. They must be notified of all laboratory charges, according to data requested and procedural code for patient billing. It is advantageous to send reports promptly so the patient can avoid late charges, which generate complaints from patients and insurance companies.

Laboratory copies of test results must be maintained in storage because data from previous days, months, or years are often requested. A copy of the combined request/report form can be easily stored and used for information retrieval. In a manual reporting system, log books are often kept in the laboratory and usually serve as duplicate recording of patient results. They can be beneficial in permitting a more rapid retrieval of a patient's previous results and aid in providing a delta check procedure. Computer systems are advantageous because they can store easily retrievable information for long periods of time, require no paperwork from laboratory personnel, be programmed to automatically display and flag delta checks, and generate management reports about workload, abnormal results, and the like.

KEY TERMS

barcodes
continuing education
CPU (central processing unit)
CRT (cathode ray tube)
cumulative summaries
e-mail
FAX machines
Hazard Communication Manual

infection control policy
medical records and charts
memoranda
material safety data sheets (MSDS)
Occupational Safety and Health Administration (OSHA)

pneumatic tube
quality control procedures
RAM (random access memory)
reference ranges
requisition form
Right to Know Act
ROM (read only memory)

STUDY QUESTIONS

1. Identify six ways to enhance the intralaboratory communications network.
2. Describe guidelines for designing a requisition/report form.
3. Name three commonly used ways to transport specimens.
4. Name areas or departments that usually receive laboratory reports.
5. What is the mechanism that formally initiates the physician–patient–laboratory communication cycle?
6. What is the most error-free method of test requisitioning and why?
7. What is the most important guideline to be followed when obtaining a blood specimen from a patient?

REFERENCES

1. College of American Pathologists: *Standards for Accreditation of Medical Laboratories.* Skokie, Ill., College of American Pathologists, 1990.

2. Becan-McBride K (ed): *Textbook of Clinical Laboratory Supervision.* New York, Appleton-Century-Crofts, 1982.
3. International Society for Clinical Laboratory Technology (ISCLT): *Physician Office Laboratory Technician Handbook,* St. Louis, Mo., ISCLT, 1989.
4. Martin BG, Viskochil KR, Amos PA (eds): *Clinical Laboratory Management, A Guide for Clinical Laboratory Scientists.* Boston, Little, Brown, 1982.
5. Slockbauer JM, Blumenfeld TA: *Collection and Handling of Laboratory Specimens, A Practical Guide.* St. Louis, J.B. Lippincott, 1983.
6. Henry J (ed): *Clinical Diagnosis and Management by Laboratory Methods.* Philadelphia, W.B. Saunders, 1990.

Interpersonal Communication Skills and Professionalism

8

COMMUNICATION IN THE PATIENT CARE ENVIRONMENT

As a vital member of the clinical laboratory team, the phlebotomist provides the link between the patient and the analytic area. The quality of the blood specimens determines the quality of the diagnostic test results. However, the ease of collection of these specimens depends upon the skills and abilities of the phlebotomist to perform the collection techniques and to interact successfully with the patient.

Bedside Manner

The climate established by the phlebotomist upon entering a patient's room begins before he or she leaves the laboratory area. The feeling of confidence that comes from the knowledge that the collection tray is clean and completely stocked is the first step in a good bedside manner. A pleasant face, neat appearance, and professional manner set the stage for a positive encounter when dealing with patients. The first 30 seconds after the phlebotomist enters the patient's room determines how that patient perceives the clinical laboratory and, in some cases, the quality of patient care offered by that hospital. Most patients admit that the procedure they dread most is being "stuck" for blood collection.

As discussed in previous chapters, the phlebotomist should introduce him or herself and then state that he or she is part of the hospital or laboratory staff. The patient should be informed that the specimen is being collected for a test ordered by the physician. A statement indicating that this is routine hospital protocol often reassures the patient. A lengthy discussion of why a certain test was ordered or what tests were ordered is not appropriate. These questions should be referred to the patient's physician. During all steps of the venipuncture, the phlebotomist should remain calm and professional. Before leaving the patient, he or she should make sure the patient is no longer bleeding and thank him or her for cooperating.

Patient Interview

Hospitals and laboratories differ slightly in their guidelines for patient interviews. All agree that proper patient identification is essential both by means of an armband and by verbal confirmation. If the patient does *not* have an armband, a positive confirmation must be made by a unit nurse who knows the patient. This process should be well documented by the phlebotomist. Special identification procedures should also be well documented for ambulatory patients. Armbands are not routinely issued in ambulatory settings; however, an identification card usually is. It may include some demographic data. Again, this should be confirmed by the patient prior to collection of specimens. The patient should always be asked "What is your name?" not "Are you Ms. Smith?" A patient on medication will often agree with anything he or she is asked. Some institutions insist that the phlebotomist ask for the patient's complete address, while others require the mention of the hometown, birthdate, or street to reinforce and confirm identity. Some prefer that patients spell an unusual last name. This portion of the specimen collection procedure assures that the remainder of the diagnostic testing protocol provides information on the correct person.

It is important for the phlebotomist to remember that verbal and nonverbal cues or body language play an important part in the communication of what the patient perceives and how he or she responds. In addition, listening skills are also a valuable part of patient communication.

Teaching Patients

For some laboratory procedures to be successful, the patient must participate and cooperate. The phlebotomist must be willing and able to provide sufficient understandable instruction to the patient for protocols to be accomplished. In some clinical situations, patients with diabetes need to be instructed on the use of mechanical aids to perform finger sticks on themselves at home to check blood glucose (sugar) levels.

Nursing staff or unit personnel may have instructed the inpatient that he or she will be fasting or have "nothing by mouth" until after the early morning blood collections. The phlebotomist should listen to patient's comments about "not having breakfast yet" or "they won't feed me." Even a question or comment about food may inspire a response to confirm that the patient was truly fasting. Even more critical are the timed tests such as the glucose tolerance test. In this test, patient understanding is essential. The patient should be informed of the following:

1. A fasting blood specimen is drawn and urine collected.
2. The fasting period is followed by a measured intake of food or a measured glucose drink.
3. After a 30-minute interval, blood is drawn and a urine specimen collected.
4. The nursing staff is advised that the time has started. Blood and urine specimens are collected at hourly intervals for 2, 3, 4, or 5 hours. *Note:* For the procedure to yield valid and reliable results the patient must: (a) stay fasting, (b) be in his or her room at the specified time, and (c) drink enough water to provide the timed urine specimens.

If the patient is a child, the parents or guardian must receive and understand the instructions. If the patient begins to feel ill or faint, the nursing personnel or phlebotomy supervisor should be notified. If the patient is an outpatient, the phlebotomist and other laboratory personnel must monitor the condition of the patient. A bed and bathroom must be convenient to the collection area to provide for the comfort and safety of the patient.

Another timed specimen often used in laboratory medicine is the 24-hour urine specimen. For the specimen to fit into most laboratory schedules, it is advisable to have the patient void at 7:00 AM and discard the urine. The next urine and all urine voided for 24 hours is saved in the container provided. The patient should be cautioned that to have good results *all* the urine must be saved or the procedure will have to be started over.

For urine cultures, the patient must be instructed in proper specimen collection techniques to ensure valid results from microbiology. Occasionally, clinic patients require instruction in collection of stool specimens for culture, examination for ova and parasites, or occult blood. Also, the Scotch tape method for diagnosis of pinworms should be available in the procedure manual if needed for outpatient teaching. Although infrequent, the need to instruct the outpatient about the collection of a 24-hour stool specimen for fecal fat may be necessary.

With the advances in the area of therapeutic drug monitoring, the physician must know not only the time and date of collection but whether the blood was collected before or after medication was given. The length of infusion time is a factor with some drug monitoring. Laboratory coordination necessitates a readily available blood collection team or a couple of designated "drug monitoring" phlebotomists. It also requires a good intradepartmental relationship with nursing service and the pharmacy.

Communication of information is essential for teaching patients and for laboratory testing. However, there are many barriers to good understanding and accurate communication. The following sections describe general concepts of communication.

Basic interpersonal communication can be depicted as a closed loop. The message must leave the sender and reach the receiver (Fig. 8–1). The receiver usually provides feedback to the sender. Without feedback, the sender has no way of knowing whether the message was accurately received or if the message was somehow blocked by extraneous factors. These factors can often filter out meaning from a message. "Filters" can be damaging to good communication. In the following sections, communication will be broken down into the more detailed components:

1. Verbal communication
2. Nonverbal communication
3. Listening skills

Verbal Communication

A basic understanding of the language is needed for any phlebotomist to communicate with all patients, young and old. However, there are filters or barriers to simple verbal communication that can interfere greatly with the patient–phlebotomist relationship.

Language Barriers.   Many members of the health care team use jargon or medical terminology to explain things to the patient. This can often be confusing to laypeople. In addition, the meaning of words varies with the context and the age of the speaker. To promote understanding, a vocabulary that is easily understood should be used with patients whenever possible. This is particularly true when dealing with children. Also, children must *not* be told "this won't hurt." Most blood collection procedures are slightly painful and

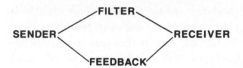

Figure 8–1. Communication loop.

therefore, it is important that the child be forewarned and prepared. It sometimes helps if the child is asked to hold something (e.g., a bandage) while the procedure is taking place. This allows the child to feel helpful and provides a distraction from the procedure.

Hearing Disabilities.   The more complex the directions are, the greater the need to communicate. Thus, the phlebotomist should be more sensitive to patients who have impaired hearing. A question like "How will you do this?" or "When will you begin to start this task?" gives better clues that the patient has heard and understood than "Do you understand?" If it is obvious that the patient did not hear, all efforts should be made to write down instructions for the patient. It is strongly recommended that writing tools be kept at the bedside of these patients and be accessible in an outpatient setting.

English as a Second Language.   Often patients will understand from nonverbal cues such as sign language, but the blood drawer must know how to locate an interpreter, if available, when the patient does not speak or comprehend English. If a large segment of the patient population speaks another language, the hospital should provide interpreters who know the basic use of that language. In the southern and western United States it is important to develop some skill in the Spanish language. For basic requests in several languages, refer to Appendix I. It is recommended that one practice the phrases with someone who can speak the language before attempting to communicate with a patient. Mispronounced words may lead to more confusion. It might also be helpful to have printed cards in different languages that can be used to transmit information. Keep in mind that English language skills and understanding may vary greatly in the United States. The country's cultural diversity lends itself to language differences. The phlebotomist should always speak respectfully, in a highly professional manner and with phrases that are clearly articulated. The dignity of the patient, whether English speaking or not, is of utmost importance. If a phlebotomist feels frustrated by an inability to communicate with a patient, the phlebotomist should seek assistance from a supervisor, translator, family member, or physician. Each patient should be treated compassionately, fairly, and with the utmost of dignity, regardless of language abilities.

Age.   The vocabulary of a teenager is different from that of someone 70 to 80 years old. The phlebotomist must be sensitive to word usage for each age.

Tone of Voice.   The tone of voice and the inflection used can change a positive sentence into a negative sounding statement. Care must be taken to be *sure* that the pitch or tone of voice matches the words that one is attempting to communicate. Sarcasm is usually communicated just by the tone of voice. Phlebotomists should make every attempt to avoid sending mixed messages to patients by practicing a calm, soothing, and confident tone of voice.

Phrases that are useful for practicing on are listed below. Using a "nice tone of voice" (calm, compassionate, professional tone with a smile on the face) and a "degrading tone of voice" (sarcastic, whiney, angry, with a frustrated look on the face), compare the ways of saying the following:

- Please . . .
- Good morning.
- How was your breakfast?
- Have you had lunch?
- May I check your ID bracelet?
- Thank you.

Practicing in front of a mirror or with a co-worker is a useful exercise for improving verbal and nonverbal skills. A simple smile can often force a change in voice tone.

Special Situations.   For patients in the surgical suite, recovery room, or emergency room, the phlebotomist should realize that the patients in these locations usually have the need for emergency or *STAT* blood collection. This requires extra speed and accuracy without jeopardizing the "personal touch." Patients that are in the hospital or come in for chemotherapy often have veins that have been damaged or must be avoided and used only for treatment. Therefore, each patient must be considered in terms of their dignity and individual needs, not as the "burn case down the hall" or "the broken leg in 3C." As long as the phlebotomist is willing to provide care in a professional, respectful manner and respond to each patient as an individual, the quality of care will improve.

Nonverbal Communication
It is often said that one of the most important parts of communication is the nonverbal component. Some educators feel that communication is comprised of 10 to 20 percent words and 80 to 90 percent nonverbal cues. These nonverbal cues or "body language" can be very positive and helpful to understanding or very negative and prevent communication. They are summarized below.

Positive Body Language
Smiling.   A simple compassionate smile can set the stage for open lines of communication. It can make each patient feel that he or she is the most important person at that particular moment. In addition, most people look better with smiles on their faces than they do with frowns.

Eye Contact and Eye Level.   The most expressive parts of the human face are the eyes. Therefore, eye contact is important in effective communication. Eye contact promotes a sense of trust and honesty between a patient and a phlebotomist. It can make the entire procedure less traumatic for the patient if he or she sees a sense of compassion and honesty in a phlebotomist's eyes.

In addition, eye level can be important. Unfortunately, bedridden patients must always look up to those in the room, including the caregivers and the phlebotomist. This can create a feeling of intimidation, being "looked down on," or weakness. It is therefore recommended that if a phlebotomist must explain a lengthy procedure to a patient, that it be done while seated at eye level with the patient. Other than this instance it is rare that the phlebotomist would have a chance to be at eye level. However, it is important to understand the concept so that one can feel what it would be like to be a bedridden patient.

Again, the phlebotomist should practice being the patient while a co-worker stands directly over him or her, looking down. Try this positioning with and without eye contact while carrying on a conversation. It is amazing what it feels like to have the roles reversed. Practice makes the phlebotomist a more compassionate member of the health care team.

Good Grooming.   Physical appearance communicates a great deal about an individual. Neatly combed hair, clean fingernails, a pressed clean lab coat, and overall tidy appearance communicate a commitment to infection control and overall cleanliness and instills confidence in a person. This is particularly important in today's hospital environment where patients and employees alike are deeply concerned about the spread of infectious diseases such as hepatitis and human immunodeficiency virus (HIV).

Erect Posture.   Most of the time phlebotomists perform their work while standing. However, there are occasions, particularly with ambulatory patients, when phlebotomists may sit down while collecting blood. In these cases, erect posture conveys a sense of confidence and pride in one's work. Slouching conveys a sense of laziness and apathy.

Good posture is helpful for both the phlebotomist and the patient. It not only minimizes the phlebotomist's back or neck strain and eases the patient's mind, but it allows the patient to feel more confident in him or her. Relaxed hands, arms, and shoulders enable the phlebotomist to work more freely and show the patient how to relax the arms and shoulders as well.

Face-to-Face.   It is important for a phlebotomist to face the patient directly when speaking. Otherwise, the patient may feel he or she is being avoided, or neglected or something is being hidden from him or her. On the other hand, if a patient turns away from a phlebotomist, it should be taken as a cue that the patient is either very frightened, angry, or in pain. The phlebotomist should try not to take it personally and do everything to make the patient feel more comfortable during the phlebotomy procedure.

Zone of Comfort.   Most individuals begin to feel uncomfortable when strangers get too close to them physically. A *zone of comfort* is that area of space around a patient that is private territory, so to speak. When a strange individual gets too close, it can cause the patient to feel nervous, fearful, or anxious. Phlebotomists must be understanding and approach nervous patients slowly and gently to avoid feelings of being threatened. This is particularly true with children, many of whom have a wide zone of comfort, that is, they do not like anyone to approach them except close relatives or friends. A skilled phlebotomist must be aware of his or her threat to a patient and approach the situation in a calm, professional, and confident manner.

In some cultures the zone of comfort may be wide, and in others people naturally speak more closely to each other. The ease with which one feels with physical closeness can also vary with gender. Some women feel very uncomfortable to have a male phlebotomist standing over them preparing to draw a blood specimen, and vice versa. It is particularly considerate if a phlebotomist recognizes this and responds accordingly. Again, respect for the patient's needs and dignity must be considered.

The phlebotomist can again practice this sensation by role reversal. This exercise should be done among co-workers who are not close friends. The phlebotomist can begin 10 feet away and, pausing between steps, should slowly approach the seated co-worker. Eye contact should be made during this exercise. The seated phlebotomist should note at what distance he or she begins to feel awkward or uncomfortable. That distance would comprise the boundary of the zone of comfort.

Another example of this uncomfortable sensation is in a crowded elevator. It is interesting to watch how often people take great measures to move so that they are not touching strangers. Notice as people exit the elevator, the remaining people move and shift to provide more space around themselves. This same sense of uneasiness is felt by patients who are approached by health care workers they do not know personally.

Negative Body Language/Distracting Behaviors
Rolling Eyes.   In most cases, when an individual rolls his eyes upward, it conveys the sense of being bored, unattentive, or unwilling to perform a duty. Because this behavior is very distracting, it should be avoided at all times when communicating, listening, or observing patients, co-workers, or supervisors.

The same can be said of gazing out the window or looking up at the ceiling. If a phlebotomist enters a patient's room and begins addressing the patient while looking out the window, the patient will feel neglected and the phlebotomist will appear unconcerned. If the window is too tempting to avoid a glance, the phlebotomist should include the patient in on the observations. The phlebotomist could make a friendly comment about the weather and so forth, then continue the specimen collection procedure when full attention can be given to the patient. Again, the objective is to make the patient feel at ease through good communication techniques so that the procedure can be successful.

Nervous Behaviors. Some nervous behaviors such as squirming or tapping a pencil or a foot can be very distracting. These behaviors can make a patient feel nervous, hurried, or anxious about an impending venipuncture. It is important to present a calm and confident image for maximum patient comfort and trust. It is also important that phlebotomists recognize these nervous behaviors in patients, particularly children, so that a special effort can be made to relieve any fear. Allowing a few extra moments of conversation or preparation may help.

Deep Sighs. A deep sigh can often transmit a feeling of being bored or a reluctance to do something. Phlebotomists must try to avoid this behavior, especially when communicating with an uncooperative or angry patient. Likewise, if a patient makes a deep sigh or moans at the mere sight of a phlebotomist, this should be a cue that a little extra attention, conversation, or a smile might ease the reluctance for the procedure.

Other Distracting Nonverbal Behaviors. There are many other actions that can convey negative, distracting, or defensive types of emotions. Among these are crossed arms, a wrinkled forehead, frequent glances at a clock, rapid thumbing through papers or a book, chewing gum, smoking cigarettes, lining up objects on a table, or yawning and stretching. It is vital for phlebotomists to realize that these behaviors can detract from their professional image when communicating with patients, families, visitors, co-workers, and supervisors. It is also important to recognize what these nonverbal cues mean if a patient happens to exhibit these behaviors (Fig. 8–2). Phlebotomists who are the most effective communicators can detect these nonverbal signs immediately and deal with them in an honest, compassionate, and professional manner. It is strongly recommended that regular in-service or continuing education programs be directed at reminding phlebotomists to be aware of positive and negative body language both in their own behavior and in that of patients. Some hospitals keep simple reminders posted on employee bulletin boards (see Table 8–1).

Listening Skills. Another key component of effective communication is the art of listening. Good listening skills help close the communication loop (see Fig. 8–1) by assuring that the message that was sent can indeed be repeated. Listening skills do not depend on intellect or educational background. They can be learned and practiced. The following tips or steps to active listening are

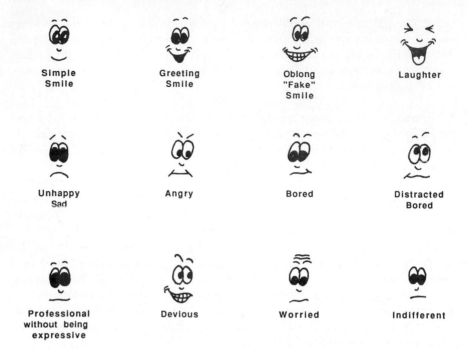

Figure 8–2. Nonverbal communication: Facial gestures.

presented as a beginning point for the development of listening skills for phlebotomists and other health care workers. Development of these skills can help an individual with professional and personal life.

Steps toward effective listening:

1. Concentrate on the speaker by "getting ready" to listen. Take a moment to clear out thoughts that can detract from one's full attention. Begin the interaction with an open, objective mind. Sometimes taking a deep breath can help clear the mind and prepare it to receive more information.
2. Use the silent pauses wisely by mentally summarizing what has been said.
3. The speaker must know someone is listening. Simple phrases such as "I see," "Oh," "Very interesting," and "How about that" can reassure the speaker and communicate understanding and acceptance.
4. Keep personal judgments to oneself until the speaker has completed his or her idea.
5. Verify the conversation with feedback. Make sure that everything was clarified. Ask for more explanation if necessary.
6. Mentally review the key words to get a summary of the overall idea being communicated.

TABLE 8–1. NONVERBAL COMMUNICATION OR BODY LANGUAGE

Positive Body Language
  Erect posture
  Relaxed hands, arms, shoulders
  Face people directly
  Eye contact
  Eye level
  Good grooming
  Maintain zone of comfort
  Smiles
Negative Body Language/Distracting Behaviors
  Slouching, shrugging shoulders
  Rolling eyes, wandering eyes
  Looking at ceiling/window, blank stare
  Rubbing eyes, excessive blinking
  Squirming
  Tapping foot, fingers, pencil
  Deep sighs, moans and groans
  Crossed arms, clenched fists
  Wrinkled forehead
  Thumbing through book/papers
  Chewing gum
  Smoking a cigarette
  Repeatedly looking at clock or watch
  Lining up objects on a desk
  Stretching or yawning
  Sitting backwards on chair, i.e. straddled
  Peering over eyeglasses
  Pointing finger at someone

7. Sense the nonverbal signs and ask for clarification. Simple prompts such as "You look sad" or "You seem upset or nervous" can add more meaning to the conversation and encourage the speaker to verbalize feelings.
8. Listen for true meaning in the message, not just the literal words. Maintain eye contact to communicate interest or concern.
9. Encourage the listener to expand his or her thoughts by the use of simple phrases such as "Let's discuss it further," "Tell me more about it," and "Really."
10. Paraphrase the idea or conversation to assure complete understanding.

FAMILY, VISITORS, AND SIGNIFICANT OTHERS

There are times in a busy hospital or laboratory day when families and visitors are much more difficult to deal with than patients. Often families and visitors make requests or demands that are not part of the accepted behavior for a phlebotomist. Patients should not be given water or food without the physician's permission. Usually, it is better to inform the nurse of the patient's request. Visitors and family can be asked to step into the hall while the blood specimen is being drawn. If the phlebotomist feels that assistance is required, a family member may be asked to assist. This can make the family members feel helpful as well as provide reassurance to the patients, particularly children.

Priests and chaplains have the right to visit privately with patients. Unless the blood specimen is timed, it is best to respect that privacy and return to that patient after completing the other draws in the unit or area. The physician may also wish to confer privately with the patient. The same procedure as with a priest or chaplain should be followed. If the procedure is timed or STAT, the phlebotomist may ask permission to collect the specimen.

Families and visitors of patients should not be permitted in the clinical laboratory areas except by prior arrangement. Their safety and the confidentiality of patient records must be considered.

APPEARANCE

One clue to a person's attitude can be general appearance and grooming. In the past, most hospitals, clinical laboratories, and physicians' offices had dress codes that carefully detailed the acceptable clothing for that health care setting. Surprisingly, today the white uniform or white laboratory coat is unacceptable in some special areas. Child Health Clinics and Children's Hospitals have decided that informal business clothing is appropriate wear when dealing with children. The white coat or smock is used to cover and protect clothing while in the technical or analytic area. However, there are clinics, hospitals, and physicians' offices that still follow the more traditional dress code. The following rules generally apply to personnel who routinely interact with patients:

1. *White uniform.* The complete white uniform should be worn with white shoes. Clogs, high heels, tennis shoes, sandals, and other casual styles are not appropriate. The entire uniform and shoes should be neat and clean. It is recommended that women wear hose without seams, that jewelry be limited to rings and a wristwatch, that nails be filed short, kept clean, and without polish. Hand lotion should be available because of drying due to frequent handwashing and prolonged use of gloves. Women should remember to apply makeup sparingly because bright or dark colors look harsh with a white uniform. Hair should be kept neatly cut, styled, and clean. Long hair, which may hide the venipuncture site or get caught in laboratory equipment, must be tied back. Men who wear moustaches, beards, or both should keep them neat,

trimmed, and clean. Many of these suggestions are also commonsense safety precautions.

2. *Smocks, tunics, or laboratory coats.* In some clinics and hospitals, phlebotomists wear white smocks, tunics, jackets, or laboratory coats with dark shoes and slacks. It is recommended that a light or white shirt or blouse be worn underneath. The sleeves of the smock or lab coat should be longer than the sleeves of the blouse.

   Supervisors should remember that the rules of dress must be applied impartially to men and women on the phlebotomy team. In all cases however, clothes should be clean and pressed.

3. "Protective" clothing (laboratory coats, etc.) and equipment must be made available by employers. Laboratories have begun laundering and maintaining a continuous supply of clean pressed laboratory coats. In this manner, employees need not take their contaminated laboratory coats home to wash with other household clothing. This keeps laboratory workers safer, emphasizes a deep regard for cleanliness, and eases patients' minds about the transmission of infectious diseases from dirty or soiled laboratory coats.

Grooming and Physical Fitness

A vital part of a nice appearance is careful attention to personal hygiene. A daily bath or shower followed by use of deodorant is recommended. Perfume or aftershave lotion should be used sparingly as patients may be allergic, or find some scents overpowering and distasteful when they are sick. It is important to maintain good health habits such as proper nutrition and exercise because the role of a phlebotomist requires physical stamina. Good health also improves the phlebotomist's appearance, attitude, and ability to cope with stress.

The proper uniform worn with the appropriate care, good grooming, and physical fitness all contribute to a professional appearance. With a pleasant smile, a positive attitude, and a neat appearance, the phlebotomist is more fully prepared to deal with patients, hospital visitors, family members, and other members of the health care team.

PATIENT RIGHTS

All members of the clinical laboratory team must recognize that their first responsibility is to the patient's health, safety, and personal dignity. Many hospitals and other health care facilities have incorporated "A Patient's Bill of Rights" as developed by the American Hospital Association into policy manuals (Fig. 8–3). Each paragraph will be examined as it relates to the role of the phlebotomist.[1]

A PATIENT'S BILL OF RIGHTS

Introduction

The American Hospital Association presents *A Patient's Bill of Rights* with the expectation that observance of these rights will contribute to more effective patient care and greater satisfaction for the patient, his physician, and the hospital organization. Further, the Association presents these rights in the expectation that they will be supported by the hospital on behalf of its patients, as an integral part of the healing process. It is recognized that a personal relationship between the physician and the patient is essential for the provision of proper medical care. The traditional physician–patient relationship takes on a new dimension when care is rendered within an organizational structure. Legal precedent has established that the institution itself also has a responsibility to the patient. It is in recognition of these factors that these rights are affirmed.

Bill of Rights

1. The patient has the right to considerate and respectful care.
2. The patient has the right to obtain from his physician complete current information concerning his diagnosis, treatment, and prognosis in terms the patient can be reasonably expected to understand. When it is not medically advisable to give such information to the patient, the information should be made available to an appropriate person in his behalf. He has the right to know, by name, the physician responsible for coordinating his care.
3. The patient has the right to receive from his physician information necessary to give informed consent prior to the start of any procedure and/or treatment. Except in emergencies, such information for informed consent should include but not necessarily be limited to the specific procedure and/or treatment, the medically-significant risks involved, and the probable duration of incapacitation. Where medically-significant alternatives for care or treatment exist, or when the patient requests information concerning medical alternatives, the patient has the right to such information. The patient also has the right to know the name of the person responsible for the procedures and/or treatment.
4. The patient has the right to refuse treatment to the extent permitted by law and to be informed of the medical consequences of his action.
5. The patient has the right to every consideration of his privacy concerning his own medical care program. Case discussion, consultation, examination, and treatment are confidential and should be conducted discretely. Those not directly involved in his care must have the permission of the patient to be present.
6. The patient has the right to expect that all communications and records pertaining to his care should be treated as confidential.
7. The patient has the right to expect that, within its capacity, a hospital must make reasonable response to the request of a patient for services. The hospital must provide evaluation, service and/or referral as indicated by the urgency of the case. When medically permissible, a patient may be transferred to another facility only after he has received complete information and explanation concerning the needs for and alternatives to such a transfer. The institution to which the patient is to be transferred must first have accepted the patient for transfer.

(continued)

Figure 8–3. Reaffirmed by the Institutional Practices Committee in 1990, *A Patient's Bill of Rights* was first adopted by the American Hospital Association in 1973. *(Courtesy of the American Hospital Association, Chicago, Illinois, 1990, with permission.)*

8. The patient has the right to obtain information as to any relationship of his hospital to other health care and educational institutions insofar as his care is concerned. The patient has the right to obtain information as to the existence of any professional relationships among individuals, by name, who are treating him.

9. The patient has the right to be advised if the hospital proposes to engage in or perform human experimentation affecting his care or treatment. The patient has the right to refuse to participate in such research projects.

10. The patient has the right to expect reasonable continuity of care. He has the right to know, in advance, what appointment times and physicians are available and where. The patient has the right to expect that the hospital will provide a mechanism whereby he is informed by his physician or a delegate of the physician of the patient's continuing health care requirements following discharge.

11. The patient has the right to examine and receive an explanation of his bill, regardless of source of payment.

12. The patient has the right to know what hospital rules and regulations apply to his conduct as a patient.

Conclusion

No catalog of rights can guarantee for the patient the kind of treatment he has a right to expect. A hospital has many functions to perform, including the prevention and treatment of disease, the education of both health professionals and patients, and the conduct of clinical research. All these activities must be conducted with an overriding concern for the patient, and, above all, the recognition of his dignity as a human being. Success in achieving this recognition assures success in the defense of the rights of the patient.

Figure 8–3. (Continued)

Review of Patient's Bill of Rights

1. The patient may be rude, ill-tempered, and uncooperative. However, it is important for hospital personnel to deliver the best quality of care they are capable of giving, being careful to show consideration, fairness, compassion, and respect for each patient.

2. Laboratory personnel are not to give misdirected or inappropriate information about laboratory tests, test results, or test procedures. This can generally be handled correctly by saying to the patient "your doctor ordered blood to be drawn for testing; it would be best to discuss the tests with him or her." The remainder of the questions should be directed to the patient's physician. It is the physician's perogative to explain medical decisions to the patient.

3. There are basically two rights incorporated in this part of the patient's Bill of Rights. First, as part of the principle of informed consent, the phlebotomist should briefly explain to the patient the procedures used to collect the blood sample. The patient also has the right to know that the blood drawing team member is part of the hospital staff and who he or she is. It is important for the phlebotomist to stress

that the physician has ordered the tests. The patient also has the right to know if someone involved in his or her care is a student.

4. If a patient refuses to have a blood specimen drawn, it is the phlebotomist's responsibility to remind the patient that the physician has ordered the clinical laboratory tests performed as part of the medical care. If the patient still refuses, the phlebotomist should inform the nursing staff and, if possible, the physician. The phlebotomist should avoid any emotional confrontation or conflict with the patient. All the actions should be documented.

5. Requests for certain laboratory tests and results on clinical laboratory tests are part of the patient's treatment and are *strictly confidential.* This rule of confidentiality extends to all areas of a health care institution and to all clinical laboratory staff. A phlebotomist should *never* discuss patient information in a public place such as an elevator, hallway, or the cafeteria. Family members or friends may overhear and be very offended. Also, patients, especially teenagers, have strong feelings about showing fear. Their need for privacy should be respected. If the patient's physician is in the room and discussing treatment or disease condition, the phlebotomist should excuse him or herself and come back later unless the physician specifically requests that the blood specimen be drawn. If the phlebotomist has a STAT request, he or she should quietly ask the physician if he or she wishes it drawn now or wants him or her to return.

6. Clinical laboratory requisition slips contain demographic data that should not be exposed to the public even if analytic results are not yet recorded. It is the responsibility of the hospital to provide security for data in electronic information storage and retrieval systems and make the information available only to those that have specific need. Any discussion of tests or test results on a specific patient are not appropriate in a public place. If the patient is a rational, responsible adult, then information given by the doctor may be shared with family and visitors by the patient or during a conference with the physician. Sometimes a very talkative patient may wish to share information of a personal and sensitive nature with the phlebotomist. It is appropriate to politely stop the patient from disclosure and continue with the collection procedure.

7. Occasionally, a patient assumes that any staff member that walks into the room is a nurse or nursing assistant. The patient may request a drink or help in moving. The phlebotomist should assist the patient in calling a member of the nursing staff to handle the request. The phlebotomist should not give food, water, or cigarettes to a patient as these items might be contraindicated because of the patient's medical condition.

8. This part of the Bill of Rights is usually applied to one physician

requesting that another physician come in as a consultant. Also, the laws and statutes require that one physician not pay another physician to become part of a case. Others feel that this applies to students. The patient has the right to know if the phlebotomist is a student. He or she has the right to refuse to be involved with students. It is important for the supervisor to reassure the patient of the student's competency to perform the procedure. In a teaching hospital or laboratory, the patient implies permission for student involvement upon admission. However, every effort should be made to have student–patient interactions be positive.[4]

9. a. A patient may feel without reason that he or she may be part of experimentation. However, in most medical teaching facilities there is a Committee for the Protection of Human Subjects that reviews any experimentation that involves human subjects in any way. On some campuses there are advertisements in the campus paper for paid subjects for research. Generally they are asked to have blood drawn to help establish the reference range for healthy people. This may vary with the project. This also holds for behavioral research and involves the decision and legal implication of deciding who to put in the group that does not participate when the gain from participating is permanent. Many research projects in medicine use numbers in large groups with no names and thus avoid having each patient in a large group provide signed consent.

   b. A patient must have the opportunity to weigh the risk factors and inconvenience against what may be learned from his or her voluntary participation.

10. Any treatment or laboratory testing ordered to aid in diagnosis or therapy will be performed in a timely manner provided the patient is willing.

11. The patient has a right to review his or her hospital bill.

12. The phlebotomist must sometimes remind a patient that special rules about test procedures are a part of hospital or diagnostic protocol and must be adhered to for successful test results.

PROFESSIONAL BEHAVIOR

Accountability

Personal *accountability* cannot be calculated in a mathematical equation. Each individual phlebotomist has a personal responsibility for providing quality assurance. For example, the phlebotomist is responsible for poor technique if a large number of separate specimens are hemolyzed on delivery to the laboratory. This is wasteful in the financial sense, not good patient care because of the need to redraw, and demonstrates poor technique. Generally, the phlebotomist is not asked to account for his or her actions unless an incident report is written or a patient or other health-care team member complains. Various time logs on patient units and in the outpatient area provide documentation of *productivity* and performance. The validity of these is based on being conscientious and honest. Personal integrity or "doing what's right when no one is looking" (i.e., washing hands between patients, observing precautions to gown and scrub in isolation, and collecting timed tests at the proper time) are reflections of a phlebotomist's personal accountability or individual responsibility for actions. In some situations, the phlebotomist may be held legally accountable or answerable for his or her actions. If a patient sues the hospital or clinical laboratory, staff members questioned about procedure will be part of a deposition. Each member of the health care team should have a personal commitment to fulfill the obligations imposed by the health care system.

Motivation and Social Behavior

Abraham H. Maslow.   In 1943 A.H. Maslow dramatically changed the theories and approaches to understanding human *motivation* by publishing his views. He summarized:[2]

1. There are at least five sets of basic needs. They are physiological, safety, love and belonging, esteem, and self-actualization. In addition, we are motivated by the desire to achieve or maintain the various conditions upon which these basic satisfactions rest and by certain more intellectual desires.
2. These basic goals are related to each other, being arranged in a hierarchy of prepotency. This means that the most basic needs (food, water) must be met before other needs can be fulfilled.

The basic model for the *hierarchy of needs* that he defined can be illustrated graphically (Fig. 8–4).

Maslow suggested that when one "need" was fairly well-satisfied, it ceases becoming a motivator. At that time the next or higher need begins to dominate the center of motivation. The lines separating the various needs should be dim or blurred as there are overlaps in each area.

Physiological Needs.   Physiological needs trigger the body's automatic efforts to maintain internal body balance or equilibrium. In the clinical laboratory, this may be expressed in the blood acid–base balance, CO_2 saturation level, glucose content, and O_2 content, to name only a few. A person who is lacking food, social contacts, security, and esteem would satisfy the hunger need first. The needs for air, food, and water are survival needs. These critical needs are met first and felt most strongly. In the hospital or laboratory setting, this helps to explain the behavior of the difficult patient who has been fasting or is just hungry. A man on the brink of starvation will dream of food, think of food, and

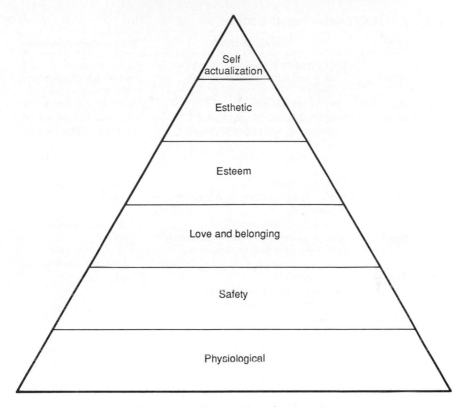

Figure 8–4. Maslow's hierarchy of needs.

work frantically to acquire food. And it is almost impossible to teach or communicate with a hungry child.

Safety Needs.   Safety needs are those needs that emerge as the center for action and thought after the physiological needs have been satisfied. Because human beings have so long ignored the consequences of air, water, and general environmental pollution, federal agencies have mushroomed in response to growing fears about human safety in relation to the environment.

In general, threats by extremes of temperature, criminal violence, or vicious animals do not occur. The usual safety need is for emotional security and support. Table 8–2 depicts another human development model based on fears and concerns at various ages. Most people feel at least a partial dependence on their employer. When an employee feels insecure, threatened, or highly dependent in his or her work situation, then he or she is not concerned with social needs, esteem needs, or self-actualization. Some employees are adaptable and do not feel threatened by new situations or procedures. However, a dependent or fearful individual may feel insecure when new computer

TABLE 8–2. HUMAN DEVELOPMENT MODEL[a]

Stage–Age	Fears/Concerns	Proper Parent Behavior
Newborn (0–12 months)	Totally dependent on parents/adults Trust that adults respond to basic needs	Parent should hold infant as an aid to collector and to comfort child
Infants and toddlers (12–24 months)	Little fear of danger Fear of separation from mother Limited language and understanding	Parent should stay in background until blood is drawn unless asked to help
Preschool (3–6 years)	Greater body awareness Play years Puppets = "play" Explain actions in language child can understand	Parent should stay in background until blood is drawn unless asked to participate
School-age Preadolescent (6–12 years)	Fears loss of self-control Less dependent on parent—autonomy Child may be willing to participate	Child may ask parent to leave room
Teenager (12–18 years)	Actively involved in anything concerning the body Embarrassed to show fear May act hostile to mask fear	May not want to have parent present
Special problems Mentally retarded	Need unhurried gentle approach	Have parent/guardian stay with child

[a]Stages 1–5 are adapted from Erickson EH: *Childhood and Society,* 2nd ed. New York, Norton, 1963.

programs are implemented in the laboratory to replace the manual method of communication. If management is arbitrary with respect to continued employment, discrimination in promotion, or favoritism in assignments, then the workplace becomes unsafe, stressful, and indeed threatening. Decreased productivity and low morale may result. However, if management has clearly defined policies that are consistently adhered to, employees become less security conscious and center on social or love needs, which become motivators of behavior.

Love Needs. Love needs include the feeling of belonging, being a part of, being accepted by one's associates, giving and receiving friendship and love. This is dramatically illustrated by the behavior patterns of most teenagers, who adhere to the dress, language, and behavioral customs of their peer group. However, healthy adults deal first with family relationships and close-knit ties. Once comfortable and secure with this group, they will turn to establish relationships with others outside the family. The absence of this support group of friends and family is keenly felt. For a child, the separation from parents and familiar surroundings for a hospital stay can be a terrifying experience.

For many people the work setting is their social group. Here, they find fulfillment of the belonging need. The predictability of this group acceptance provides each person with support and a sense of recognition as an important group member. The belonging need expands beyond the internal person to the external with time. As an example, the group pressure at work may either inhibit productivity or facilitate productivity to meet the goals of the organization.

Ego or Esteem Needs.   There are two facets to the level of ego or esteem need; one is internal, and the other is external. Essential is the individual's need to think well of and believe in him or herself. Esteem needs can be defined by how competent one feels to meet current and future needs; by perceived self-image as either a success or failure; and the impression of ability to acquire knowledge and skills for future situations.

The external aspect of ego needs are provided by others in terms of reputation, feedback from others about work or technical skills, ability to receive respect or trust from others, and the continuity of respect and reputation over time. Satisfaction of ego and esteem needs may be generated in the workplace or the outside environment. When a person has a "positive" or "winning" image, he or she can strive to move into the next need level.

Self-actualization.   Self-actualization or self-fulfillment is an ongoing continuum or cyclical set of needs to reach some internally defined personal goal. Projects are begun and completed; new projects are undertaken.

Esthetic.   Esthetic needs are those for beauty and artistic creation. Some individuals need to maintain order and beauty in their lives through art, music, theatrical expression, and the like.

In summary, at any one point in time, a person may be fulfilling social ego and self-actualization needs in overlapping layers of concern. It is important to remember that "Thus man is a perpetually wanting animal. Ordinarily, the satisfaction of these wants is not altogether mutually exclusive but only tends to be. The average member of our society is most often partially satisfied and partially unsatisfied in all his/her wants."[2]

Motivation has been defined as inducing people to act in a desired manner. People either perform of their own choice or they are persuaded to perform. Attitude, however, is the personal feeling expressed in words or behaviors. Some behavioral scientists feel that an internal stimulus moves us to be motivated. However, feelings that are expressed either verbally or in activities are a portrayal of attitudes. Others theorize that attitudes are expressions of how people feel and see themselves in terms of any given situation. A specimen control supervisor may say that a phlebotomist has a negative attitude about a patient because of observed behavior on the part of the employee that exhibits unacceptable actions. Attitudes may be vague or concrete and defined. The work setting should provide a climate that makes positive motivation and attitude development possible. Some people use personality to express what is meant about attitude. The right personality for the health care field can be defined as a caring personality coupled with a willingness to help and do things for others. A cheerful disposition, even temper, methodical manner, and reliable nature are valuable assets in any setting, particularly in dealing with patients. If the phlebotomist can be polite, tactful, efficient, and calm in emergencies, then the interpersonal relationships on the phlebotomy team can be pleasant and work can be performed with little friction.

Ethics

The principles of right and wrong conduct as they apply to professional problems are the *ethics* for that profession. Professions set standards of conduct for members and expect those standards of performance to be adhered to in their work. In the health care field, the ideal of behavior for physicians continues to be expressed in the *Hippocratic Oath.*

While somewhat antiquated and controversial it includes the following:

> I will prescribe regimen for the good of my patients according to my ability and my judgment and never do harm to anyone. To please none will I prescribe a deadly drug, nor give advice which may cause his/her death. Nor will I give a woman a pessary to procure abortion. But I will preserve the purity of my life and my art. I will not cut for stone, even for patients in whom the disease is manifest; I will leave this operation to be performed by practitioners (specialists in this art). In every house where I come I will enter only for the good of my patients . . . all that may come to my knowledge in the exercise of my profession or outside of my profession or in daily commune with men, which ought not to be spread abroad, I will keep secret and never reveal.[3]

Written about 400 BC this oath is still taken by physicians around the world before entering practice. Standards of behavior are implied in the oath for each member of the health care team. The major points are:

1. Do no harm to anyone intentionally.
2. Perform according to sound ability and good judgment.
3. Do that for which training has occurred, not more.
4. Do not become involved in anyone's care out of curiosity; only deal with those to whom assigned.
5. Facts about patients are not to be part of conversation but kept confidential.

The American Society for Medical Technology.   Just as physicians and nursing personnel have developed a Code of Ethics, the laboratory professionals known as Medical Technologists or Clinical Laboratory Scientists have developed a standard of performance and expressed these expectations in a code (Fig. 8–5)[3,4] The major themes of the code are:

1. Accuracy and reliability of laboratory test results
2. Confidentiality[3]

Preamble

The Code of Ethics of the American Society for Medical Technology (ASMT) sets forth the principles and standards by which clinical laboratory professionals practice their profession.

The professional conduct of clinical laboratory professionals is based on the following duties and principles:

I. Duty to the Patient

Clinical laboratory professionals are accountable for the quality and integrity of the laboratory services they provide. This obligation includes continuing competence in both judgment and performance as individual practitioners, as well as in striving to safeguard the patient from incompetent or illegal practice by others.

Clinical laboratory professionals maintain high standards of practice and promote the acceptance of such standards at every opportunity. They exercise sound judgment in establishing, performing and evaluating laboratory testing.

Clinical laboratory professionals perform their services with regard for the patient as an individual, respecting his or her right to confidentiality, the uniqueness of his or her needs, and his or her right to timely access to needed services. Clinical laboratory professionals provide accurate information to others about the services they provide.

II. Duty to Colleagues and the Profession

Clinical laboratory professionals accept responsibility to individually contribute to the advancement of the profession through a variety of activities. These activities include contributions to the body of knowledge of the profession, establishing and implementing high standards of practice and education, seeking fair socioeconomic working conditions for themselves and other members of the profession, and holding their colleagues and the profession in high regard and esteem.

Clinical laboratory professionals actively strive to establish cooperative and insightful working relationships with other health professionals, keeping in mind their primary objective to ensure a high standard of care for the patients they serve.

III. Duty to Society

Clinical laboratory professionals share with other citizens the duties of responsible citizenship. As practitioners of an autonomous profession, they have the responsibility to contribute from their sphere of professional competence to the general well-being of the community, and specifically to the resolution of social issues affecting their practice and collective good.

Clinical laboratory professionals comply with relevant laws and regulations pertaining to the practice of clinical laboratory science and actively seek, within the dictates of their consciences, to change those that do not meet the high standards of care and practice to which the profession is committed.

(continued)

Figure 8–5. Code of Ethics of the American Society for Medical Technology. *(Courtesy of the American Society for Medical Technology, Washington, D.C.; 1992)*

As a clinical laboratory professional, I acknowledge my professional responsibility to:

- Maintain and promote standards of excellence in performing and advancing the art and science of my profession;
- Safeguard the dignity and privacy of patients;
- Hold my colleagues and my profession in high esteem and regard;
- Contribute to the general well-being of the community; and
- Actively demonstrate my commitment to these responsibilities throughout my professional life.

Figure 8–5. (Continued)

Hospital Code of Ethics. Many hospitals across the country have estab lished individual codes of ethics. Often they deal more specifically with specialty care for the hospital or with the specific mission of the hospital. An example is shown in Figure 8–6.

The National Phlebotomy Association. The National Phlebotomy Association has also designated responsibilities for the phlebotomist. As a defined subgroup in the area of providing laboratory service, the phlebotomist will:

1. Represent the Clinical Laboratory or Department of Laboratory Medicine.
2. Become knowledgeable in the behavioral sciences and apply that knowledge to human relationships with patients and fellow health care team members.
3. Maintain accuracy, reliability, and reproducibility of results.
4. Respect the Patient's Bill of Rights.
5. Serve within the specified framework of skills as defined by the hospital or laboratory standards of performance and phlebotomist job description.[5]

The phlebotomist, as in other areas of the laboratory, must continue to upgrade and maintain quality of skills. He or she must know about new techniques, new tubes, changing time constraints on tests, computer data, and changes in scientific knowledge. The phlebotomist must accept the concept that patient safety and quality care come before saving time. He or she should also be willing to ask for assistance when dealing with a difficult patient or procedure. A phlebotomist collects only those specimens ordered by the physician and the ones that he or she has been trained to collect.

In summary, ethical conduct can be expressed in routine behavior by the phlebotomist if he or she

1. Is polite to patients, regardless of the circumstances
2. Does not discuss patients' ailments with them
3. Does not discuss the respective merits of the various forms of therapy

Preamble

Our institution is a specialized center devoted to the care of patients with cancer and to the prevention and eradication of malignant disease. We strive to combine the activities of patient care, education, and research to benefit not only patients currently receiving care but also future generations. In this diversity, there is often tension; therefore, we hold before us this Code of basic moral principles against which to measure our service and to bond patients and staff together in the difficult task of contending with cancer.

Principle 1

Reverence for the patients for whom we are privileged to care is our primary concern. Such reverence affirms the value and dignity of life.

Principle 2

Acknowledging the value and dignity of life, we dedicate ourselves to provide our best care and to use our knowledge to attempt cure of the disease in each patient while pursuing understanding of the basic biologic nature and eradication of cancer.

Principle 3

The presence of cancer may justify, but not demand, heroic measures. Curing disease, reducing suffering, and sustaining an acceptable quality of life, as defined by the patient with the help of health care professionals, are central goals of this institution.

Principle 4

All who serve in this institution have specific tasks and roles, yet all are equal as potential friends to patients. Because of these vocational and personal bonds, each of us bears individual moral obligations to each patient.

Principle 5

Knowledge-seeking research and knowledge-disseminating instruction are valued institutional goals. These pursuits require at least three conditions: participants who are informed about risks and benefits; actions that do not undermine the patients' therapeutic needs; the transmission of truthful information that is based on sound evidence.

Principle 6

The diagnosis of cancer is not just an identification of a disease but also carries with it a potential burden for patients, who may feel stigmatized, and for those close to them, who share the impact. We must understand their perceptions and help them to come to terms with their altered lives.

Principle 7

Patients justly expect personal information to be confidential, yet their medical records are accessible to all health care providers. All information must be recorded responsibly. Access also confers a moral obligation. Access must be justified and not harmful to the patients' interests.

(continued)

Figure 8–6. The University of Texas M.D. Anderson Cancer Center Code of Ethics. *(Courtesy of University of Texas M.D. Anderson Hospital, Houston, Tex., 1992, with permission.)* Adopted June 1984.

Principle 8
Since our specialized roles result in varying levels of function and decision making, we affirm the need to demonstrate mutual respect and to acknowledge interdependence as co-workers responsible for the welfare of patients.

Principle 9
The immediacy of patient care tends to obscure the relevance of basic biologic research. We affirm that research, responsibly conceived and scientifically sound, establishes an environment of learning, encourages exacting practice, fosters new knowledge, and creates realistic prospects of eradicating cancer, thus promoting a favorable balance of risks and benefits.

Principle 10
Cancer therapy and research are expensive endeavors demanding conscientious stewardship; however, financial considerations should never dictate the quality of care offered to each patient.

Figure 8–6. (Continued)

4. Never prescribes
5. Does not discuss the physician with the patient
6. Keeps appropriate records of specimen collection as described in institutional policy
7. Is alert to hazards for patient and other members of the health care team.[5]

When considering the implications of ethical behavior, the concepts of *honesty, integrity,* and *regard for the dignity of other human beings* continue to be the personal foundations for professional codes. Only the phlebotomist dealing with patients on a one-to-one basis knows for sure whether the work he or she performs each day is based on tenets for optimum behavior.

DEALING WITH STRESS

Stress is very prevalent in the workplace. In studies funded by the United States Department of Labor, it was reported that nonphysician laboratory personnel ranked third in terms of stress level experienced in the workplace. Because of rapid technological progress, personnel have been forced to make rapid behavioral adjustments to a faster-paced and more pressured life, which tends to induce stress.

Figure 8–7 shows the possible daily interactions that occur to the phlebotomist and also the patient in a health care setting.

Some people prefer to cope with the stress of illness by retreating from

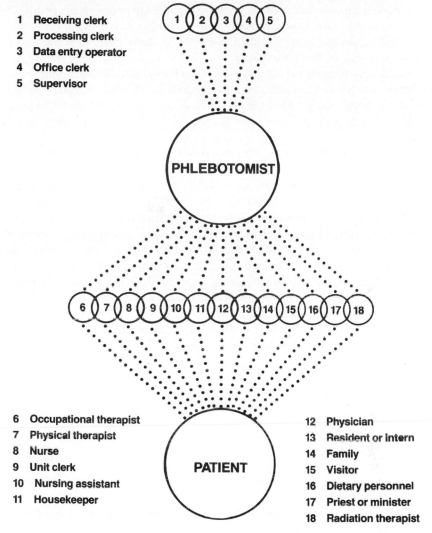

1 Receiving clerk
2 Processing clerk
3 Data entry operator
4 Office clerk
5 Supervisor

6 Occupational therapist
7 Physical therapist
8 Nurse
9 Unit clerk
10 Nursing assistant
11 Housekeeper

12 Physician
13 Resident or intern
14 Family
15 Visitor
16 Dietary personnel
17 Priest or minister
18 Radiation therapist

Figure 8–7. Interaction pathways.

personal interaction. In the clinic or hospital setting, this is not possible. Thus, stress for health care professionals and patients can increase. What is stress? Usually, it is defined by physiological changes such as:

1. Elevated blood pressure
2. Increased heart rate
3. Increased breath rate
4. Increased body metabolism
5. Increased blood flow to muscles

When there is constant stress, chronic high blood pressure can result. This is significant because it is a predisposing factor to heart attack and stroke. These diseases of the heart and brain account for more than 50 percent of the deaths each year in the United States.[6]

Stress may happen because of constant change with little escape from it. Too often, the trauma associated with change is overlooked. For the phlebotomist, the change may be a shift in work hours, the route covered, the people one works with, the supervisor, new techniques and policies, or some or all of these.

Hans Selye, in *The Stress of Life,* discusses what stress can be to the human condition.[7] Selye said, "Stress is not even necessarily bad for you; it is also the spice of life, for any emotion, any activity causes stress." A certain level of stress pushes people to achieve, to win, and to compete. However, too much may incapacitate or make a person ill. Selye's research into the impact of stress on the body led him to conclude that rest can *almost* restore the body to the prior level of fitness. Like a piece of elastic pulled too tight for too long, when stress is relieved the body does not quite return to the original level of fitness.

Selye also concluded that exposure to stress does not necessarily make it easier to withstand greater stress. It may make the body even more vulnerable. Wear and tear on the body caused by stress may lead to premature aging.[8]

Bettina Martin in a lecture entitled "Dealing with Stress and Making It Work for You," suggested some rules for low-stress living.

1. Make time your ally, not your master.
2. Associate mostly with gentle people who affirm your personhood.
3. Learn and practice the skill of deep relaxation.
4. Use aerobic exercise to improve health.
5. Engage in satisfying, meaningful work.
6. Don't let your work dominate your entire life.
7. Find some time in every day for complete privacy.
8. Open yourself up to new experiences. Find self-renewing opportunities.
9. Read interesting books and articles to freshen your ideas and broaden your point of view.
10. Don't bite off more than you can chew.
11. Seek rewarding experiences in all dimensions of living.
12. Surround yourself with cues that affirm positive thoughts and positive approaches to life and that remind you to relax and unwind occasionally.[8]

Keith Schnert, MD, described some additional coping ideas in his book *Stress/Unstress.* He suggested that by using visualization (see a favorite place vividly in the mind), relaxation, and fun the level of stress can be dramatically reduced. Also, each person should sing in the shower, do bend and stretch exercises, and take time to relax.[9] By using appropriate techniques to deal with stress, doing some reasonable planning, and being aware of the importance of time management, the phlebotomist can cope more successfully with the stress of working as part of the health care team. In the work setting, knowing the job skills to perform the techniques and procedures well, having good interpersonal relationships, and understanding more about human behavior can aid the phlebotomist in approaching each day more positively and productively.

PROFESSIONAL ORGANIZATIONS

Three national organizations that recognize the phlebotomist as a definitive and vital part of the health care team are listed below. All are sponsors of certification examinations.

1. *The American Society for Medical Technology (ASMT)* has recognized clinical laboratory personnel for over 50 years. There are several types of memberships available depending on the education and experience of the individual. Currently, most phlebotomists are joining ASMT as associate members as part of the Phlebotomy section. The National Certifying Agency (NCA) offers a certification examination for phlebotomists.
2. *The National Phlebotomy Association* was established in 1978 to recognize the phlebotomist as a distinctive and identifiable part of the allied health team. This organization also offers a certification examination for phlebotomists.
3. *American Society of Clinical Pathologists* allows nonphysician members to gain Associate membership status. Through their Board of Registry a Phlebotomy Technician Examination (Pbt (ASCP)) is offered annually. This is a criterion-referenced examination model. It includes coverage of entry-level skills of a phlebotomist and uses taxonomy levels that assess recall (recognize facts), interpretive skills (use knowledge to interpret numeric data), and problem-solving skills (use applications of specific information to solve problems).

KEY TERMS

accountability	motivation	professional
distracting behaviors	negative body	organizations
ethics	language	STAT
hearing disabilities	Patient's Bill of Rights	zone of comfort
listening skills	positive body	
Maslow's hierarchy of	language	
needs	productivity	

STUDY QUESTIONS

1. In identifying the alert adult inpatient, what are the major steps for the phlebotomist to follow?
2. After an outpatient has had a venipuncture performed, what techniques should the phlebotomist follow before dismissing the patient?
3. Identify and describe four barriers to simple verbal communication.
4. List five behaviors that exhibit "positive body language."
5. List five behaviors that exhibit "negative body language." Describe how each of these is interpreted by patients.
6. Describe the 10 steps to effective listening.
7. List five of the major topics in the "Patient's Bill of Rights" that are important for the phlebotomist to remember.
8. Outline Maslow's hierarchy of needs.

REFERENCES

1. Patient's Bill of Rights, American Hospital Association, 1990.
2. Maslow AH: *Motivation and Personality,* 2nd ed. New York, Harper & Row, 1970.
3. *Code of Ethics.* American Society for Medical Technology, Bethesda, MD, 1992.
4. American Society for Medical Technology, Passport to Success (Brochure).
5. National Phlebotomy Association, Guidelines, 1980.
6. Benson H: Your innate asset for combating stress. *Harvard Business Review* 74402, July–August, 1974.
7. Selye H: *The Stress of Life,* 2nd ed. New York, McGraw-Hill, 1978.
8. Martin BG: Dealing with Stress and Making It Work for You. Lecture at a meeting of American Society of Clinical Pathologists.
9. Schnert KW: *Stress–Unstress,* Minneapolis, Augsburg Press, 1981.

Total Quality Management and Continuous Quality Improvement

9

DEVELOPMENT OF TOTAL QUALITY MANAGEMENT/CONTINUOUS QUALITY IMPROVEMENT IN HEALTH CARE

In 1986 the Joint Commission on the Accreditation of Healthcare Organizations (JCAHO) initiated an Agenda for Change as a strategic plan for the future of health care organizations. A vital part of this plan was based on Juran's model of Total Quality Management (*TQM*) and Deming's principles of Continuous Quality Improvement (*CQI*).[1,2] The first strategy of the JCAHO plan took place in the mid and late 1980s when they instituted the *10-step process* for quality assessment of clinical indicators (Table 9–1).

Since then, JCAHO has focused the accreditation process on concrete attempts for improving the quality of health care services. Different terms have been coined to imply the same basic premise for improving the quality of

TABLE 9–1. JCAHO 10-STEP PROCESS FOR QUALITY ASSESSMENT

1. *Assign responsibility.* The director or chairperson is responsible for monitoring and evaluating service quality. A written plan should describe responsibilities, the laboratory setting, the populations served, and the QA activities.
2. *Delineate the scope of care.* All major sections of the laboratory must be covered.
3. *Identify key aspects of care.* These include high-volume procedures, high-risk procedures, problematic procedures, and high-cost procedures.
4. *Construct indicators.* Indicators should specify which activities, events, or patient outcomes will be monitored.
5. *Define thresholds of evaluation.* Thresholds specify the lower limits of acceptable quality. Exceeding them should stimulate further evaluation and problem resolution.
6. *Collect and organize data.* Two basic types of monitors should be used, i.e., scanning monitors (to provide important statistics about the laboratory's operations) and focused monitors (to periodically collect data to determine causes, nature, or scope of a problem).
7. *Evaluate data.* This includes comparing performance to standards, analyzing patterns and trends, evaluating statistical significance and clinical relevance, and analyzing causes.
8. *Develop a corrective action plan.* The plan should detail who or what is to change, what specific actions will be taken and when, and should focus on improving the system or behavior.
9. *Assess actions and document improvement.* The corrective actions must be monitored until the problem is resolved.
10. *Communicate relevant information.* Complete reports (including objectives, findings, conclusions, corrective actions, and follow-up results) must be forwarded to the appropriate officials in a timely manner.

From Martin BG: *The CLMA Guide to Managing a Clinical Laboratory.* Clinical Laboratory Management Association, Malvern, Penn., 1991, with permission.

services. These include "total quality management," "continuous quality improvement," "quality assurance," "integrated quality assurance," to name a few. This second phase of the Agenda for Change is more visionary and includes wider accountability for the actual improvement process. This chapter will highlight some of the basic concepts behind quality improvement and the tools and methods to assess quality and will provide some examples of how phlebotomists can play a vital role in the improvement process. [3,4,5]

The health care industry has been relatively late in joining the quality revolution that has been occurring for the past two decades in other service industries. Much of the credit for initiating this quality revolution goes to *Dr. W. Edwards Deming,* an American statistician who spent time in Japan and helped develop modern Japanese management theories. His work focused on minimizing variation in the manufacturing process, similar to a laboratory's goal of minimizing the variations in laboratory testing. Deming had his greatest impact on manufacturing companies such as the automotive industry. However, now many hospitals and health care organizations are adopting his management principles. Other noted quality innovators are Drs. Joseph Juran, Avedis Donabedian, Donald M. Berwick, and Philip Crosby. The JCAHO's plan is based on Juran's model of TQM and Deming's principles of CQI. Key elements of these theories are briefly summarized in Table 9–2. Of the individuals listed, only Dr. Donabedian, a physician, had a background in health care. Using

TABLE 9–2. SUMMARY OF THEORETICAL APPROACHES TO QUALITY IMPROVEMENT

Author	Approach
Deming	Do not tolerate poor service.
	Constantly improve production and service.
	Institute training for all workers.
	Institute effective leadership.
	Drive out fear. Create a climate of trust and innovation.
	Break down barriers between departments.
	Eliminate slogans.
	Eliminate numerical quotas.
	Remove barriers to pride of workmanship.
	Take action.
Juran	Promote customer satisfaction.
Donabedian	Structure
	Process
	Outcomes
Crosby	Zero defects
	Strive to be error free
Berwick	"Kaisen," which is the Japanese term for continuous search for opportunities for all processes to get better.
	Shift away from a regulatory model or seeking out the "bad apples," and move to seeking opportunities for improvement through mistakes.
	Learn from the mistakes.

his expertise, he pinpointed key aspects (structure, process, outcomes) of health care functions that needed to be monitored for quality improvement. His contributions are also briefly summarized in Table 9–2.

TOTAL QUALITY MANAGEMENT

Total Quality Management is a process aimed at continuous quality improvement, not just meeting the minimum standard. The focus is on improving the entire process of health care. It includes, but is not limited to reducing outliers, variations, or errors in all types of health care settings. It involves all levels of the health care team, including the phlebotomist. And, perhaps most importantly, it focuses on customer satisfaction. Customers include patients and other health care workers such as technologists, nurses, students, pathologists, and all physicians who use or are a part of the laboratory service. Examples of customers might include a ward clerk responsible for charting a result, a patient who needs blood drawn for surgery the next morning, an anesthesiologist waiting for a STAT blood gas result, or a pathologist who needs to review an abnormal blood smear. Even the JCAHO current accreditation guidelines recognize the need for "customer input through patient feedback."[4]

The major characteristics of hospitals with successful TQM are as follows:

1. The organized total quality management approach must permeate the hospital horizontally and vertically through the organizational chart.
2. The objectives of TQM must be continuous improvement instead of meeting fixed, predetermined standards.
3. Groups, teams, or quality circles must include multidisciplinary individuals, preferably experts from the major groups that contribute to the process being studied.
4. The groups or teams must be accountable to customers (patients and other members of the health care team).
5. The professional standards must improve over time.
6. There must be an incredible commitment to customer satisfaction.[1,5,6]

Refer to Table 9–3.

Success of the hospital, a team, a service, or an entire laboratory can then be measured by the rate of improvement, not just by compliance with preexisting standards. This way of thinking is relatively new to health care providers and sometimes very difficult and time consuming to put into practice. However, the laboratory areas are ideal settings for implementing TQM because most laboratory personnel are already familiar with some of the assessment tools such as charts, flow diagrams, check lists, log sheets, among others.

Total quality management is an umbrella concept that encompasses assessment of structure, process, outcome, prevention, and customer satisfaction. Traditionally, clinical laboratory services have focused primarily on quality control (QC) or monitoring the testing process, and secondarily on quality assurance or outcomes assessment. Chapter 10 will review QC, and this chapter will cover the other aspects of TQM. Table 9–4 highlights some differences between traditional laboratory QC and CQI.

TABLE 9–3. WHO ARE THE CUSTOMERS?

Internal inpatients
Outpatients
Patients' families and friends
Patients' support groups
Blood donors
Clinical laboratory scientists
Clinical laboratory technicians
Secretaries and clerks
Pathologists
Nurses
Administrators
Human resources personnel
Attending physicians
Students
Research staff
Research grantors
Anyone who provides financial support (insurance companies, taxpayers, foundations)

TABLE 9–4. CONTINUOUS QUALITY IMPROVEMENT AND QUALITY CONTROL: SIMILARITIES AND DIFFERENCES

Continuous Quality Improvement (CQI)	Quality Control (QC)
CQI is a theoretical framework and management commitment to improve health care structures, processes, outcomes, and customer satisfaction. It is ongoing and involves all levels of the administrative structure of an organization.	QC monitors process. It adjusts the analytical process to meet specific standards. It includes activities such as developing technical policies and procedures, assuring that supplies are functional and not outdated, calibrating and maintaining equipment, and performing functional checks. It involves running QC samples in parallel with patient samples and participating in proficiency testing programs.

Structure

Assessments of structural components include the following examples:[7]

- *Physical structure.* Facilities where services are provided, adequacy of supplies, safety measures, availability, and condition of equipment such as computers, sterilizers, autoclaves, and glucose monitoring devices.
- *Personnel structure.* Numbers of personnel and support staff for each service, ratios of staff to patients, and qualifications of staff, availability of the medical director or supervisors.
- *Management/administrative structure.* Updated, available procedure manuals, composition of committees, adequacy of systems for record keeping, open lines of communication throughout the organizational chart.

Most assessments of structural issues are done by a multidisciplinary team who can determine the adequacy of environmental and physical conditions. Structural components in quality assessment may reveal potential problems that other assessments (process and outcome) cannot. For example, use of outdated blood collection tubes may cause faulty laboratory results, even though the blood collection, testing, and reporting processes are perfect and the treatment plan for the patient (outcome) is appropriate.

Process

Process assessments are very common throughout the specimen collection and clinical testing arenas. This is where traditional quality control measures are applicable. However, in addition to the normal laboratory data collection routines, other methods are effective for monitoring process. These include evaluation of patient records for complications, direct observation of practices, videotaping health care interactions and practices, patient interviews, and questionnaires. Chapter 10 will provide more detail on the QC procedures for specimen collection services.

Outcome

The ultimate goal of CQI is to improve patient outcomes. Most outcomes assessments rely on information in the patient's medical record. Chart reviews usually evaluate the health status after services are provided. Timing is usually an important component of these measures. Outcome assessments are typically the most difficult to measure and often relate to recovery rates, cure rates, return to normal functions, and so on. Poor patient outcomes have been described as the "5 Ds":[8]

- Death
- Disease
- Disability
- Discomfort
- Dissatisfaction

Unfortunately, phlebotomists can have negative impacts in each of these categories. For example, misidentification of a patient can result in an erroneous crossmatch and blood transfusion, which could be fatal to a patient (Death). Inappropriate cleansing techniques or hand washing could result in transmitting nosocomial infections (Disease). Poor venipuncture techniques such as improper needle insertion or excessive probing could result in nerve damage (Disability) or severe pain (Discomfort). And lengthy waiting times, rude behavior, or messy work sites can contribute to an overall feeling of patient dissatisfaction. Even though these examples are extreme, they do exist in reality and need to be improved.

Satisfaction

The study of satisfaction among patients and health care providers is usually accomplished using questionnaires, mail-outs, and telephone or personal inter-

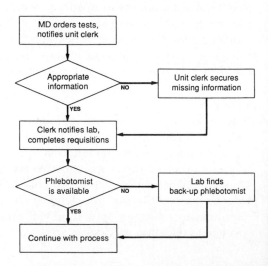

Figure 9–1. Flow chart. *(Adapted from Martin BG (ed): The CLMA Guide to Managing a Clinical Laboratory. Malvern, Penn., Clinical Laboratory Management Association, 1991.)*

views. While the information gathered using these techniques may be subjective, knowing *why* customers are dissatisfied and *which* customers are unhappy is extremely valuable. This information can be used to improve targeted services or aspects of a service.

Tools and Trends for CQI

In a laboratory, check sheets, run charts, and statistical tests can be used to review both the analytical and nonanalytical parts of the laboratory. In an analytical sense, clinical laboratory scientists and technicians use data collection to assure test sensitivity, specificity, precision, and accuracy. In a nonanalytical sense, data can be used to assess timeliness of response to requests, turnaround time for reporting test results, and effective communication.

Tools for implementing CQI include the following[6]:

Flow charts. Useful for breaking a process into its components so one can understand how it works (Figure 9–1).

Pareto charts. Bar charts that show the frequency of problematic events; the Pareto principle suggests that "80 percent of the trouble comes from 20 percent of the problems" (Figure 9–2).

Cause and effect (Ishikawa). Diagrams that identify interactions between equipment, methods, people, supplies, reagents (Figure 9–3).

Line graphs, histograms, scatter diagrams. Pictoral images representing performance trends.

Brainstorming. Used to stimulate creative solutions in a group.

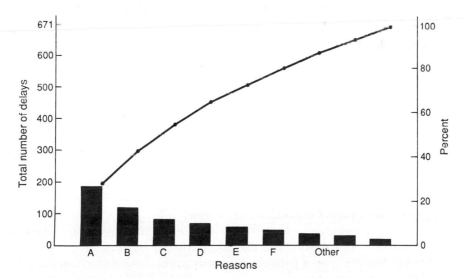

Figure 9–2. Pareto chart. *(From Martin BG (ed): The CLMA Guide to Managing a Clinical Laboratory. Malvern, Penn., Clinical Laboratory Management Association, 1991.)*

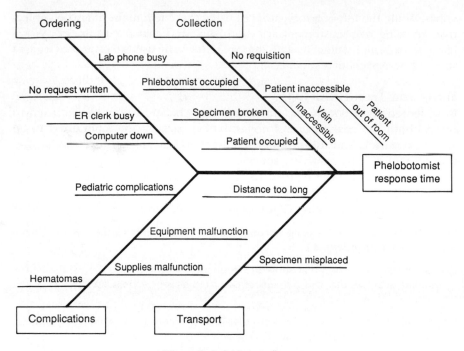

Figure 9–3. Ishikawa diagram.

Westgard et al. suggest a *"5 Q" framework* for clinical laboratories that focuses on:[9]

- Quality Planning (QP)
- Quality Laboratory Practices (QLP)
- Quality Control of Processes (QC)
- Monitoring performance, Quality Assessment (QA)
- Quality Improvement when problems occur (QI)

This is a self-perpetuating, cyclical process that should become a way of life for all employees in the laboratory. However, each health care institution has different characteristics and the laboratory's quality management program will vary based on philosophy, mission, and tools selected for use.

CQI for Specimen Collection Services

CQI studies for specimen collection services can be very revealing for laboratory employees, supervisors, and managers. A study by Howanitz, et al. indicated that 98.6 percent of patients in a study group from numerous different hospitals were satisfied with many aspects of the phlebotomy services they received. In this group, 97.3 percent of patients had blood collected on the first phlebotomy attempt, 16.1 percent of punctures resulted in ecchymosis, and in 25 percent of patients the time required for the phlebotomy procedure was 5 minutes or less. Each of these factors, in addition to numerous others, was analyzed and areas for targeted improvement were identified. One of the general areas sited for suggested improvement was in reduction of discomfort or pain caused by the puncture.[8] Examples of CQI *monitors* that should be considered in specimen collection services are listed in Table 9–5.

Monitors for quality assessment should fit specific criteria in order to be useful and valid. The *RUMBA model* is an easy check for determining the feasibility of a QI monitor.

- R—Relevant
- U—Understandable
- M—Measurable
- B—Behavioral
- A—Achievable

Before beginning a study of a particular monitor (or problem), the RUMBA criteria should be applied. The following questions should be asked:

- Are the problems or variations in practices relevant to laboratory services or patient care?
- Are the items to be monitored understandable by those who will be collecting the data?
- Can measurable objective data be collected?
- Are there behavioral aspects that can be changed if necessary?
- Is the project realistic and achievable?

An important factor that can sometimes become a stumbling block for quality assessment is the actual data-collection process. Most of the data can be collected from information already available in the laboratory or by adding a brief tally or list to forms already in existence. In addition, there are many

---

TABLE 9–5. CQI MONITORS FOR SPECIMEN COLLECTION SERVICES

Phlebotomist response time (for inpatients)
Patient waiting time (for outpatients)
Time for phlebotomy procedure to occur
Percentage of successful phlebotomies on the first attempt
Number of phlebotomy attempts beyond the first attempt
Phlebotomy attempts per patient by medical service
Number and size of hematomas
Number of patients who faint
Amount of time spent and number of phone calls needed to acquire appropriate identification
Number of redraws requested due to inadequate specimens
Contribution of phlebotomist to turnaround times of designated laboratory tests
Number of incomplete forms, documents, logs, and so on
Number of therapeutic drug monitoring tests that have incorrect documentation or timing
Number of specimens received in incorrect tubes

TABLE 9–6. SOURCES OF INFORMATION FOR QUALITY ASSESSMENTS

Medical records
Incident reports
Accident reports
Written complaints
Patient questionnaires
Customer focus groups
Quality circles
Committee reports
Staff meetings
Marketing agents
Pathologists
Attending physicians
Direct observation
Laboratory employees

other accessible sources of information (Table 9–6) though use of some of these may require special permission.

KEY TERMS

brainstorming	histograms	QC
cause and effect	JCAHO's 10-step	RUMBA model
CQI	process	structure
customer satisfaction	monitors	TQM
Dr. W. Edwards	outcomes	Westgard's "5 Q"
Deming	Pareto charts	framework
flow charts	process	

STUDY QUESTIONS

1. Describe JCAHO's 10-step process for quality assessment.
2. List five characteristics of TQM for a phlebotomy service.
3. Name 10 "customers" served by members of the phlebotomy team.
4. List the "5 Ds" that relate to patient outcomes. Give examples of how the phlebotomy service might adversely affect these outcomes.
5. Draw a flow chart of the patient identification process.
6. Give five examples of possible monitors for specimen collection services.
7. List eight sources of information for quality assessment data.

REFERENCES

1. Simpson KN, Kaluzny AD, McLaughlin CP: Total Quality and the Management of Laboratories, *Clinical Laboratory Management Review,* 448–462, Nov/Dec 1991.

2. Clark GB: Quality assurance, an administrative means to a managerial end: Part III; *Clinical Laboratory Management Review,* 463–475, Nov/Dec 1991.
3. Maffetone MA: TQM: passion and process; *Clinical Laboratory Management Review,* 476–478, Nov/Dec 1991.
4. JCAHO: *Accreditation Manual for Hospitals, 1992.* Oakbrook Terrace, Ill., 1992.
5. Martin BG (ed): *The CLMA Guide to Managing a Clinical Laboratory.* Malvern, Penn., Clinical Laboratory Management Association, 1991.
6. Uniker WO: Achieving the customer-oriented laboratory, *MLO,* Dec 1991.
7. Graham NO (ed): *Quality Assurance in Hospitals,* 2nd ed. Rockville, Md., Aspen Publications, 1990.
8. Howanitz PJ, Cembrowski GS, Bachner P: Laboratory Phlebotomy-CAP Q-Probe Study of Patient Satisfaction and Complications in 23,783 Patients. *Arch Pathol & Lab Med,* 115, 867–872, Sept 1991.
9. Westgard JO, Barry PL, Tomar RH: Implementing TQM in Health Care Laboratories. *Clinical Laboratory Management Review,* 5(5), 354, 1991.

10 Quality Assurance and Safety in Blood Collection

CHAPTER OUTLINE

Clinical laboratory test results are increasingly used by physicians for diagnosis and treatment of their patients. Thus, every step in the formulation of these results must be of superlative quality. Clinical laboratories are responsible for the methodology that assures reliable, accurate test results. The method used to assure reliable, accurate data is referred to as *quality assurance.* Quality assurance plays a major part in the laboratory in (1) patient preparation and specimen collection, (2) specimen transportation and processing, (3) instrumental and technical performance of clinical laboratory assays, (4) laboratory safety, and (5) in-service training and education of laboratorians and other health care professionals.

Laboratory professionals have developed quality assurance guidelines for specimen collection and processing, record keeping, preventive maintenance of laboratory instruments, proficiency testing, laboratory personnel, and day-to-day quality control. These guidelines are formally adopted into a laboratory as a quality assurance program. Professional agencies and governmental agencies [e.g., College of American Pathologists (CAP), American Association of Bioanalysts, Institute of Clinical Scientists, Joint Committee on the Accreditation of Healthcare Organizations (JCAHO)] have intensified efforts to improve quality of laboratory performance through the establishment of quality assurance accreditation standards. These organizations provide accreditation to those clinical laboratories that maintain a proper quality assurance plan and program. The steps that are included in such a program are

1. Identification of potential problems in such a program
2. Providing objective evaluation of the cause and extent of the problem
3. Establishment of priorities to confront the problem
4. Providing activities to correct the problem
5. Providing procedures to continually monitor the activities that have been established to correct the problem
6. Documentation to demonstrate that the quality assurance plan is effective and efficient in providing quality patient care

The term "quality assurance" implies a program that guarantees quality patient care. "*Quality control*" implies operational procedures used to implement the quality assurance program.

The quality control officer, clinical laboratory supervisor, or laboratory director usually regulates the quality assurance program in the clinical laboratory. The size of the laboratory and number of staff generally dictate who handles the quality assurance policies and tasks.

All laboratory personnel must follow all quality assurance policies and procedures to assure quality patient care. Because specimen collection is the first step in the process of acquiring quality results, the phlebotomist must provide the laboratory with perfect specimens. All of these efforts can markedly improve the precision and accuracy of information produced by the clinical laboratory.

COLLECTION PROCEDURES TO ENSURE QUALITY

Quality assurance in the clinical laboratory begins before the sample is collected from the patient. In order to obtain perfect specimens, first the patient and the specimen container must be prepared. If the patient is not adequately prepared, the laboratory procedures and instrumentation cannot compensate for the shortcomings. Thus, the clinical laboratory must provide the nursing staff with a floor book (Table 10–1) that describes laboratory services, preparation of the patient, and special handling of patients' specimens. The phlebotomist should be aware of the protocol that is necessary to prepare patients and specimen containers for laboratory assays in order to instruct the nursing staff in this capacity and thereby lead to quality specimen collection. Thus, a monthly review of the laboratory's collection procedures and policies is recommended to reduce collection errors and hopefully lead to perfect specimen collection. Examples of the types of collection procedures that the phlebotomist should review include

1. Collection of blood specimens by skin puncture
2. Isolation techniques
3. Microcollection techniques on newborns
4. Capillary blood gases
5. Collection of blood specimens by finger stick
6. Intensive care blood collections
7. Pediatric blood collection techniques
8. Collection of specimens for intravenous glucose tolerance tests
9. Inability to collect blood specimen
10. Patient identification

Also, the phlebotomist should have access to a pocket-sized collection booklet that contains the same information as in the floor book (e.g., laboratory test, laboratory section in which procedure is performed, required collection container, amount of required sample, preservatives for sample handling).

Some examples of patient preparation and specimen container preparation include

1. The patient must ingest at least 300 g of carbohydrates daily for at least 3 days prior to glucose tolerance test.
2. The patient must be fasting for 12 to 16 hours before a glucose analysis.
3. The mechanics of the glucose tolerance test should be explained to the patient before the test so that he or she will understand the reason for fasting prior to the test. The fasting blood specimen is collected in the morning rather than at a random collection time to avoid the following laboratory test results:
   a. The effects of exercise

TABLE 10–1. SAMPLE PAGES FROM FLOOR BOOK

	Surgical Service Laboratory	Emergency Center Laboratory	Critical Care Laboratory	Perinatal/UCHH Laboratory
Open	2:00 AM–7:00 PM (Mon–Fri)	24 hours (closed Sat/Sun 7–3 shift)	24 hours	open except 3:00 PM–11:00 PM
7–3 break AM/PM	none	8:30 AM–8:50 AM	none	9 AM–9:20 AM
7–3 lunch AM/PM	none	11:00 AM–11:30 AM	none	12:30 PM–1 PM
3–11 break PM	5:00 PM–5:20 PM	9 PM–9:20 PM	none	none
3–11 lunch PM	1:00 PM–1:50 PM	6 PM–6:30 PM	none	none
11–7 break PM/AM	none	2 AM–2:50 AM	none	1 AM–1:50 AM
Tests Performed:	Blood gas Coox WB Na/K WB glucose CBC Spun Hct	Blood gas Electrocytes BUN Creatinine Glucose Calcium CBC UA Pregnancy test	Blood gas Coox COP Osmo (bl/ur) WB Na/K Ur Na/K WB glucose Spun Hct TSP (refrac) Ion Calcium	Blood gas COP TSP (refrac) WB glucose CBC Spun Hct

Code	Test	Specimen Requirements	Analysis & Reporting Times	Reference Range	Lab
2105	Cholesterol, total	serum: 1 mL blood, speckled top; prefer fasting specimen.	Performed 24 hr/day, 7 days/week; results in 4 hr.	150–200 mg/dL; 200–240 mg/dL marginal risk for CHD; >240 mg/dL substantial risk for CHD	C

288

Code	Test	Specimen	Schedule	Normal value	Lab
3150	Cholesterol, high density lipoprotein (HDL-Cholesterol)	4 mL blood, speckled top; obtained 14 hr after fasting.	Performed on Monday and Thursday, 9 AM cutoff. Results in 8 hr.	Average risk of coronary heart disease: M ≥ 45 mg/dL F ≥ 55 mg/dL	C
	Cholesterol, low density lipoprotein (LDL-Cholesterol)	10 mL blood, speckled top; obtain 14 hr after fasting.	Performed on Monday and Thursday, 9 AM cutoff. Results in 8 hr. Results calculated from HDL-cholesterol, total cholesterol, and triglycerides.	Not established	C
5105	Chromosome analysis	Call cytogenetics ext. 4523.	Results in 3 to 4 weeks.	Interpretation by cytogeneticist	R
	CMV antibody (Ab)	3 mL blood, speckled top.	Performed Tuesday and Thursday, 9 AM cutoff. Results in 2 weeks.	≤ 1:16	I
80076	Coccidiomycosis (fungal titer)	4 mL blood, speckled top.		Nonreactive	R
5180	Cold agglutinin	3 mL blood, speckled top placed in warm water, deliver immediately.	Performed Mon–Fri; results in 8 hr.	Negative <1:16	I
20060	Colloid osmotic pressure (COP)	1 mL blood in a heparinized syringe, mix well to prevent clotting; remove needle, use stopper or 3 mL blood, speckled top tube.	Performed 24 hr/day, 7 days/week; results in 30 minutes.	20–25 mm Hg	CCL PNL
	Compatibility testing (crossmatch)	Adult: 5–10 mL blood, red top or purple top Child: 3 mL blood, red top or purple top Neonate: Consult Blood Bank.	Performed 24 hr/day, 7 days/week. Available in 1 hr if no antibodies present.	NA	BB
5060	Complement: C_3	3 mL blood, speckled top.	Performed Mon–Fri, 9 AM cutoff; results in 8 hr.	55–120 mg/dL	I
5065	Complement: C_4	3 mL blood, speckled top.	Performed Mon–Fri, 9 AM cutoff; results in 8 hr.	20–50 mg/dL	I
84210	Compound S, plasma (11-deoxycortisol)	4 mL blood, speckled top. Deliver immediately.	Results in 5 days.	0.05–0.25 mcq/100 mL post metyrapone <7 µg/100 mL	R

From Hermann Hospital Clinical Laboratories, Houston, Tex., with permission.

b. The effects of changes in posture
c. The effects of diurnal variation
4. A fasting specimen is desirable for triglyceride and cholesterol analysis.
5. Ten milliliters of concentrated hydrochloric acid (HCl) must be added to a 24-hour urine collection container prior to collection in order to preserve the clinical constituents to be analyzed in the laboratory.

Anticoagulants and Preservatives: Quality Assurance

As discussed in Chapter 3, the phlebotomist uses various anticoagulants and preservatives in the collection of blood specimens. These tubes containing anticoagulants must be inverted promptly after blood is drawn to assure mixture of the anticoagulant and blood and thus provide quality assurance of a perfectly collected specimen. As reviewed in Chapter 4, when several evacuated tubes of blood are collected on a patient, tubes containing anticoagulants should be filled last so that proper inversion can occur and carry over of anticoagulants to clotted tubes will not occur.

In order to assure quality, the anticoagulants and preservatives should meet the requirements established by the National Committee for Clinical Laboratory Standards.[1] The manufacturer of the anticoagulants and preservatives must provide the shelf-life of these additives on the packages so that the user will know how long these additives are effective. When restocking the supply of collection tubes, the tubes with a shelf-life (expiration date) nearest to the current date should be placed in front on the shelf so that they are used first. In addition, for blood collection tubes, the manufacturers must test and verify draw and fill accuracy until the stated expiration date. The phlebotomist should be cognizant of expiration dates on any item used in specimen collection. Quality assurance accreditation standards require the health care institution to establish quality control procedures for proper inspection of new lot numbers of evacuated blood collection tubes. Each time a new lot number of tubes is placed into use, the tubes must be checked for the designated factors, as shown in Table 10–2.

In addition, quality can be obtained in specimen collection only with fresh specimens. If the blood specimen is not to be run immediately, the phlebotomist must make certain that it is stored properly until the test is run.

Quality Assurance in Shipping Specimens to Reference Laboratories

If the specimen is to be shipped to a reference laboratory, the phlebotomist should review the laboratory procedure on the "Handling of Samples for Reference Laboratory Work" (Table 10–3) to prepare the specimen in the proper manner and maintain a suitable specimen for the laboratory test. In order to avoid additional expense and inconvenience to the physician, the patient, and the laboratory, it is very important to verify the specific specimen requirements for the reference laboratory. Thus, for reference laboratory specimens,

TABLE 10–2. QUALITY CONTROL ON EVACUATED BLOOD COLLECTION TUBES

Date _____   Lot no. _____

Tube size _____

Tube color _____

Expiration date _____

Checked by: _____

Each time a new lot number of tubes is placed into use, tubes must be checked as indicated below. Please sign off after checking the new lot number.

Vacuum draw at 760 mm Hg and 20°C:	Result:
Visual inspection for anticoagulants	
Sterility of tube (if indicated)	
Check for clots by straining anticoagulated blood through gauze	
Sample spin down	
Stopper pull-off	
Breakage from Spinning	
Taking cap off	
Metals contamination	
Check for Sodium	
Potassium	
Ammonia	

the phlebotomist must make certain to submit the quantity specified by the reference laboratory for the laboratory test. As a rule of thumb, the volume of blood drawn should equal $2^{1}/_{2}$ times the amount of serum or plasma required. For example, to obtain 4 mL of plasma, draw at least 10 mL of blood.[1]

In addition, the patient must be properly prepared prior to the blood collection. Since many specimens are sent to reference laboratories for hormone assays, the blood must be collected at specified times according to the circadian rhythms of the hormones. Also, the patient's position (lying down or seated) has a major impact on many reference laboratory studies. Other fluctuations caused by the physical status of the patient (diet, emotional state, prior medications) can be a determining factor in the overall utility of the laboratory results. It is important for the phlebotomist to be aware of proper patient preparation for these referral laboratory specimens.

TABLE 10–3. HANDLING OF SAMPLES FOR REFERENCE LABORATORY WORK

Principle

Specimen Control will have responsibility for the receipt, record keeping, and dispatch of all clinical specimens to be sent to reference laboratories. This will ensure adequate centralized control over the entire process from specimen collection to reporting.

Order Entry of Tests

1. All specimens to be sent to reference laboratories will be ordered into the computer system in the same manner as any other request by Specimen Control personnel.
   a. Five digit test codes and mnemonics for ordering can be found in the Handling Inquiry. Also in this Inquiry are instructions for processing, specimen type, reference lab assigned, minimum volume, and usually the turnaround time expected.
   b. If a test code cannot be found, or there are questions about the specimen received, the slip and specimen should be taken to the Reference Lab area on weekdays, 6:00 AM to 2:30 PM. After hours and on weekends, the slip and specimen should be placed in the Reference Lab refrigerator for further action.
   c. Tests not found in the Handling Inquiry will require the attention of the Manager or Supervisor. The consultation with the appropriate technical director and laboratory administrator may be required.
2. Infrequent or special tests not defined in the computer system will be ordered as miscellaneous tests built for each approved reference lab. On special approval, a different reference may be used and a miscellaneous test is available for this situation.
   a. These test codes will ask for "source" at order entry. At this prompt, the requested test is entered for documentation.

Processing of Specimens

1. At the start of each working day in Reference Lab, the refrigerator will be checked for requests that have not been ordered for varying reasons. These will be researched and order entered.
2. A Referred Out Test Log will be printed for at least a 36-hour period of time, or greater on Mondays. All outgoing specimens will be checked off the log as they are packaged to send out.
3. A manual log will contain specimen number, name of patient, name of test requested, and the Mayo control number if sent to that lab.
4. The pending list for each reference lab/worksheet will be reviewed for any missed procedure on a daily basis.
5. A weekly printing of the Referred Out Test Log for all reference labs will be printed and kept for auditing of invoices.

Processing Billing Information

1. Each reference lab test defined in the system is billed at order entry and included on the billing tape.
2. Tests not defined in the system must be order entered as a miscellaneous test.
   a. Each miscellaneous test code has the miscellaneous CDM code of 40199993 with no price attached in the file maintenance.
   b. These tests will "kick" out of the billing tape onto the error log.
   c. Charting personnel will fill out a manual debit slip for the account number and test ordered.
   d. Reference lab personnel will complete the debit slip, supplying the test name and price and return to Charting.
   e. Charting will monitor a manual log to assure the debit is sent through on a timely basis.
3. For every test referred, one handling fee will be charged. The test code is 88888 (CDM 40199977).

(continued)

TABLE 10–3. (*Continued*)

---

    a. Each procedure code defined in the system is built as a profile that includes the Handling test code. Billing for the handling is therefore automatically generated when the procedure test code is ordered.

    b. When a debit slip for a miscellaneous test code is completed by Reference Lab personnel, the test code for handling and delivery must be included.

  4. If there is no charge for a test from a reference laboratory, only the handling fee will be charged.

  5. Any fees charged by a reference laboratory for performing a test on requested STAT basis will be billed to the patient.

Processing Results

  1. As results are received from reference laboratories, the results will be entered into the computer system.

  2. Worksheets are designated by reference laboratory when a test is assigned.

  3. Each test result is entered, along with date specimen was sent out and date report was received. Each report was designed to follow the report format of each reference laboratory. The name of the reference lab performing the test is included in the report header on the report.

  4. Tests whose results are too long and complex or include graphs or pictures are charted under separate cover. Date sent and date reported are resulted in the system, which in turn generates the message on the report that "results are reported under separate cover."

  5. Computer procedure for computer resulting.

    a. Log on the Result System: c HHAAR

    b. Manager: "H,S"

    c. Worksheet: enter worksheet number or mnemonic

    d. Default workload methodology: "RETURN"

    e. Print workload warning message (N): "RETURN"

    f. Specimen number: enter specimen number to be resulted

    g. As result codes appear, enter the information and result until complete.

    h. Release results: enter "A" for all.

  6. A copy of the original report from the reference laboratory will be filed in Reference Laboratory. Files are retained for two years.

Workflow of Pretransplant Tissue Typing Procedures

  1. No direct patient billing is involved in Pretransplant tissue typing.

  2. Reference Lab is responsible for monitoring reports for completeness and audits the invoices received from MSRDP to Hermann Hospital for accuracy in billing.

  3. A manual logbook is maintained. No computer order entry is performed.

    a. Data processing copies of tissue typing requests are logged in the Pretransplant book indicating date of service.

    b. As reports are received from the Histocompatibility laboratory, they are checked for completeness and date report is received is written in the logbook.

    c. A copy of the finished report is filed in a folder assigned to each pretransplant recipient in the file room in Reference Laboratory.

    d. As the test is approved for payment on the invoice, a notation is made in the logbook.

Tests Referred for Other Laboratory Sections

  1. Tests referred out for other laboratory sections due to technical problems with an in-house procedure:

    a. The sections sending out the test will prepare the specimen according to the specifications for the particular Reference Laboratory.

(*continued*)

TABLE 10–3. *(Continued)*

b. The test will be reported by the section; no record will be kept in the Reference Laboratory computer log.

c. When the outside laboratory report is received in the Reference Laboratory, it is forwarded to the technical section to report out the results. A copy of the outside laboratory report is then returned to Specimen Control and retained in the file. The cost of the procedure will be charged to the appropriate section on the Expense Transfer Report at the end of the month. Those tests are not counted in the Reference Laboratory monthly workload report. No handling fee is charged.

Verifying Invoices

1. All invoices from reference laboratories must be checked against the Referred Out Test Log and, as necessary, other file documents to verify that all reports have been received and recorded and that all charges are legitimate.

2. Copies of approved invoices are filed in Laboratory Administration.

Notes

1. All requests for clinical procedures not performed in the Department of Pathology and Laboratory Medicine must be submitted to Specimen Control with appropriate specimens request slips and billing documents. The Laboratory will not handle the reporting of or billing for any procedure unless protocol is followed.

2. Samples will be sent only to the reference laboratory designated for the particular test. Recommendations for permanent addition to or changes of this list must be submitted to the Assistant Laboratory Director. For rare tests, a laboratory may be designated on an emergency basis by the Administrative Laboratory Director or Assistant Laboratory Director after consultation with the appropriate doctorate staff.

3. Special research procedures performed by various laboratories in Hermann Hospital and/or the University of Texas Medical School will not be considered as clinical laboratory procedures and the laboratories performing these procedures will not be treated as reference or billing for such procedures.

4. All questions concerning the status of Reference Laboratory work should be referred to Reference Laboratory or Specimen Control.

From Hermann Hospital Clinical Laboratories, Houston, Tex., with permission.

Breakage and leakage may also result during shipping if the specimen is not packaged properly. For interstate shipment of biohazardous specimens to a reference laboratory (see Chapter 6 for further discussion of biohazardous specimens), the federal government requires that the labeled specimen be placed in a securely closed, watertight container (primary container— Vacutainer tube, for example), which shall be enclosed in a second, durable watertight container (secondary container). The label must include all necessary patient identification information. The space at the top, bottom, and sides between the primary and secondary container must contain sufficient absorbent material (e.g., paper towels) to absorb the entire contents of the primary container in case of breakage or leakage. The set of primary and secondary containers should be enclosed in an outer shipping container constructed of corrugated fiberboard, cardboard, or wood. The mailing package must include the properly completed laboratory request form. The outer shipping container for this biohazardous specimen must bear a label (Fig. 10–1) stating

1. Etiologic agent
2. Biomedical material

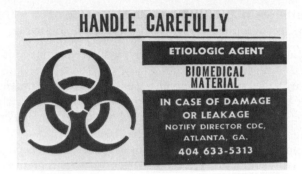

Figure 10-1. Label for shipment of biohazardous specimen to reference laboratory.

3. In case of damage or leakage, Notify Director, CDC, Atlanta, Georgia 404-633-5313

Also, on a separate label on the outer container, the address label must be affixed. For further information regarding regulations regarding shipment of biologic specimens, the Centers for Disease Control (CDC) at the following address should be contacted:

Centers for Disease Control
ATTN: Biohazards Control Officer
1600 Clifton Road
Atlanta, GA 30333

Since certain air and overland transportation services do not accept medical specimens for shipment, it is important to call the transportation service before shipping the specimen to verify that it can be transported by the company. In addition, the request for picking up the specimen should occur as early as possible after the blood is collected to avoid any delays.

If frozen specimens are required for a particular laboratory procedure to be performed at the reference laboratory, the serum or plasma should be separated from the cells as soon as possible. The frozen specimen should be shipped in a polyform or similar type of insulated package. Dry ice can be packaged with the specimen to extend the utility of the specimen for up to four days.[7] The insulated package needs to (1) be large enough to accommodate the specimen and dry ice and (2) include thawproof materials. The specimens should be frozen in plastic vials only. Since extreme cold may cause ordinary plastic labels to become brittle and detach from the specimen tube, it is recommended to use cloth, paper, or special plastic labels. Also, submit a *separate* frozen specimen for *each* test requested since blood constituents are sensitive to thawing and refreezing for the performance of several types of assays.[1]

Requirements for a Quality Specimen

The requirements for a quality specimen include the following:

1. The patient is prepared properly and medication interference is avoided, if possible.
2. The correct specimens are collected from the correct patients with the proper labeling. Because it is the policy of most clinical laboratories to discard specimens that are unlabeled or labeled incorrectly, the phlebotomist must abide by the written laboratory policy describing acceptable identification of specimens to ensure perfect specimen collection. The potential errors in after-the-fact reidentification of a specimen by floor personnel can be extremely detrimental to the patient in question and must be avoided. (See Chapter 4 for identification and labeling procedures.)
3. The correct anticoagulants and preservatives are used with the sufficient amount collected. (See Chapter 3 on Anticoagulants and Preservatives.)[1]
4. The specimens are not hemolyzed.
5. The fasting specimens are collected in a timely fashion and are actually fasting samples.
6. Timed specimens are correctly timed and documented.
7. Specimens without anticoagulants need to stand a minimum of 30 minutes for clot formation to occur completely. (Gel separator tubes will shorten the time for clot formation, dependent upon manufacturer's tubes.)
8. Specimens are transported to the clinical laboratory in a timely fashion to maintain freshness.

In order to conform to these requirements, the phlebotomist should review the clinical laboratory's procedures to identify the designated delivery times (Table 10–4) for each laboratory procedure. If the laboratory does not have *designated delivery times* for specimens, the phlebotomist may wish to suggest to his or her laboratory supervisor that such a system would ensure fresh specimens and, thus, high-quality laboratory results. NCCLS states that specimens should be received by the laboratory within 45 minutes from the time of collection.[4] A list of the specimens that are delivered after the designated time limits should be maintained in a Problem Log for Quality Assurance in Specimen Control. Such a list can usually help detect the source of the problem so that quality assurance can be maintained in the specimen control section. The list reveals the number of specimens that were delivered after the allowable limits and how late they were. The supervisor of specimen control usually decides whether the late specimen should be discarded and recollected.

In addition to ensuring that the delivery times for specimens are maintained, the phlebotomist and the nursing staff should be aware of the test procedures that must be scheduled with the specimen control section in the

**TABLE 10-4. EXAMPLES OF DESIGNATED DELIVERY TIMES
FOR LABORATORY SPECIMENS**

Clinical microbiology	
Routine bacterial culture	45 min
Swab with holding medium	20 min
Swab without holding medium	40 min
Body fluids	
Parasitology	
Feces for amoeba identification	Immediately
Clinical chemistry	
Glucose	20 min
Enzymes	30 min
Na^+, K^+, Cl^-, HCO_3^- (electrolytes)	30 min
Chemical profile	45 min
Coagulation	
Prothrombin time (PT)	45 min
Partial thromboplastin time (PTT)	45 min
Clotting time	Immediately
Urinalysis/clinical microscopy	
Routine urinalysis	45 min

laboratory. For example, to ensure that enough phlebotomists are available for glucose tolerance tests, it is advisable to have the glucose tolerance test scheduled with specimen control at least 24 hours prior to the test. The persons scheduling the test should be entered into a glucose tolerance test log book. A cutoff number of scheduled glucose tolerance tests should be determined for the specimen control section to ensure that the phlebotomists will be able to obtain every specimen at the proper time. Other frequently encountered laboratory assays that must be scheduled in advance include blood specimens drawn for drug monitoring. This scheduling process is another means to assure quality specimen collection.

Number of Blood Collection Attempts

Another way the specimen control section of the laboratory can provide quality assurance to the patients is by logging the number of unsuccessful collection attempts. If the phlebotomist has had consecutively unsuccessful attempts to draw blood from different patients, the supervisor and phlebotomist will know that the problem in blood collection must be identified and solved to avoid future unsuccessful attempts. Most clinical laboratories have a written procedure on the "Documentation of Specimen Collection" including a section entitled Inability to Draw Specimen (Table 10-5), which describes the steps that should be taken by the phlebotomist in (1) unsuccessful collection attempts, (2) patient unavailability, and (3) patient refusal.

Also, a log should be kept on the number of times that blood has been collected from pediatric and newborn patients (Fig. 10-2). Due to their blood volume, it is best to collect the minimum required amount of blood for each laboratory assay to avoid significant blood loss during their hospital stay. Each

TABLE 10–5. DOCUMENTATION OF SPECIMEN COLLECTION ON NURSING UNIT LOGBOOKS

Principle

The logbook on any hospital unit for which the laboratory routinely performs phlebotomy is the only record of what has been actually drawn on a given patient. It is critical to patient care that this documentation be complete whether successful or unable to draw.

Procedure

Documentation of Successful Phlebotomy

1. All requests for laboratory tests should be stamped and written on the unit's logbook prior to run times specified in the "Laboratory Floor Book." 6 AM requests will be entered on the logbook by unit, prior to sending requests to the laboratory for order entry. Add-ons will be allowed if postponement to next scheduled run would affect patient care. Any abuse of the system will be brought to the Manager's attention.

2. Requests on computer-generated labels that serve as requests for phlebotomy are checked against the logbook prior to drawing of blood. Any discrepancy should be brought to the attention of the unit secretary or nurse for resolution of orders. Any test deleted from the log by request of unit will be circled and explanation of deletion along with requestor's name will be written on the log. Any tests added to requests should be added to logbook. If any tests are added but not requested on computer labels, a stamped request must be made by nursing unit.

3. After the appropriate specimens have been collected, each patient that is complete will be initialed by phlebotomist and time of draw entered in appropriate box on logbook. At the bottom of the list of patients, a line is drawn and EOR or End of Run will be written to signify all is complete.

Inability to Draw Specimen

1. A maximum of two laboratory employees will attempt to obtain blood from a patient.

2. Any unsuccessful attempt to obtain blood *must* be documented on the logbook and request.

3. Patient Unavailable:

    a. If you are unable to obtain blood when requested because a patient is unavailable (gone to x-ray or surgery, out of room), hold these slips until you have completed all other patients on that nursing unit. Check the patient's room again before leaving unit.

    b. If patient is still unavailable, notify his primary nurse if available or unit secretary. Leave the slip(s) at the desk, circle the orders, and with the following write on the logbook:

    1) Reason patient unavailable
    2) Time and initials of collector/technologist
    3) Name of nurse notified

    The patient will then be drawn on the next scheduled run.

4. Patient Refused:

    If patient refuses to be drawn, notify his primary nurse. Often the nurse can convince the patient to cooperate. If not, leave slips at the unit desk with the following information on the logbook:

    a. Patient refused
    b. Time and initials of collector/technologist
    c. Name of nurse notified

5. Patient Missed:

    a. If at any time the person collecting blood is unable to obtain the blood, he or she should check to see if there is another collector/technologist to help.

(continued)

TABLE 10–5. *(Continued)*

   b. If no other laboratory employee is available, notify the patient's nurse that the patient was missed and that another person from the laboratory will try on the next run unless nurse requests attempt be made sooner. Leave the slips at the desk with the following information on the logbook:

     1) Patient missed

     2) Time and initials of collector/technologist

     3) Name of nurse notified

   c. Upon returning to the laboratory, notify Specimen Control. A collector will then attempt to obtain the specimen at the next collection run unless otherwise requested.

   d. If the second person is unavailable to obtain the specimen a nurse is again notified and the above information is again documented on the requisition and the logbook. At this time request that a physician draw the blood.

  6. In cases where an adult patient is combative or verbally abusive of laboratory personnel and nursing staff is unavailable, the phlebotomist should notify his supervisor in Specimen Control. If the phlebotomist is instructed by the supervisor to refuse, the primary nurse should be notified of the refusal and it must be documented on the logbook noting:

   a. Reason for refusal

   b. Name of the nurse notified

  7. If the phlebotomist has a test requested that cannot be found in the specimen requirement book, the nurse should be asked to consult the chart for clarification and then the doctor should be contacted to clarify if still not clear. The phlebotomist, meanwhile, can call Specimen Control or other sections of the lab for a more familiar name for the test and test requirements. If no other name can be found and no clarification offered to the phlebotomist, he *must* refuse to draw the test. The logbook should be marked "no such test" and the primary nurse notified and her name recorded on the logbook. The supervisor in Specimen Control or Technologist in charge of the laboratory should also be notified before the phlebotomist leaves the floor.

Note

If computer-generated labels were used as a request for the early morning run, bring the labels with the written reason for not drawing back to Specimen Control. Put the labels on the logging clipboard. These will be taken back up for the next collection run unless otherwise requested.

From Hermann Hospital Clinical Laboratories, Houston, Tex., with permission.

laboratory should have a table of maximum amounts of blood that can be drawn on these patients, as shown in Table 10–6. The log book provides a check on the amount of blood that has been drawn from these patients to avoid problems in significant blood loss.

Quality Control in the Collection of Blood Cultures

As discussed in Chapter 5, the phlebotomist's main concern when obtaining a blood culture specimen is to prevent contamination of the blood culture by skin organisms. The quality control procedures that should be adhered to by the phlebotomist in order to prevent contamination include

1. The venipuncture site should not be touched after it has been prepared for needle insertion.

2. Unsterile gauze should not be put over the venipuncture site until after blood is drawn.

Week ___1___   Month _October_   Year _1992_
Collection Log on Pediatric and Newborn Patients

Date	Patient	Age	Patient Number	Floor	Test Requested	Amount Collected
10/4/92	Rubinoff, Baby	4 days	1650421	NB Nur	Chemistry screen	3 microtainers
10/4/92	Gustafson, H.	5 yrs	177482	6B	electrolytes	2 × 250 μL
10/4/92	Benson, J.	12 mo	185621	6B	Hb & Hct	2 × 20 μL

Figure 10–2. Blood collections on pediatric and newborn patients. *(Courtesy of Hermann Hospital Clinical Laboratory, Houston, Tex., with permission.)*

3. The requisition must show the date and time of the blood culture collection and the initials of the phlebotomist who collected it.

Sometimes, even with all of the precautions in blood culture collection, contamination occurs. To determine the rate and possible source of blood culture contamination, the clinical microbiology section may maintain a written or computer *collection log* to tabulate negative and positive culture results

TABLE 10–6. MAXIMUM AMOUNTS OF BLOOD TO BE DRAWN ON PATIENTS UNDER 14 YEARS

Patient's Weight		Maximum Amount to Be Drawn at Any One Time (mL)	Maximum Amount of Blood (Cumulative) to Be Drawn During a Given Hospital Stay (1 month or under) (mL)
lb	*kg (approx.)*		
6–8	2.7–3.6	2.5	23
8–10	3.6–4.5	3.5	30
10–15	4.5–6.8	5	40
16–20	7.3–9.1	10	60
21–25	9.5–11.4	10	70
26–30	11.8–13.6	10	80
31–35	14.1–15.9	10	100
36–40	16.4–18.2	10	130
41–45	18.6–20.5	20	140
46–50	20.9–22.7	20	160
51–55	23.2–25.0	20	180
56–60	25.5–27.3	20	200
61–65	27.7–29.5	25	220
66–70	30.0–31.8	30	240
71–75	32.3–34.1	30	250
76–80	34.5–36.4	30	270
81–85	36.8–38.6	30	290
86–90	39.1–40.9	30	310
91–95	41.4–43.2	30	330
96–100	43.6–45.5	30	350

From Hermann Hospital Clinical Laboratories, Houston, Tex., with permission.

and contaminated specimens. This log can detect the contamination rate of blood cultures and the particular shift when the blood culture was collected. Many laboratories use 3 percent as their threshold for blood culture contamination.[2] Thus, high contamination rates may be traced to an individual with poor collection practices, such as inadequate cleaning of the venipuncture area. High contamination rates may also be traced to specific areas of the health care institution (i.e., emergency room, intensive cardiac care). The emergency room personnel may inadequately disinfect the puncture site due to concern for speed, whereas in the intensive cardiac care unit, the indwelling catheters may have to be used instead of venipuncture, which can lead to an increased contamination rate for blood cultures.

Quality Control and Preventive Maintenance on Specimen Collection Instruments

The phlebotomist should be aware that quality control and preventive maintenance occurs on certain instruments and equipment in the specimen control section. For example, as shown in Table 10–7, thermometers are one type of instrument that must be maintained by blood collection personnel. The sphygmomanometer is another instrument used in blood collection procedures that must be maintained and checked for quality assurance. Table 10–8 shows an accuracy check for a sphygmomanometer that should be used by a phlebotomist if he or she uses one during blood collection procedures.

Another instrument frequently used and maintained by phlebotomists is the centrifuge. The *centrifuge* that is used to spin down the blood must be checked for accurate speed in addition to the preventive maintenance procedures. The speed of the centrifuge can be checked by a *tachometer,* which indicates the speed in *revolutions per minute (RPM).* The relative centrifugal force or *g value* is then determined from a nomogram as shown in Figure 10–3. The g value gives the efficiency of the instrument by determining the true force exerted by the centrifuge.[3]

A g force of approximately 1000 for 10 minutes is usually efficient for good separation of cells or clotted blood from plasma or serum. However, it is imperative to follow the manufacturer's directions when separating blood specimens using gel separator devices. These collection tubes usually require a specified, higher force than 1000 g for complete separation. The NCCLS publishes a manual entitled "Procedures for the Handling & Processing of Blood Specimens," which the phlebotomist may want to review for more information on centrifugation of blood specimens.[4]

Quality Assurance in Bedside Glucose Testing

The control of blood glucose levels is extremely important in the care of diabetic patients. In many health care institutions, phlebotomists are now performing *bedside glucose testing* with small, compact blood glucose monitoring instruments. These instruments use reagent strips that are read in the

TABLE 10–7. QUALITY CONTROL AND PREVENTIVE MAINTENANCE OF THERMOMETERS

Standards to Be Achieved and Maintained
Prior to placing in service, all thermometers must meet the following specifications:

Location	Usual Temperature Range (°C)	Allowable Deviation from NBS Standard (°C)
Refrigerators	0 to 6	1
Freezers	−5 to −20	2
Incubators	20 to 40	1
Heat blocks	Above 100	2

Thermometers that fail to meet requirements cannot be used and should be referred to the Supervisor for return to manufacturer.

Calibration Procedure
1. Thermometers should be tested against an NBS certified thermometer within or near the temperature ranges intended for use. Refrigerator thermometers should be calibrated near 0°C, freezers near − 10°C, and so on. Both the standard thermometer and thermometer being tested should be held in water, mineral oil, or other suitable fluid to avoid rapid changes in temperature while reading.
2. Recalibration is required (a) when a thermometer calibrated in one temperature range is to be used in another temperature range, (b) when a thermometer is suspected to be damaged (dropping or other accidents), and (c) on an annual basis to assure continued accuracy.
3. Each thermometer will be given a number and this number will be recorded in a quality control book and kept in the office of the Quality Control coordinator. This book must be signed out and returned by supervisors to record calibration data each time new thermometers are installed in service.
Calibrated thermometers may be obtained from the Quality Control coordinator in case of an emergency need.

Quality Control Procedures
1. Record each morning in the QCPM Book the highest (H) and lowest (L) temperature from the Maximum–Minimum thermometer maintained in the refrigerator and the freezer compartments. The procedure for using the Taylor Maximum–Minimum thermometer is as follows:
   a. To record the minimum index (L), refer to the left-hand side of the thermometer. *Read the bottom edge of the index.*
   b. To record the maximum index (H), refer to the right-hand side of the thermometer. *Read the bottom edge of the index.*
   c. Record the minimum index in the QCPM Book under "Low," and the maximum index under "High." Initial all entries.
   The upper left-hand side of the thermometer is in minus degrees. The upper right-hand side of the thermometer is in positive degrees.
2. After taking the two readings, reset each index by placing the ceramic magnet across the U-tube in a horizontal position and draw downward slowly, until the indices come to rest on the tops of the mercury columns.
3. If mercury becomes separated, grasp the thermometer firmly at the upper end giving a number of forceful downward swings, until the columns are reunited.

Person(s) Responsible
Medical technologist or collector to be designated by the supervisor.

(continued)

TABLE 10–7. *(Continued)*

Preventive Maintenance

Keep thermometers clean and handle with care. Turn in any broken thermometers to the Safety Coordinator.

Abbreviations: NBS, National Bureau of Standards
From Hermann Hospital Clinical Laboratories, Houston, Tex., with permission.

---

instrument. Examples of these bedside glucose monitoring instruments include Accu-Check II (Boehringer Mannheim Diagnostics, Indianapolis, Ind.); Glucocheck (Larken Industries, Ltd., Lenexa, Kan.); Diascan (HDI—Home Diagnostics Inc., Eatontown, N.J.); and Glucometer II (Ames Division, Miles Laboratories, Elkhart, Ind.). Since over half of laboratory errors are clerical rather than instrument, reagent, or procedural failure, a bedside glucose instrument with a printed report is preferable.

In order to perform the blood glucose determinations, phlebotomists need to be aware of the quality assurance procedures that are required to obtain accurate and precise results. A skin puncture is customarily performed to obtain the blood for these bedside glucose assays. The patient's finger should be cleansed with alcohol and allowed to dry. A microcollection lancet is used to puncture the finger and cause the blood to form a drop. The first drop is wiped away and the next drop is applied by allowing the drop to fall from the finger upon the strip or reagent pad. After the specified time indicated with the instrument's instruction sheet, the blood is removed by blotting or by washing and the strip is placed in the instrument to obtain a glucose reading. The timing of the reaction is critical, and in most of these instruments, the time is called to the attention of the operator by a buzzer or alarm.

TABLE 10–8. ACCURACY CHECKS FOR SPHYGMOMANOMETER

Sphygmomanometers should be checked quarterly, or more often if handled roughly during transportation or if any defects are suspected.

1. The aneroid gauge is guaranteed to be accurate throughout the scale as long as it is within the "0" reading in the absence of pressure. If ever out of "0," the gauge is returned to the factory for repair and recalibration.

2. The inflating system, exhaust valve, and tubing should be checked for significant leaks in pressure. It should not exceed more than 5 mm Hg/s. Inflate cuff to 250 mm Hg. Hold the pressure for 1 min as a test for slow leaks.

3. Test the gauge for accuracy by testing against a "calibrated gauge." Lay the cuff of the "calibrated gauge" flat on a table. Pump air (bulb) into the bag until the dial reads between 40 and 60 mm Hg. Clamp the tube leading to the bulb so that it is airtight. When air is unable to escape, remove the bulb and adapter from the tube and insert another gauge in its place. Unclamp the tube. Both gauges should read the same pressure. The pressure inside the bag is then raised by pressing down on the bag and the increase in pressure should read the same on both gauges. A difference of more than 5 mm Hg in the reading is not acceptable. The gauge in question is returned to the factory for recalibration.

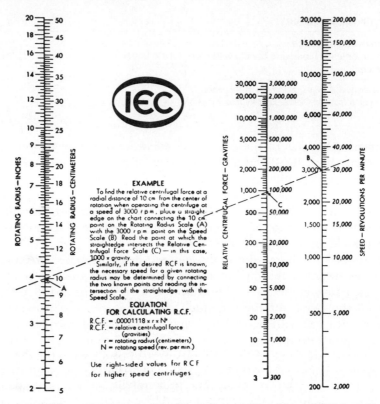

Figure 10–3. Nomogram for calculation of relative centrifugal force (RCF) in g. *[From Henry J (ed): Clinical Diagnosis and Management by Laboratory Methods. Philadelphia, W.B. Saunders, 1979, with permission.]*

These instruments should be calibrated with glucose standards (calibrators). The glucose values need to be regularly monitored with quality control material. This control material should be similar to the patient's specimen to inform the phlebotomist if the analytical system is working properly. For example, the glucose control should be based on the use of whole blood since this type of body fluid is used for measuring with bedside glucose monitoring instruments.

As the phlebotomist performs the glucose assay each day on the patient's blood, control material must be analyzed. The control value obtained on each day is plotted on a chart under the appropriate date (Fig. 10–4), and the daily plots are joined neatly with a straight line. The interpretation of this chart is based on the fact that for a normal distribution, 95 percent of the values about the mean or average (x) should be between ± 2 standard deviations (SD) from the mean (average) and that 99 percent of the values are between ± 3 SD from the mean.

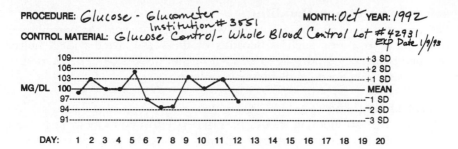

Figure 10–4. Clinical chemistry quality control chart.

Some bedside glucose testing instruments are capable of storing and downloading calibrators, controls, and patients' results and can thus provide a complete instrument log for quality assurance interpretation. Table 10–9 provides a list that will help lead to quality results through *avoidance* of these problems.

SAFETY IN SPECIMEN COLLECTION

The goal of safety in the health care institution is to recognize and eliminate hazards and provide information on safety education so that employees can have a healthy work environment. The responsibility for safe working conditions must be assured by the employer and has been mandated by law under the Occupational Safety and Health Act (OSHA) of 1991.[5] Knowledge of OSHA requirements and cooperation between the employer and employee concerning these requirements are necessary in health care facilities to achieve a safe working place. Thus, the phlebotomist needs to become aware of safety policies and procedures in his or her health care institution.

TABLE 10–9. Problems to Avoid in Bedside Glucose Testing

Specimen is inappropriately stored.
Wrong volume of specimen is collected.
Specimen is collected at wrong time.
Instrument blotting/wiping technique is not performed according to manufacturer's directions.
Reagents are outdated.
Timing of the analytical procedure is incorrect.
Reagents are not stored at proper temperature, leading them to deterioration.
Patient has not dieted properly for procedure.
Patient's result/time/date/etc., are mislabeled.
Recording of result is incorrect.
Battery for instrument is weak or dead.
Calibrators and/or controls are not properly used.
Results are not sent to appropriate individuals in timely manner.

Safety in Specimen Handling

Patients' specimens should be handled with caution to avoid the possibility of acquiring an infection such as hepatitis or those associated with Acquired Immune Deficiency Syndrome (AIDS). For further discussion of precautionary measures for specimen handling, see Chapter 6.

Personal Hygiene

While on the job, nothing should be inserted into one's mouth (e.g., food, pencils). Hands should be washed frequently during the day, before and after contact with patients or patients' specimens, before and after eating, drinking, or smoking, and before and after using the restrooms. Cosmetics should not be applied while on the job (Fig. 10–5). The phlebotomist should avoid biting his or her fingernails or rubbing his or her eyes. Eating, drinking, or smoking within the specimen control section and other laboratory sections must be avoided. No food should be placed in any laboratory refrigerator unless a refrigerator is designated "FOR FOOD ONLY." A laboratory coat should be worn completely buttoned while collecting specimens and removed prior to coffee breaks or lunch. Loose clothing such as scarves that might become entangled in the centrifuge should never be worn. Long hair must be tied so that it cannot come in contact with specimens or become entangled in the centrifuge. Open-toed shoes are usually prohibited in most clinical laboratories due to the hazards from chemicals and glassware.

Laboratory Safety

Laboratory safety includes a variety of policies. However, the phlebotomist should remember a few key safety rules at all times. The patients' specimens should be covered at all times during transportation and centrifugation. Centrifuging specimens is best performed within a biohazard safety hood (Fig. 10–6). All waste from specimen collection must be disposed of in the

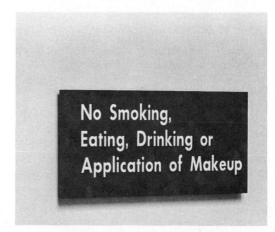

Figure 10–5. Required safety in specimen collection.

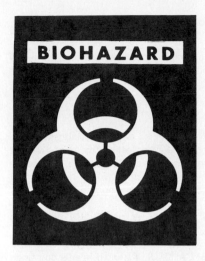

Figure 10–6. Sign for biohazardous material.

correct containers. One container is usually a heavy double plastic bag that is used for blood specimens disposal, another container for gauze and general trash, and a special container for needles, syringes, and lancets. Urine specimens are usually flushed down the drain with water or flushed down the toilet. Waste should be disposed of gently so that liquids do not splash on other objects. In addition, the work area within the specimen control section should be disinfected periodically according to the clinical laboratory schedule.

If an accident occurs such as sticking oneself with a needle after performing venipuncture on a patient, the phlebotomist should (1) immediately cleanse area with isopropyl alcohol and apply a Band-Aid and (2) contact the immediate supervisor and the necessary forms, laboratory tests, and vaccinations should be completed.

If an emergency or STAT call is made or received, the phlebotomist should not hang up the receiver until all the necessary information has been obtained and the other party has hung up his or her receiver. Table 10–10 gives a summary of precautions for the protection of laboratory workers based upon the 1991 OSHA rule.[5]

Fire Safety

Fire safety is the responsibility of all employees in the health care institution. Phlebotomists, therefore, should be familiar with the use and location of fire extinguishers and procedures to follow during a fire. They should be knowledgeable of the exact locations of fire extinguishers and fire blankets. The blankets should be available to smother burning clothes or to use as a fire shield if fire is blocking the exit. Health care institutions usually have periodic safety education programs in which the phlebotomist can participate and become skillful and knowledgeable in the use of fire safety equipment.

TABLE 10–10. Safety Precautions that *Must* Be Followed by Phlebotomists

Universal Precautions
1. Gloves must be worn during *all* phases of blood collection procedures (inpatient or outpatient facilities). Extremely important to avoid blood and body fluid exposure
   a. with non-intact skin
   b. from aerosols from centrifuging specimens
   c. with difficult patients
   d. when training in phlebotomy techniques
2. Gloves must be changed between patients and hands washed after removing gloves.
3. A laboratory coat, smock, or gown must be worn during blood collection procedures and left at laboratory/clinic when leaving work area. The laboratory coat should be cleaned by health care facility.
4. If possibility of body fluid or blood splashing, facial protection must be provided by health care facility and used by phlebotomist.
5. Accidental needlesticks must be avoided. NO RECAPPING BY HAND! Use resheathing device and/or rigid needle container for disposal.
6. Do not handle any needles.
7. All sharps, including lancets must be disposed of CAREFULLY in rigid needle container.
8. Perform proper biohazardous disposal of patient's blood collection items.
9. Avoid mouth-to-mouth resuscitation contact.
10. A personal respirator should be used if possible exposure to aerosolized *Mycobacterium tuberculosis*.
11. THINK to avoid accidental injuries.
12. Decontaminate blood collection devices and surfaces after use.

Fire Extinguishers.   The components of fire are fuel, oxygen, and heat, plus the necessary chain reaction. Four general classifications of fires have been adopted by the National Fire Protection Association.[6] The classifications are

1. *Class A fires,* which occur with ordinary combustible material such as wood, rubbish, paper, cloth, and many plastics
2. *Class B fires,* which occur in a vapor–air mixture over flammable solvents such as gasoline, oil, paint, lacquers, and flammable gases
3. *Class C fires,* which occur in or near electrical equipment
4. *Class D fires,* which occur with combustible metals such as magnesium, sodium, and lithium and are infrequently encountered in health care institutions

Fire extinguishers correspond with each class of fire.

1. *Class A extinguishers.* Soda and acid or water is used to cool the fire.
2. *Class B extinguishers.* Foam, dry chemical, or carbon dioxide are used to combat fires composed of vapor–air mixtures over solvents.
3. *Class C extinguishers.* Dry chemical or carbon dioxide (nonconducting extinguishing agents) can be used to combat electrical fires.
4. *Multipurpose (ABC) extinguishers.* This type of extinguisher is frequently installed in health care institutions because it reduces the confusion that operation and maintenance of various types entail.

Proper Use of Fire Extinguishers

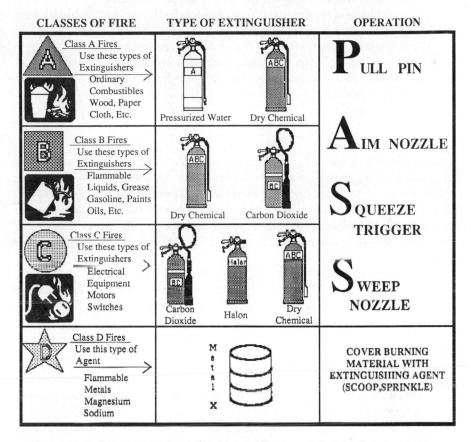

Figure 10–7. Proper use of fire extinguishers. *(Courtesy of Risk Analysis and Loss Control—Institutional Affairs, The University of Texas Houston Health Science Center.)*

As shown in Figure 10–7, the phlebotomist should learn how to use the various kinds of fire extinguishers in the workplace. Use of the wrong type of extinguisher may not only fail to put out the fire but can actually spread it.

Some "do's" and "don'ts" relating to fire safety in health care institutions are[3]:

1. Immediately pull the alarm box located nearest the area you are in.
2. Then call the fire number assigned. It should be posted on or near every phone.

3. If the fire is small, attempt to extinguish it, using the proper extinguisher.
4. Should evacuation be necessary, use only stairwells for exiting.
5. Close all doors and windows before leaving the area.
6. If clothing is on fire, drop to the ground and roll, preferably in a fire blanket.
7. If caught in a fire, crawl to the exit. Because smoke rises, breathing is easier at floor level. Breathing through a wet towel is helpful.
8. Do not block entrances, and do not reenter the building.
9. Do not panic.
10. Do not run.

Electrical Safety

A major hazard in any area of a health care institution is the possibility of electrical current passing through a person. In the clinical laboratory, the phlebotomist sometimes operates electrical equipment such as a centrifuge. He or she should be aware of the location of the circuit breaker boxes in order to assure a fast response during an electrical fire or electrical shock. The phlebotomist should not use electrical equipment if power cords are frayed or if control switches and thermostats are not in good working order.

The centrifuge or other electrical equipment must be unplugged before maintenance is performed. An electrical instrument that has had liquid spilled on or in it or has had liquid come in contact with the wiring should be immediately unplugged and dried out prior to any further use.

If an electrical accident occurs involving electrical shock to some employee or patient, the phlebotomist should be aware of the following:

1. The electrical power source must be shut off. If this is impossible, carefully remove the electrical contact from the victim using something such as asbestos gloves that does not conduct electricity or place one's hand in a glass beaker and push the power supply away from the victim. The rescuer should not attempt to touch the victim without the above precautions!
2. Medical assistance should then be called and cardiopulmonary resuscitation (CPR) started immediately. The victim should not be moved prior to medical assistance. A fire blanket or other warm clothing should be put over the victim to keep him or her warm until medical help arrives.

Radiation Safety

The three cardinal principles in protecting oneself from radiation exposure are time, shielding, and distance. Radiation exposure is cumulative and, thus, the length of exposure at any one time is one major factor in minimizing the

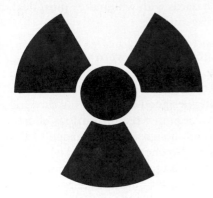

Figure 10–8. Sign for possible radiation hazard.

hazard. Areas where radioactive materials are in use and stored must have warning signs (Fig. 10–8) posted on the entrance doors. All radioactive specimens and reagents must also be properly labeled with the radioactive sign.

Probably the phlebotomist will encounter possible hazards from radiation exposure only if he or she must collect specimens from patients in the nuclear medicine or x-ray departments, or take specimens to the radioimmunoassay section in chemistry. Thus, the phlebotomist should be cautious in entering an area with the radiation sign and be knowledgeable of the institution's procedures pertaining to radiation safety.

Mechanical Safety

Because the centrifuge is probably the most frequently used instrument by the phlebotomist, he or she should learn how to maintain this instrument and become familiar with the parts. For example, the phlebotomist should know if the carriers are in the correct position prior to use. If the carriers are not in the correct position, they can swing out of the holding disks into the side of the centrifuge. Also, the wrong head, wrong cups, or imbalanced tubes can lead to the same dangerous problem. If this particular type of accident occurs, patients' specimens or chemicals that are spinning may be propelled onto the side of the centrifuge, be broken, and create a dangerous, hazardous problem. Thus, it is of utmost importance to abide by the *preventive maintenance* schedule and procedures for the centrifuge.

Chemical Safety

Because the phlebotomist must sometimes pour preservatives such as HCl into containers for 24-hour urine collections and transport these to the patients' floor, he or she should be knowledgeable of *chemical safety.* Labeling may well be the single most important step in the proper handling of chemicals. Laboratorians should be able to ascertain from appropriate labels the contents of the container and the nature and the extent of hazards with which they must deal. Carefully read the label before using any reagents.

Eye Wash and Showers.   The proper clothing must be worn when working with chemicals. A buttoned laboratory coat, safety glasses, and gloves provide protection and prevent skin contact. When transporting acids or alkalis, an "acid carrier" should be used. It is a specially designed container for carrying large quantities of hazardous solutions. Any room in which hazardous chemicals are in use or in storage must have a caution sign at the entrance of the room specifying the type of chemicals present. No chemicals should be stored above eye level, because of the danger of breakage or spillage involved in reaching. All explosives should be stored in an explosion/fireproof room separate from the flammables stored there.

Safety showers should be nearby for use if an accidental chemical spill occurs. Because permanent damage to the skin can result from chemical burns, the victim of a chemical accident must immediately rinse for at least 15 minutes after removing contaminated clothing.

In case of a chemical spill in the eye, the victim should rinse his or her eyes at the eyewash station for a minimum of 15 minutes. Contact lenses must be removed prior to the rinsing in order to thoroughly cleanse the eyes. The victim should not rub the eyes because this may cause further injury. If someone is hurt in a chemical spill, he or she should be taken to the Emergency Department for treatment after rinsing the eyes for 15 minutes.

Chemical Spill.   If a chemical spill occurs, the phlebotomist should obtain a spill clean-up kit from the clinical chemistry section. The kit includes absorbents and neutralizers to clean up acid, alkali, mercury, and other spills. The absorbent and neutralizer used depend upon the type of chemical spill. The absorbent and neutralizer have an indicator system that identifies when the chemical spill has been neutralized and can be considered safe for sweep up and disposal. The phlebotomist should become familiar with the procedures for cleaning up chemical spills in his or her place of employment.

Disposal of Chemicals.   Chemical waste such as acids and alkalis that are soluble in water can be disposed of by flushing them down the sink with cold water. Acids and alkalis should be poured into a large amount of water before flushing down the sink. The acid *must* be added to water and not vice versa to prevent a violent chemical reaction.

Disaster Emergency Plan

Many health care institutions have developed procedures in case of a hurricane, flooding, earthquake, bomb threat, and other disasters. The phlebotomist should become familiar with these procedures because he or she must be prepared for an immediate course of action if conditions warrant it.

EMERGENCY PROCEDURES

The phlebotomist should become knowledgeable of emergency care procedures because accidents do occur even though precautionary measures are in place. He or she must be able to detach him or herself from the emergency situation to a degree in order to perform well and deliver the best possible health care.

In an emergency situation, the following objectives must be met for the victim: prevent severe bleeding, maintain breathing, prevent shock and further injury, and send for medical assistance.

Bleeding Aid

Severe bleeding from an open wound can be controlled by applying pressure directly over the wound. A clean handkerchief or other clean cloth (compress) should be placed over the wound before applying pressure by the hand. In an emergency, in the absence of any clean cloth, the bare hand should be used until a cloth compress becomes available. Bleeding of an extremity such as an arm or leg can be decreased by elevation. The injured portion should be raised above the level of the victim's heart unless the injured portion is broken. However, even with elevation, pressure to the wound should be maintained until medical assistance arrives. A tourniquet should not be used to control bleeding except for an amputated, mangled, or crushed arm or leg, or profuse bleeding that cannot be stopped otherwise.

Breathing Aid

When breathing movements stop or lips, tongue, and fingernails become blue, immediate mouth-to-mouth resuscitation is needed. Delay in using this technique may cost the victim's life. Directions for mouth-to-mouth breathing include the following:

1. See if victim is conscious by *gently* shaking the victim and yelling "ARE YOU OKAY?" If there is a possibility of neck injury, do not shake the victim! If there is no response to the gentle shaking and yelling, call out for help and start aid immediately.
2. First step is to place the victim on his or her back on a firm, flat surface. Caution must be exercised if the person has a spine or neck injury. No twisting should occur to the victim's body.
3. Next, open the airway by checking for obstructions: tongue, chewing gum, vomitus, and so on. Then place one hand on the victim's forehead and, applying firm, backward pressure with the palm, tilt the head back (Figure 10–9). Place the fingers of the other hand under the bony part of the lower jaw near the chin and lift to bring the chin forward with the teeth almost to occlusion. The jaw should be supported as the head is tilted back. This position is called the head-tilt/chin-lift.

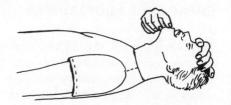

Figure 10–9. Head-tilt/chin-lift for emergency care.

4. Listen and feel for return of air from the victim's mouth and nose for approximately 3 to 5 seconds. Also, at the same time, look for the victim's chest to rise and fall.
5. If there is no breathing, maintain the head-tilt/chin-lift and pinch the victim's nose shut with the hand to prevent air from escaping. Open mouth widely, take a deep breath and seal mouth over the victim's mouth (Fig. 10–10). Blow into victim's mouth. Watch for the victim's chest to rise. (If it does not, airway is blocked and must be cleared.)
6. Give two full ventilations. If this still does not start an air exchange, reposition the head and try again. After two more ventilations, again look, listen, and feel for breathing. Improper chin and head positioning is the most common cause of difficulty with ventilation.

Circulation Aid

In order to maintain circulation in a victim, the phlebotomist must know the techniques of basic cardiopulmonary resuscitation (CPR). Thus, he or she should check with the supervisor about the availability of CPR classes at the health care institution because this emergency technique has to be demonstrated to the learner for proper skills to be obtained.

Preventing Shock

Shock usually accompanies severe injury. It may result from bleeding, extensive burns, insufficient supply of O_2, and other traumatic events. Early signs include pale, cold, and clammy skin, weakness, rapid pulse, increased and shallow breathing rate, and, frequently, nausea and vomiting.

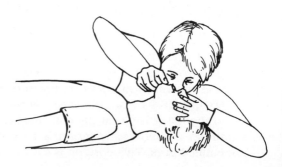

Figure 10–10. Breathing aid in emergency situation.

The main objectives in treating a shock victim are to improve circulation, provide sufficient oxygen, and maintain normal body temperature.

The following actions are recommended if first aid is given to a shock victim.

1. Correct the cause of shock if possible (e.g., control bleeding).
2. Keep victim lying down.
3. Keep the victim's airway open. If he or she vomits, turn head to the side so that the neck is arched.
4. In the absence of broken bones, elevate the victim's legs so that the head is lower than the trunk of the body.
5. Keep the victim warm.
6. Call for emergency assistance.

Actions that are definitely *NOT* recommended include

1. Do not give fluids to a victim who has abdominal injury; the person is likely to require surgery or a general anesthetic.
2. Do not give fluids to an unconscious or semiconscious person.

KEY TERMS

bedside glucose testing	designated delivery times	quality control
bleeding aid	g value	radiation safety
breathing aid	mechanical safety	revolutions per minute (RPM)
centrifuge	preventing shock	tachometer
chemical safety	preventive	
circulation aid	maintenance	
collection log	quality assurance	

STUDY QUESTIONS

The following questions may have one or more answers.

1. A fasting blood specimen for glucose analysis is collected in the morning rather than at a random collection time for which of the following reasons?

   a. To avoid the effects of exercise.
   b. To avoid the effects of changes in posture.
   c. To enhance the effects of diurnal variation.
   d. To enhance the phlebotomist's schedule.

2. A fasting blood specimen is needed for which of the following clinical laboratory assays?

a. complete blood count (CBC)   c. cholesterol
b. triglyceride   d. glucose

3. Which of the following instruments are usually in the specimen control area and must have preventive maintenance and quality control checks?

a. blood gas analyzer   c. centrifuge
b. thermometer   d. sphygmomanometer

4. If a fire occurs in or near electrical equipment, which of the following fire extinguishers should be used?

a. class A extinguisher   c. class C extinguisher
b. class B extinguisher   d. ABC extinguisher

5. What are the major principles in protecting oneself from radiation exposure?

a. distance   c. combustibility
b. time   d. shielding

REFERENCES

1. Standard for Evacuated Tubes for Blood Specimen Collection: NCCLS Approved Standards, 3rd ed. Villanova, Penn., National Committee for Clinical Laboratory Standards, 1991.
2. Reller LB, Murray PR, MacLowray JD, et al: Blood Cultures II. Cumitech 1A. Washington DC, American Society for Microbiology, 1982.
3. Lorimor K, Collins F: Monitoring quality control in the clinical laboratory, in Becan-McBride K (ed): *Textbook of Clinical Laboratory Supervision.* New York, Appleton-Century-Crofts, 1982.
4. National Committee for Clinical Laboratory Standards: Procedures for the Handling and Processing of Blood Specimens, H18-T. Villanova, Penn., NCCLS, 1984.
5. Department of Labor, Occupational Safety and Health Administration. Occupational exposure to bloodborne pathogens; final rule (29 CFR 1910.1030). *Federal Register,* Dec. 6, 1991, pp. 64004–64182.
6. National Fire Protection Association: National Fire Codes—Vol. 1. Quincy, MA: National Fire Protection Association, 1990.
7. Nelson JC: How to get the best service from a referral laboratory. *MLO* Aug 1991, pp 63–69.

11 Liability and Risk Management

GENERAL LEGAL PRINCIPLES

The laws governing medicine and medical ethics complement and overlap each other. For many years, even centuries, the decision of the physician or health care professional was unquestioned. This has changed. Health care consumers and patients have become more aware, more critical, and much more willing to sue anyone that their lawyer feels has been at fault, including phlebotomists.

In reality, the legal system in the United States has 52 systems. Each state, the District of Columbia, and the Federal Government have separate systems. The courts are places where disputes are settled by judicial decision. Both federal and state courts generally have three levels.

1. Trial courts—some have limited and some have wide jurisdiction.
2. Intermediate—are generally courts of appeal.
3. Supreme court—of each state and of the federal system will hear only specific cases.

General state courts hear more serious civil cases in which damages of over $10,000 are in suit and in criminal actions. The law can be viewed as a system of social control,[1] or the law can be described as common sense influenced by political and public policy considerations. Lawyers have become advisors to health care professionals and institutions in matters ranging from termination of treatment to approval of experimental protocols. Some lawyers specialize in hospital law or food and drug law; personal injury lawyers handle malpractice claims, and others are especially knowledgeable about Medicaid and Worker's Compensation benefits. No lawyer can master all of these areas. William J. Curran defined "health law" as a "speciality area of law and law practice related to the medical and other health fields—such as dentistry, nursing, hospital administration, and environmental law."[1]

Legal Terminology

To grasp the legal implication of health care, some knowledge of basic terminology is important. A few major definitions follow.[1,2]

Assault. The unjustifiable attempt to touch another person or the threat to do so in such circumstances as to cause the other to believe that it will be carried out, or to cause fear.

Battery. The intentional touching of another person without consent; unlawful beating of another, or the carrying out of threatened physical harm.

Breach of duty. An infraction, violation, or failure to perform.

Civil law. Not a criminal action; the plaintiff sues for monetary damages.

Consent. Legal authorization to perform medical procedures or provide care.

Criminal actions. Deal with the acts or offenses against the public welfare; can lead to imprisonment.

Defendant. The health care provider against whom the action or law suit is filed.

False imprisonment. The unjustifiable detention of a person without a legal warrant.

Felony. Varies by state but generally is defined as public offenses where, if defendant is convicted, he will spend time in jail or prison.

Invasion of privacy. The physical intrusion upon a person; the publishing of confidential information, though true, but of such objectionable or personal nature as to be offensive.[3]

Liable. Under legal obligation, as far as damages are concerned.

Litigation Process. The process of legal action to determine a decision in court. Many malpractice cases are negotiated and settled out of court.

Malpractice. Improper or unskillful care of a patient by a member of the health care team or any professional misconduct, unreasonable lack of skill, or fidelity in professional or judiciary duties.

Misdemeanor. The general term for all sorts of criminal offenses not serious enough to be classified as a felony.

Negligence. Failure to act or perform duties according to standards of the profession.[4]

Plaintiff. The claimant who brings a lawsuit or action.

Respondeat superior. The concept whereby actions of one individual may be imputed to another person having control. This suggests that a technician's negligent act can be imputed to a laboratory corporation. Under this concept, supervisors and directors may be held liable for the negligent actions of their employees. This concept is also referred to as *vicarious liability.*

Tort. A legal wrong in which the person who commits it is liable for damages in civil action.

Negligence.   In the past decade there has been a noticeable increase in the number of legal cases in which the laboratory is directly or indirectly involved. Negligence is "a violation of a duty to exercise reasonable skill and care in performing a task." There are four factors or key points that must be considered in alleged negligence cases.[2,4]

1. *Duty*—relates to what duties or responsibilities the hospital or health care worker had toward the patient; also includes all the individuals who had a duty toward the patient.
2. *Breach of duty*—relates to whether or not the duty was breached and if it was avoidable.
3. *Proximate causation*—relates to whether or not the breach of duty actually contributed to or caused injury; also concerns all the parties involved in contributing to the alleged injury.
4. *Damages*—relates to whether or not the plaintiff was actually injured and when these injuries were discovered.

There are many circumstances that could be considered negligence if phlebotomists are not extremely careful. There have been legal cases in which confusion of patient samples led to a patient's death.[3] Misidentification of patient's sample for sexually transmitted disease studies has also led to legal action.[5]

Patient Confidentiality.   Negligence cases can also arise out of violation of the right to privacy. "No one except the patient may release patient results without a clinical need to know."[4] Patient or employee laboratory results must be considered *strictly* confidential. Negligence can be sought if employees' or patients' drug abuse results are released to anyone other than the attending physician or other authorized individuals. This is particularly true when referring to employee or athlete drug or alcohol abuse screening and for HIV testing. Confidential materials include communications between the physician and the patient, the patient's verbal statements, and nonverbal communications such as laboratory test results.

Malpractice.   The relationship between doctor and patient is, in the legal sense, a contractual one. The basic elements involved are common with other contracts. The elements of contracts are:

Offer. The physician offers to provide service either by opening an office or being on a hospital staff or both. Thus he or she has made herself available to patients who seek care.

Acceptance. The patient visits the physician for treatment of a disease or disorder and may agree to accept medical care.

Consideration. The patient accepts treatment and pays for the care provided by the physician.[6]

By completing these steps, there is a contract that implies obligations on the part of *both* the physician and the patient. The physician is obligated to provide medical care to the patient if he or she follows directions and pays for the service. There is even a question about the length of grace period in terms of payment. Also, the patient generally has to refuse treatment before the physician is legally freed from his or her obligation. By agreeing to provide service, the physician is required to provide a standard of care.

If the physician is a pathologist and medical director of a medical clinical laboratory, in most cases he or she is responsible under the law for the standard of care and performance of the laboratory staff. Therefore, a breach of standard on the part of a phlebotomist could place both pathologist and phlebotomist at risk.

The trend toward medical malpractice is not as new as most people seem to believe. The first case was reported in London in the 1300s. In the 1850s, Abraham Lincoln tried and won three medical malpractice cases before he was elected President. It is estimated that 5 to 10 percent of the physicians in the United States are involved in medical malpractice lawsuits, that is, negligence cases. Malpractice, in the usual sense, implies that the health care provider did something wrong; it usually involves improper or unskilled care where the practitioner has not exercised judgment or performed to the expected standard of care.

Physicians, however, do not guarantee cures, only treatment or therapy. The patient bringing the lawsuit (plaintiff) must have been injured or damaged by the health care professional's breach of duty (failure to use standard of care). Damage or injury may be either physical, mental, or financial.

Informed Consent.   If the patient requires treatment that is of potential risk, the physician must explain risks and alternatives prior to asking the patient to sign an "Informed Consent" form. This form is required for surgical, experimental, or other invasive procedures. Health care providers have become more cognizant of informed consent principles since this is the largest area of litigation.[2] This is one reason the phlebotomist should state in simple terms what the procedure for blood collection will be. Under the law, there are special consent rules for children, unconscious adults, and emergency situations.

Expert Witnesses. For a jury of laypeople to judge negligence, they must hear from expert witnesses concerning practice patterns and levels of skill. To win the case, the patient's expert witness must be willing to testify in court that the defendant health care professional was negligent, that is, that he or she did not provide the standard of care that other physicians of that speciality in that community would provide.[1] In the *Small* v. *Howard* case in 1880, the court ruled that a village practitioner would be required to have only knowledge and skills of other practitioners in "similar localities." This rule of community standard held until *Brune* v. *Belinoff,* in which the court held that all specialists in anesthesiology should be aware of advanced practices of their profession regardless of location.[6]

MEDICAL RECORDS

Medical records are vital. A phlebotomist or any other member of the health care team cannot be expected to remember a patient from whom blood was drawn 3 to 4 years ago. The medical records must be neat, legible, and accurate. They are extremely important if a medical malpractice case goes to court. Medical records have 4 basic purposes:[2]

1. Allows for continuity of patient's care plan.
2. Provides document of the patient's illness and treatment.
3. Documents communication between the physician and the health care team.
4. Provides a legal document that can be used by patients, hospital, or health care workers to protect their legal interests.

Medical records are also used for nonmedical reasons that are not directly tied to medical services such as billing, utilization review, quality improvement, and so on. It is important to remember that many cases are not in the literature because often the health care institution or health care provider negotiates, arbitrates, and settles out of court.

However, the following are cases that are of interest for laboratorians:

1. *Requests by police.* Nurses, technologists, and phlebotomists are concerned about drawing a blood sample when requested by police on an unconscious patient or lacking the patient's consent. The United States Supreme Court ruled in *Schmerber* v. *State of California* that tests performed on a blood sample drawn by a physician in a hospital from a person arrested by the police were admissible in a court action.[6] This may vary by state.

2. *Laboratory report case.* A patient who was pregnant for the first time had her blood typed in January 1971. The report sent to her physician was that her blood type was A-positive. The patient gave birth to her second child on June 29, 1977. The child was brain damaged with paralysis on the right side of the body as a result of hemolytic blood disease of the newborn. The laboratory records in 1971 and 1977 showed the mother's blood type to be O-negative. In a malpractice suit, the parents charged that the physician's and his employees' negligence caused the child's injuries. The physician who was chief of the laboratory when the blood test was performed was found liable, as was the phlebotomist. *Lazernick* v. *General Hospital of Monroe County* (PA 1977).[7]

3. *Respondeat superior or vicarious liability.* The doctrine of *respondeat superior* is applied to employees. Even though the employer is liable for the employee, both can and generally will be sued. The plaintiff's lawyers generally go after the employer because of the possibility of a larger settlement. However, employers may be cleared, leaving the employee to stand or fall alone. In the mind of some professionals, the *deep pockets concept* tends to minimize the risk for laboratory employees. Generally, organizations and individuals best able to pay are the most likely candidates for suit. Job descriptions that commonly define laboratorians' duties as administrative and procedural rather than judgmental have kept technicians, technologists, and phlebotomists at low legal exposure levels.

4. *Proper technique is vital.* A malpractice suit was filed against a physician for negligence in drawing a blood sample. The patient claimed that the physician damaged the radial nerve of the right wrist by failing to use a sterile needle for blood specimen collection. The site of venipuncture became swollen, tender, and inflamed. The patient testified that the needle was laid near a used tongue depressor. The same needle was used for several attempts to redraw. The patient, after retrial, was awarded monetary damages. *McCormick* v. *Auret* (GA 1980).

5. *Proper use of equipment.* A patient was admitted for treatment of pneumonia. On the second day, the patient complained of cold and numbness in his right hand. On the fourth day, a vascular surgeon examined the hand and ordered 4000 U of heparin in hopes of restoring blood flow. The hand had to be amputated. In court, the expert witness testified that a blood pressure cuff had been left on for an extended period. He was awarded $40,000. *Walton* v. *Providence Hospital.*[6]

6. *Consent to treatment.* The US District Court for the Southern District of Texas upheld a state judge in ordering temporary removal of an infant from her parents' custody to that of a child welfare unit and empowering the unit to provide necessary emergency medical treatment. The parents, who were Jehovah's Witnesses, refused to consent

to a blood transfusion needed because of the Rh-negative factor in their child's blood. The court said that the parents could not choose to make martyrs of their children. *Lacy* v. *Judge Robert Lowry.* Harris County Hospital district.[9]

7. *Confidentiality.* Blood bank laboratories are continually faced with problems regarding notification of donors, patients, or both who have given or received blood that is positive for the human immunodeficiency virus (HIV). In addition, there have been cases in litigation where blood from a seronegative donor transmitted AIDS. However, one must continually remember that results of these tests must be considered *strictly* confidential.

8. *Drug screening for employees and athletes.* Many sports associations and major companies are requiring urine drug screens for athletes and employees. Oftentimes this is without prior notice and therefore the procedures for specimen collection, processing, analysis, and reporting results can be very strict and well defined. The National Institute on Drug Abuse (*NIDA*) defines requirements for collection, processing, and testing. The following steps are usually involved:

   a. Sterile, airtight specimen containers that can be sealed are strongly recommended. Special preservatives may be required for the analyses.

   b. A "proctor" should be present during the urine collection process to ensure that the specimen was obtained from the appropriate person. Specialized facilities should be maintained for specimen collection, particularly for urine collections.

   c. The specimen must be properly labeled to establish a "*chain of custody.*" A split sample may be required for parallel testing, confirmation, or both.

   d. Specimens should be sealed and locked in a transport container during transfer from the collection site to the testing site to prevent tampering.

   e. Careful documentation of who received the specimen must be maintained. The number of personnel handling the specimen should be minimized.

Phlebotomists who are involved in the specimen collection process must adhere to every detail of established procedures to avoid anything that would jeopardize the validity of results. This is also true with specimens collected as a result of criminal or forensic investigations.

MALPRACTICE INSURANCE

Since hospitals are places where seriously ill patients are admitted and treated with highly sophisticated medical technology, the likelihood for problems is greater here than in other health care settings. Often, the health care staff in the hospital or clinic laboratory are part of a blanket malpractice insurance policy. However, if the phlebotomist is employed by a pathologist who has a contract with an institution or owns a clinic, the staff may be protected by the pathologist's malpractice insurance policy.

Malpractice insurance rates for pathologists are generally the lowest premiums charged because of their low risk level. At the bench and administrative levels, laboratories have rarely been named in malpractice suits. Part of the reason for so few cases is that under the legal concept of respondeat superior, responsibility for wrongful acts of the employee (agent–servant) rests on the employer (principal–master). Also, another reason for not being named in a suit is the "deep pocket" concept. The phlebotomist with less money or no insurance in the past has not been a target for suit. However, the advances in technology and increased complexity of health care have increased legal exposure for allied health professionals. Often, laboratorians feel safe from legal responsibilities because of limited interaction with patients. However, the phlebotomist and any other staff member that routinely deals with the public in patient–health provider relationships are indeed liable. Therefore, each individual should examine the possibility of malpractice suits and the need for malpractice insurance from a personal standpoint.[8]

If the phlebotomist decides to purchase malpractice insurance, there are several factors that should be carefully considered.

1. Is adequate dollar value coverage provided? Recent lawsuits have totaled $1,000,000 damages against physicians.
2. What are the limitations of coverage?
3. What are the procedures that must be followed for the policy to provide coverage? Some state that divulging the amount of coverage or the fact that he is covered voids the policy.
4. The phlebotomist should not assume that the lawyers representing the hospital, laboratory, or clinic will have his or her best interests at heart. The attorney's first obligation is to serve those who have hired him or her. There have been cases in which the hospital was cleared of all charges but the allied health professional was held liable for damages. For the phlebotomist, if an adult patient seems alert and does not object to the blood specimen collection, then consent is implied. Proceeding without consent may give rise to assault and battery, as well as civil suits.

With the purchase of malpractice professional liability insurance, the attorney's fee and court costs usually are covered. Some of the professional organizations offer professional liability insurance at a reasonable or reduced rate. With the advent of organ transplantations, renal dialysis, and hyperbaric care, the avenues of liability are widened. A genuine concern for others and careful attention to technique are good investments of the phlebotomist's time. A record of continuing education courses, seminars, workshops, or academic credits should be a part of each phlebotomist's personal file.

MANAGEMENT OF RISK

Concepts of Risk

Risk can be described as "exposure to the chance of injury or loss."[2] There are many risks facing health care workers on a daily basis. It is important for phlebotomists, supervisors, and managers to reflect on their personal risk and that of their employers. Active steps should be taken to understand risk factors and minimize areas of risk for the benefit of patients and protection of employees and employers. Risk can be managed using carefully planned objectives that can be categorized as preloss (to reduce or prevent losses) and postloss (how the facility can recover from a loss). The goals and objectives of the institution or department can guide the risk management program. A generic model of *risk management* might involve the following levels:[2,10]

- *Risk identification and analysis*—analysis and measurement of identified risks.
- *Risk treatment*—use of tools (safety manuals, policies and procedures, public relations tactics) to prevent harm or losses.
- *Education*—of patients, employees, and visitors.
- *Risk transfer or postponement*—shift risk to other parties (liability insurance, contract services, and employees).
- *Risk evaluation*—assessment of what should be done.

One way to identify risk is to review "*incident*," "*accident*," or "occurrence" reports that involve laboratory or phlebotomy services. Employees must be continually encouraged to use these tools because without an effective reporting system, proper investigations and risk assessments cannot be made. An "incident" or "occurrence" does not have to result in injury. The older term "accident report" is not often used anymore because it implies that an error occurred, which may not always be the case. Trends of events that deviate from normal, but fortunately do not harm any patients are most revealing and controllable.

Risk treatment has two elements, loss/risk control, and risk financing.[2] Loss/risk control means that the department should attempt to reduce the frequency of errors or events that can potentially cause financial loss. Similar to quality improvement programs, the aim would be to reduce adverse outcomes such as excessive venipunctures on the same patients, reducing the number of hematomas, and so on. Risk financing refers to how to pay for losses once they have occurred (liability insurance or other means). If a patient faints during venipuncture and injures himself, care should be taken to assist and provide free services for the person to recover. Documentation should clearly indicate the details of the accident and each step of the follow-up.

Education and communication are also vital to the risk management process. If employees do not know about new procedures, they cannot be expected to follow them.

TABLE 11–1. TIPS FOR MINIMIZING RISK

Follow up on all incident reports.
Participate in continuing education.
Know the extent of liability coverage.
Provide highly professional, courteous behavior.
Follow established procedures.
Maintain documentation.
Obtain proper consent.

Risk transfer through the use of liability insurance is also an important part of the risk management process. Contracting for services has also traditionally shifted some of the liability to other parties. However, federal and state laws are changing to include contract personnel and contract services (i.e., laboratory reference labs, diagnostic radiology services) under the respondeat superior concept. This would suggest that health care facilities might be held liable for services performed by those with whom they have contracts.

Evaluation of all the elements of risk management above may show a need for changes in procedures, employee counseling, or educational programs. Table 11–1 indicates some commonsense tips for minimizing risk in a phlebotomy setting.[2,10]

KEY TERMS

accident	deep pocket concept	misdemeanor
assault	defendant	negligence
battery	felony	NIDA
breach of duty	incident	plaintiff
chain of custody	informed consent	respondeat superior
civil law	invasion of privacy	risk management
confidentiality	liable	tort
criminal action	malpractice	

STUDY QUESTIONS

1. Describe the four factors that are considered in negligence cases.
2. Define the following terms: informed consent, invasion of privacy, liable, malpractice.
3. Describe the basic purposes of the medical record.
4. Explain the generic model of risk management.

REFERENCES

1. Curran WJ: Titles in the medicolegal field: A proposal for reform. *Am J Law Med* 1:10, 1975.
2. Troyer GT, Salman SL: *Handbook of Health Care Risk Management,* Rockville, Md., Aspen Publications, 1986.
3. *Parker* v. *Port Huron Hospital,* 105, N.W. 2d 854 (1981).
4. Steindel SJ: Legal issues associated with physicians office testing. *J Med Technol* 4(3), 104, 1987.
5. *Hensley* v. *Heavrin,* 282 S.E. 2d 854 (1981).
6. Creighton H: *Law Every Nurse Should Know,* 4th ed, W.B. Saunders, Philadelphia, 1981.
7. *Lazernick* v. *General Hospital of Monroe County* (PA1977).
8. Zeiler WB: How your laboratory can minimize malpractice risks, *MLO,* May 1982.
9. *Lacy* v. *Judge Robert Lowry,* Harris County Hospital District, et al, USDT No 74H-124, Mar 16, 1977.
10. Bunting RF: Risk management and prevention in the clinical laboratory. *Clin Lab Science,* 5:1, 35–37, Jan/Feb 1992.

12 Management, Strategic Planning, and Education

CHAPTER OUTLINE

The health care system is changing rapidly because of the dynamics of financial reimbursement, changing demographics and patient populations, and shifts from inpatient to ambulatory settings and home health care. As a result, health care professionals must be knowledgeable of trends and how to make managerial and operational adjustments that do not compromise quality but are cost effective. Health care facilities continue to face pressures to reduce costs and improve services. Managers and supervisors must know how to guide their staff through frequent and often difficult changes.

Management has been described as a dynamic process. When applied to phlebotomy services, it has both technical and interpersonal components. Objectives of the clinical laboratory are accomplished through appropriate practices and human resource use.

Management process includes, but is not limited to, the following functions:[1]

- *Planning*—short and long range.
- *Organizing*—human resources (recruitment, training, retention).
- *Decision making*—assessing options and exploring opportunities.
- *Motivating and providing feedback*—effectively communicating and implementing policies and procedures.
- *Establishing standards*—policies and procedures.
- *Evaluation*—assessing successes/failures.

There are many management theories that describe supervisory styles of managers. Generally, these depict management styles as points on a continuum or in a matrix. For example, Figure 12–1 depicts decision-making styles; at one end of the spectrum is the democratic style and at the other end is the autocratic style.

The democractic style relates to having groups make their own decisions as a concensus. The autocratic end is exemplified by the managers who make all decisions themselves and dictate policy or decision results to subordinates. In reality, laboratory supervisors should create a flexible environment whereby decisions can be made by one individual if time and circumstances do not allow consensus building. An example would be for authorization of an emergency request that calls for special handling. On the other hand, if employees

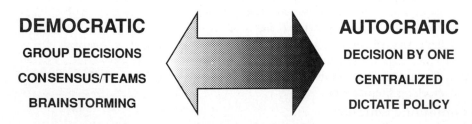

DEMOCRATIC		AUTOCRATIC
GROUP DECISIONS		DECISION BY ONE
CONSENSUS/TEAMS		CENTRALIZED
BRAINSTORMING		DICTATE POLICY

Figure 12–1. Decision-making continuum.

TABLE 12-1. POSITIVE TRAITS OF EMPLOYEES AND SUPERVISORS

Communicates positively
Helps people
Communicates with credibility
Demonstrates proficiency and competence
Takes pride in work and accomplishments
Conveys a positive impression
Works effectively with co-workers
Maintains eye contact with patients
Makes good use of verbal and nonverbal skills
Displays excellent attention to technique
Constantly sharpens and updates skills
Remains calm in difficult situations
Follows up on assignments
Is dependable and punctual
Is conscientious and prepared
Shows flexibility in decision making
Is self-motivated
Is trustworthy
Is ethical

are allowed to participate in decisions and planning, they are more likely to be motivated to support the resulting product. Other positive characteristics of a well-rounded employee and supervisor are suggested in Table 12-1.

The specimen collection or phlebotomy unit provides the interface between physicians, patients, nurses and the administrative and technical units of the clinical laboratory. Therefore effective management, planning, and educational objectives for phlebotomy services are vital to the success of any health care facility. This chapter will cover basic management concepts as applied to phlebotomy services, key functions of strategic planning, and strategies for phlebotomy educational opportunities.

MANAGEMENT OVERVIEW

Management of phlebotomy services involves a technical component and a nontechnical component. A successful manager will set objectives for her/himself and seek to accomplish them within targeted time periods by involving, teaching, or managing other people (Table 12-2). Objectives can be set for groups or individuals. All objectives should be reasonable, attainable, measurable, acceptable, and understandable and should involve people. The technical components involve the use of correct procedures and practices so that complications or laboratory testing errors do not result. The nontechnical components can relate to minimizing risk, interpersonal communication, and professionalism.

TABLE 12–2. OBJECTIVES OF A HOSPITAL PHLEBOTOMY UNIT

It is the goal of the Department of Laboratory Medicine to establish a service program in support of hospital policy that will enable it to provide experienced technicians in patient care areas to provide the following services:

1. To draw and collect clinical specimens as required by the responsible physicians, to facilitate both the diagnoses and treatments of our patients.
2. To provide a liaison service between the responsible physician and the Department of Laboratory Medicine with regard to the scope and level of services available.
3. To deliver specimens to the appropriate laboratory section, and to promptly communicate results of examinations performed.
4. To maintain respect for the dignity and feelings of all patients.
5. Under the direction of the responsible physician or nurse, to aid in the delivery of patient care as required.

Adapted from Division of Laboratory Medicine, The University of Texas, M.D. Anderson Cancer Center, Houston, Texas.

Four major objectives of specimen collection identified by Lorimor and Collins are:[2]

1. Specimens are collected from the proper patient.
2. Specimens are properly identified with the correct information.
3. The necessary specimens are collected in the appropriate containers, in sufficient amounts, and with proper technique.
4. Specimens are available in the laboratory at a time that allows maximum efficiency in determining the result.

An example of the objectives of a phlebotomy unit in a large hospital is given in Table 12–2.

In planning a phlebotomy unit, the goals and mission of the hospital, agency, clinic, or company must be considered first. Generally, those goals start with a statement such as "provide efficient and effective patient care" with the understanding that if this goal is met, the corresponding reward of recognition, status, and financial solvency or gain will also be achieved. However, the manager of the phlebotomy unit looks beyond this type of goal or mission to more specific ones that may or may not be recorded as those of the institution. For example, some health care institutions also have research and educational goals as well as those of patient care. Prior to setting objectives for the phlebotomy unit there are many pieces of information that the manager needs. Most of this information may be obtained by investigating the environment in which the unit operates. The persons who can furnish this information are those who direct the hospital, who own the facility, who direct the patients to the unit (physicians), and who serve the patients (medical technologists, nurses, dieticians, and other health personnel).

STRATEGIC PLANNING

Planning with Administrators

Prior to beginning any planning session, accurate information is needed. Senior administrators may be the best sources for the following information:

1. The source and number of patients needing the services of the phlebotomy unit (e.g., inpatients, outpatients, patients from health promotional programs in industry, physician-requested analyses on individual patients, or patients in mass screening programs). If the directors or owners do not have this information, it may be necessary to ask physicians, administrators in other settings, directors of the health promotion programs in industry, or directors of the mass screening programs. This type of information is useful in planning for equipment, supplies, and personnel for a phlebotomy team.

2. The age and sex distribution of the bed patients (inpatients) and ambulatory patients (outpatients). The type of phlebotomy equipment and the scheduling may be dictated by the location of the phlebotomy unit (e.g., in a children's hospital, a nursing home, a women's hospital with primarily obstetric cases).

3. The socioeconomic, religious, and/or ethnic background of the patients. Special communication skills and considerations by the phlebotomist may be necessary for a specific population of patients.

4. The proportion of inpatients to ambulatory patients. This information is useful in planning for personnel and space requirements of the unit. If patients are to come to the phlebotomy unit, consideration should be made on the space and furniture arrangement to accommodate all types of patients, including the physically handicapped.

5. Availability of space and proximity of the phlebotomy unit to the laboratory that is to perform the analyses on these specimens. Some phlebotomy units in hospitals are responsible for distributing the specimens to the various laboratories: microbiology, chemistry, serology, hematology, clinical microscopy, blood bank, or specialty reference laboratories across the city or out of the city. This information is important in planning transportation time, specimen preservation techniques, the number of personnel needed to transport the specimens to the laboratories, the need for mailing containers, and special mailing or shipping instructions for specimens.

6. The availability of a computer to maintain data files on the patients, their physicians, names and addresses, the date and time of specimen collections, and transportation of specimens. Often, in a hospital setting the collecting lists of patients, names of tests, patients' room numbers, and specimen labels are generated by a computer. The inventory

of supplies, collection schedules, and other administrative uses of the computer add to the efficiency of the phlebotomy unit.

7. What types of computer systems are being planned for the future, e.g., hospital information systems, laboratory information systems, or PC networks.

Planning with Doctors, Nurses, Laboratory Personnel, and Other Allied Health Professionals

When the phlebotomy unit is placed in a hospital or a matrix environment of other professionals who are performing a service to the same patients and specimens, it is important to learn about their expectations of the phlebotomy unit.

The doctors, nurses, respiratory therapists, radiographers, and physical therapists require time with the patient. It is not uncommon for the phlebotomist to arrive at a patient's room to find that the patient has been transported to the x-ray department or is out of the room for physical therapy. On other occasions, the physician or nurse may be changing a dressing or working with the patient in a way that makes it impossible for the phlebotomist to perform his or her job. Identifying a protocol for these situations helps avoid conflict.

Some physicians have certain protocols for their patients. For example, a presurgical protocol may include the following tests: prothrombin time, partial thromboplastin time, blood count, and urinalysis. Another physician may require additional laboratory tests. It is useful to learn from the physicians which types of patients they expect the phlebotomy unit to serve and which kinds of test batteries they usually request. This information provides some indication of the time required to collect the specimens and the kinds of collecting tubes and supplies that are necessary. The medical specialties of the physicians (e.g., pediatrics, oncology, obstetrics, infectious disease) indicate to some extent the types of supplies that are needed. The planning of a phlebotomy unit is improved if the kinds of specimens can be anticipated.

Medical technologists in clinical laboratories begin to prepare for the analysis of specimens as early as 6:00 or 7:00 AM. They usually expect the phlebotomy specimens to arrive at 8:00 AM or as early as 7:30 AM. It is necessary to coordinate the phlebotomist's schedule with the other health care responsibilities.

Food service schedules by the dietary service are important to know so that fasting specimens can be collected before the patient's meal tray arrives. A frequent complaint by patients is that their meal trays are delayed or their food becomes cold while they await the phlebotomist.

Coordination of the schedules and expectations of the other health professionals is important to the planning of a phlebotomy unit. After considering the information that can be obtained in advance, the objectives of the phlebotomy unit are outlined and recorded.

Scheduling should be done by supervisors in a fair and consistent manner for all employees. There are several computerized scheduling systems that can be used routinely to schedule full- and part-time employees. If the computerized versions are not available, there are scheduling boards similar to bulletin boards with columns and rows that correspond to times, dates, and people. Even a simple matrix on paper with time slots and weekdays can suffice as a schedule. Sometimes it is cost beneficial for the health care facility to have people on-call, particularly for evenings, nights, weekends, and holidays. This usually relates to people who are not paid unless they come into work. However, supervisors should be advised of state and federal laws that govern the amount of responsibility the health care facility has on private lives of employees, even if they are on-call.

Planning for Staff

The *staffing* of a phlebotomy unit depends upon the factors discussed above. Unless the duties of the phlebotomy section are assumed by evening and night personnel of the clinical laboratory or another unit, staffing for 24 hours is necessary in a hospital setting. Most specimens are collected in the morning; therefore, the largest staff is usually required at that time. However, if a large surgical patient population is served and these patients are admitted for pre surgical workup in the afternoon, the phlebotomy staff would need to accommodate these patients.

In order to maintain a core of staff and also meet increased workloads at these certain hours, some phlebotomy units employ a core of full-time equivalents, full-time employees (FTEs) and several part-time employees at the peak hours. A method for estimating the number of needed personnel is given later in the discussion of budget preparation.

In many hospitals with large trauma centers or emergency rooms, a phlebotomist may be stationed in that area to provide a liaison to the laboratory and to handle the large volume of specimens to be collected there. Phlebotomists may be regularly assigned to a specific patient unit so that the rapport with the patients, nurses, and physicians is strengthened and an effective communication within the laboratory exists.

Thus, phlebotomy staffing requirements depend on:

1. Volume of specimens to be drawn
2. Permanent assignment of phlebotomists on daily assignments
3. The number of times that blood collections are made on any one floor or patient unit
4. Other duties of phlebotomists besides collecting blood, for example, collecting other specimens from the patient unit (cultures, urines, etc.), discussing specimen collections that require special information, interpreting the phlebotomy procedure book, or transmittal of specimens from the phlebotomy unit to the laboratories for analyses

5. The special nature of the patient population (e.g., children, burn patients)

The qualifications of the employees of the phlebotomy unit need to be determined. These qualifications are best based on job performance requirements and level of expertise and knowledge required for the service that the phlebotomy unit must provide. The personal qualities expected of a phlebotomist are:

1. Neat appearance
2. Confidence
3. Concern for patient
4. Courteousness
5. Adherence to rules of conduct of the department

If phlebotomists who have successfully completed a formal phlebotomy training program are employed, the need for long orientation and instruction periods at the beginning of employment is markedly reduced. In addition, trained or experienced phlebotomists have already made a commitment to this work and are not as subject to leave after a few days of employment as are trainees on the job who had little understanding of the work. If non-English-speaking patients are anticipated, consideration should be given to at least one employee who can converse in those languages. Figure 12–2 depicts a departmental organizational chart for a laboratory service.

Planning for Safety and Quality

Precautions are necessary in handling specimens to prevent the infection of phlebotomists and transmittal from one patient to another. These precautions are similar to those taken in the areas of the clinical laboratory. They include using acceptable biohazard disposable methods and infection control procedures. These safety precautions are discussed in Chapters 3, 6, and 9.

Quality assurance is indeed a significant aspect of managing a phlebotomy unit. The first three categories in which quality control plays a part in the total quality assurance in the clinical laboratory are (1) patient preparation, (2) specimen collection, and (3) the transportation, handling, and processing of

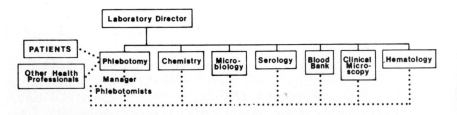

Figure 12–2. Organizational chart for phlebotomy matrix.

specimens.[2] Discussions of quality control requirements for specimen collection are discussed in Chapter 9.

Planning for Space and Facilities

The phlebotomy unit should be readily accessible to ambulatory care facilities, elevators and corridors to inpatient units, and the trauma center. In addition to specimen collection, this division records the requisition, patient data, and information about the patient that are pertinent to the interpretation of test results. Examples of such information are time of last meal, medications, pregnancy, presumptive diagnosis, age, and sex. This concept places the phlebotomy unit as the first data gathering and entry to the information center of the clinical laboratory. Most often this data collection occurs with the use of a computer.

Adequate areas, preferably private cubicles, must be provided for the collection of blood from ambulatory patients. These areas are generally furnished with a table on which to keep collecting supplies and a chair with a specially designed armrest. Cubicles that also accommodate stretchers or wheelchairs should be provided. Many facilities have begun using blood donation chairs for ambulatory phlebotomy services. They are very comfortable and minimize the risk of injury from fainting.

There must also be adequate storage space for phlebotomy supplies, including collecting trays. The disposable nature of most of the supplies of the phlebotomy unit requires the availability of a large storage space. There must be collecting trays for each phlebotomist. The phlebotomist's collecting tray becomes personalized by the individual arrangement of supplies, the cleanness, and orderly stocking of supplies. Few phlebotomists elect to share collecting trays.

The supplies are generally ordered a week or two in advance and an inventory of one week's usage is maintained. Because other departments in the hospital may also use tubes, needles, and phlebotomy supplies, it is necessary that these stocks be kept secure and inventory records be maintained.

Within the phlebotomy or specimen collection unit, the equipment generally required includes refrigerators, centrifuges, sinks (preferably with foot pedals), and puncture-proof biohazard disposal waste containers.

LEADING, ORGANIZING, BUDGETING, AND MONITORING

Leadership

The manager of the phlebotomy unit should act as a leader and role model. He or she needs to have the phlebotomy skills, the time, and the expertise required to manage effectively. He or she should also be expected to serve as a role model in dealing with patients and other health professionals. The leadership qualities of the manager should be expressed tactfully, openly, fairly, and with good humor in dealing with all employees. The basic aspects of leadership include the following:[1]

- Understanding of others
- Respect for others
- Knowledge of situations
- Adaptability/Flexibility
- Enthusiasm
- Objectivity
- Communication skills
- Confidence in oneself and one's subordinates
- Proper use of authority
- Providing recognition
- Courage
- Dependability
- Integrity
- Ethical and moral values

Types of leadership styles have been described by McGregor,[3] Blake and Mouton,[4] and Likert.[5] All have described styles ranging from authoritarian to a more participative management style. The participative type or style of concern for people and production (Blake and Mouton) is generally agreed to be the best leadership approach.[6] In this style, the employees are involved in the planning and organizing of the work. In any case, the manager has the authority and power to assure an acceptable performance by the unit. The judicious and wise use of authority and power are the marks of a good manager.

In managing a phlebotomy unit, it is possible to develop an opportunity for the advancement of those employees who wish to advance. This advancement may be fostered by allowing a change of shift hours or assisting in securing financial assistance for employees to enroll in formal academic courses. Another type of advancement is provided by developing several levels for phlebotomists in the unit. For example, at The University of Texas Cancer Center M.D. Anderson Hospital in Houston, Texas, the phlebotomist with experience or 2 years of formal education is classified as a Laboratory Liaison Technician (LLT). This individual enters a program offered in the hospital that prepares him or her to advise nurses and physicians on the preparation of the patients for laboratory testing and on the interference of some procedures with the laboratory analyses. LLTs have access to patients' charts so that specimen collection can be coordinated with the total health care of the patient. This level of responsibility for phlebotomists has improved the quality of care provided to the patient by eliminating multiple venipunctures and repeat collections and creating an effective working relationship with nurses, physicians, and other allied health professionals.

Organizing

Some of the aspects of managing discussed in the sections on planning are closely related to organizing. The formal organizational structure is representative of the activities and functions necessary to carry out the objectives and goals of the phlebotomy units.

When the phlebotomy unit is in an institution that also has a clinical laboratory, the phlebotomy unit is customarily a part of the clinical laboratory. A formal organization structure is shown in Figure 12–2. The span of supervision and the additional position of an assistant manager of the phlebotomy unit depends upon the skill, knowledge, and experience of the employees and the variety of different tasks these people are expected to perform. The most important resource in accomplishing the objectives of the unit are the employees. It is important in the management operation of monitoring to be certain that each employee fully understands what is expected and the criteria that will be used to evaluate his or her performance.

Schedule of Phlebotomy Collections.   Collections of specimens are usually done at specified times in the hospital. The schedule for the collection of specimens that are to be analyzed that day usually begins with a collection at 7:00 AM followed by others at 11:00 AM, 3:00 PM, and 7:00 PM The early collection gathers specimens that must be collected while the patient is fasting or before surgery. The others provide collection of specimens ordered by the physician after the early collection or after the patient becomes available for specimen collection (e.g., returns from physical therapy). Information gathered by a supervisor of a phlebotomy unit for use in planning, staffing, and scheduling is shown in Table 12–3.

Additional or different collection times may be necessary for critical care units. Individual collection trips are made to patients' rooms, surgery, or emergency or trauma room for emergency (STAT) requests.

One of the most difficult problems facing the director and manager of a phlebotomy unit is to achieve a plan to restrict the designation of STAT to truly life-threatening instances. This type of planning requires the most effective communication and cooperation with the hospital administration and medical staff.

Budgeting

Types of Budgets.   Zero-base budget is one in which all items are justified anew as if no previous budget existed. All items are evaluated and priorities are given. The budget, line by line, is to be justified to the administration. During times of fiscal restraint and possible retrenchment, this type of budget is popular.

Typically, the "forecast budget" has been used in budget preparation. The

TABLE 12-3. AREA HOSPITAL SAMPLE OF PHLEBOTOMY MANAGEMENT CHARACTERISTICS

Institution	Size (beds)	Technologists Collect	Part-time Employees	Mode of Supervision	Comments
A.	270	5 PM–6 PM only	No	Supervisor of Specimen Collection unit	30 daytime technicians, changing shifts and rotations; also staff clinics, do hearing tests, x-rays, and other tests, in addition to blood collection
B.	550	No	Yes	Technical Laboratory sections responsible for own collection	Strict attendance policy; technicians are given some supervisory experience
C.	1200	No	No	Supervisor of Specimen Collection unit	Morning collections: 5 AM–7:30 AM, 9 full-time phlebotomists, no regular collections after morning runs
D.	1200	No	Yes	Supervisor of Specimen Collection unit	10–11 part-time employees, 10 full-time phlebotomists; absenteeism and tardiness are problems
E.	850	Yes 2 per floor	No	Supervisor of Specimen Collection unit	Morning collection at 7 AM–8:30 AM, 15 technologists on patient floors

manager reviews the current budget and adjusts the line item allocations as he or she expects changes to occur over the period of the new budget. The adequacy of the budget prepared in either way is highly dependent upon the information, knowledge, and the synthesis of the information into a scenario involving the phlebotomy unit.

Direct and Indirect Costs.   Costs considered in the preparation of a budget for a phlebotomy unit include direct costs (e.g., supplies, equipment, etc.) and indirect costs. Indirect costs consist of the rental space, laboratory and institutional administrative costs, maintenance and janitorial service, and utilities. These indirect costs are customarily allocated to a department or unit based upon a formula. The formula may use the number of personnel, the square feet serviced, or the number of revenue-producing departments to share the allocation.

Fixed and Variable Costs.   Fixed costs in a budget are those that remain stable over a period of time. These are costs of space, utilities, and administration that do not necessarily fluctuate with a change in workload. The variable costs, which include supplies, change in proportion to the volume of work. Fixed costs are larger because almost two thirds of the fixed costs in a hospital are due to personnel salaries and benefits.

Revenue.   The costs of collecting specimens may or may not be charged as an item to the patient. Generally, it is an addition to the total cost of the analysis to be performed. In some instances when the phlebotomy unit is to collect specimens on a STAT basis or on animals or is to engage in some special screening programs, a charge for the collection is made. The revenue for collecting specimens is anticipated and planned in the overall planning of the clinical laboratory or institutional budget.

Considerations in Budget Preparation.   Customarily, the cost of operating the phlebotomy unit has been allocated among the other accounting centers or units and has not been totally evaluated or financially planned as a separate "cost center" or "revenue center." However, as administrative skills are sharpened and accountability is increased, the identification of costs and the planning of budgets in this unit are going to increase in importance.

The items to be considered in the preparation of a budget for phlebotomy are:[7]

1. Historical workload, volume of specimens and other work to be done
2. The human hours required and the skill level needed
3. Materials, supplies, and outside services
4. Equipment and maintenance
5. Revenue collected and rate setting

Once the budget is prepared, it must be presented to the administration for approval and monitored regularly after it is implemented.

Workload and Human Hours Required

The volume of specimens that are to be collected per month can be anticipated from the information gained in planning the phlebotomy unit. This figure improves as experience is gained and records are available for identifying trends. Other services that are to be performed are also considered, for example, mailing, specimens distribution to laboratories for analyses, and record keeping.

Although there are several ways to calculate productivity and workload, the *College of American Pathologists (CAP) Workload Recording Method* (WLR) is most widely used by clinical laboratories. It is published annually with the latest revisions and updates. Therefore it is important to reassess annually the methodology used to calculate workload statistics. The WLR Method uses a 5-digit coding system for each laboratory procedure, identifies what should be counted, and assigns a unit value for each. By calculating the number of procedures performed, along with personnel time, standards, controls, and repeats, the supervisory or administrative staff can make informed decisions about scheduling, budgeting, planning, and staffing.[8]

A "unit value" is the number of minutes of technical, clerical, and side time required to perform all of the activities to complete the defined procedure once. "One workload unit represents one minute of personnel time."[8]

Some of the CAP units are designated in Table 12–4. The "workload" describes the total units or minutes during a specified time period. Some laboratories

TABLE 12–4. CAP WORKLOAD UNITS FOR SPECIMEN COLLECTION PROCEDURES

CAP Code	Procedure Name	Unit Value
89335	Capillary Puncture: Travel and collection time	e14.0
89336	Capillary Puncture: Outpatient	e 8.0
89341	Venipuncture: Travel and collection time	e10.0
89342	Site prep sterile venipuncture (blood culture)	e 1.0
89343	Venipuncture: Outpatient	e 4.0
89350	Arterial puncture: Travel and collection time	12.0
89140	Report delivery within hospital	e 3.0
89142	Report charting	e 2.5
89143	Gowning/degowning for complete isolation (includes hand-washing, gloving, masking)	e 5.0
89145	Gowning/degowning only (with or without handwashing)	e 0.5
89340	Urine collection by laboratory personnel	6.0

e: Extrapolated value determined by CAP but not an "assigned value." Units without the "e" are "assigned values."
From CAP: *Workload Recording Method & Personnel Management Manual, 1992 Edition,* Northfield, Ill. CAP, 1991.

tabulate monthly data, with special reviews on a quarterly basis. Others tabu-late data by 4-week periods, which are not necessarily synchronized with the calendar months. Whatever the time cycle chosen, each laboratory section within a health care facility should use the same time frame. It is also helpful if the workload cycle is synchronous with budgetary or financial reporting peri-ods. The WLR Method suggests collection of data in nine categories to allow for differences in the reimbursement rates of procedures. These categories are as follows:

- Inpatient
- Outpatient
- Quality controls and standards
- Repeats
- Emergency room specimens
- Referrals (specimens received)
- Interstate (specimens received)
- Regional laboratories
- Others

A test can have the same workload and staffing needs but be reimbursed or paid for at different rates. By collecting workload data in these categories, labora-tory directors can make more educated decisions about future directions, staffing services to be referred to other laboratories, and which services are most cost beneficial. According to CAP WLR, work in the clinical laboratory is categorized as timed activities (workloaded) and support activities (non-workloaded time). The workloaded activities are specimen collection, testing, and manipulation of instruments during testing. Support or non-workloaded activities are answering the telephone, recording, reporting results, purchasing supplies, doing inventory, computer activities, accounting, billing, charting, delivery of specimens, glassware washing, periodic calibrations, writing or reading procedure manuals, cleaning, equipment maintenance and repair, su-pervision, teaching, educational activities, training new employees, checking the quality control information, and so on. These data also allow for four types of productivity assessments[8]:

- *Paid productivity*—workload units per paid hour
- *Total productivity*—hourly total of workload units plus time for sup-port activities
- *Worked productivity*—workload units per hour worked; accounts for holiday, sick, vacation, and other paid time away from work
- *Available productivity*—quantifies workload units and support activity per worked hour.

All measures are used for identification of management problem areas, staffing, and scheduling decisions. For example, when comparing work productivity with paid productivity, one can see the impact of "paid time off." Also, to analyze "idle or standby" time, the available productivity is assessed. The ideal productivity (100 percent or 60 minutes per hour) is not achievable in reality because of the necessary support activities mentioned above and other factors such as paid time off. However, using CAP productivity measures, a good manager cannot only monitor his or her own section but compare productivity among other sections of the laboratory and even other similar services in outside facilities. The CAP holds periodic workshops for new supervisors who wish to learn more about the CAP WLR method.

Each test or specimen-collection procedure should have a thorough cost analysis performed so that supervisors and managers can maintain a resonable knowledge about how expensive the specimen-collection process is and whether or not it is reimbursible. They should know how much Medicare or other third party payers are reimbursing hospitals. If the process is not cost beneficial, supervisors need to try to adjust and maximize cost efficiency without sacrificing quality.

A cost analysis procedure may include the following cost assessments:

- *Direct costs*—cost of the tube, needle, gloves, alcohol, tray (cost depreciated over 3 to 5 years), request slip, tourniquet gauze bandages, labor discard buckets, and so on.
- *Indirect costs*—cost of utilities, space, maintenance, janitorial services, laundry for laboratory coats, administration, research, or educational costs.

Estimations of revenue that include the direct and indirect costs are made in collaboration with the departmental and institutional administration.

Monitoring

Monitoring the resources and performance of the phlebotomy unit is a management activity that points to adjustments needed in budgeting, planning, or organizing. It also gives the manager an opportunity to catalog the progress and successes of the unit and its employees.

Equipment and Supplies. An inventory of the equipment and supplies in the phlebotomy unit is necessary. A list of each piece of equipment by name, institutional identification tag number, and location should be maintained by the manager and a copy should be given to the laboratory administrator. A review of the accuracy of this list should be made at least annually, with notations and additions made as equipment is discarded, updated, or added. When equipment is discarded or relocated, a record of this must be kept on file. Records of maintenance service on the equipment are also kept. Maintaining a supply inventory represents a more complex operation. From experience or calculation, volumes of the various kinds of supplies that are needed can be ordered in advance and kept in stock. Space for the storage of supplies is valuable and stocking of large volumes of supplies ties up capital. For these reasons, supplies are generally purchased on a contract basis whereby a designated volume is expected to be purchased over a year's time. The phlebotomy unit requests a certain portion of these supplies to be delivered each week or each month and the institution is billed at that time. Many hospitals maintain approximately 2 weeks' phlebotomy supplies on hand. A long delivery time on orders increases the stock that must be kept on hand or the timing of the ordering.[1]

Monitoring Performance.   The importance of employees and the leadership abilities of the manager have been discussed. The performance of employees is evaluated according to the standards established by the phlebotomy unit, described in the phlebotomy manual, and provided to the employee at the time of employment. Without standards or definitions of how to do a job well, the performance review is meaningless. It is very difficult to determine standards of performance, and many variables have an effect. These include:

- Ownership of the facility (nonprofit vs. for profit)
- Ambulatory vs. hospital services
- Primary, secondary, or tertiary care providers
- Educational mission
- Research mission
- Managerial climate: autocratic vs. democratic
- Professionalism
- Technical competence
- Productivity

When situations occur indicating that an employee has failed to meet the criteria, a record should be made and kept in the employee's file. This file should also hold records of all performance appraisals, even those that showed extra devotion or unique contribution to the job. It is important to document the positive aspects of performance. At regular intervals, the manager meets with the employee and reviews the employee's performance by the established criteria. This meeting should also afford the employee an opportunity to discuss problems or concerns with the manager. Both employee and supervisor can learn from mistakes and turn them into constructive situations.

There are ways to use language in a positive way for constructive criticism. Table 12–5 gives examples of phrases that encourage and strengthen a performance appraisal.

There are also errors that managers or supervisors make when evaluating employees. These include the following:[9]

Halo effect. One performance factor outweighs all other factors in a negative or positive bias

Leniency. "Good guy syndrome": supervisor avoids controversy

TABLE 12-5. EFFECTIVE PHRASING FOR CONSTRUCTIVE PERFORMANCE EVALUATIONS

Performs with a high degree of accuracy	Recognizes importance of appearance
Performs with consistent accuracy	Takes pride in personal appearance
Recognizes the importance of accuracy	Gives attention to personal hygiene and dress
Strives for perfection	Wears protective clothing when appropriate
Avoids mistakes and errors	Excels in interpersonal communication
Keeps accurate records	Displays good posture
Gives meticulous attention to detail	Projects a positive image
Develops and maintains 2-way communications	Excels in nonverbal and verbal communication
Effectively communicates with coworkers	Uses proper oral and written language
Demonstrates high level of expertise	Constantly updates skills
Combines technical competence and loyalty	Devotes time and effort to developing skills
Keeps abreast of computer applications	Minimizes wasting of supplies, equipment
Can be relied upon to be present at work	Is reliable and supportive
Is consistently punctual, regular in attendance	Attains results to assigned tasks
Seeks personal growth and development	Understands personal strengths and weaknesses
Constantly strives to improve professionalism	Displays eagerness to improve
Provides suggestions for department improvement	Monitors improvement
Is a self starter	Displays eagerness to try new approaches
Is a solution seeker	Requires minimum supervision
Does things without being told	Takes action without delay
Understands all aspects of job	Shares knowledge with coworkers
Promotes harmony and teamwork	Demonstrates respect for patients
Builds team spirit	Shows compassion for others
Displays ability to learn quickly	Is loyal to the organization
Makes use of learning opportunities	Takes pride in job

From Neal, JE: *Effective Phrases for Performance Appraisals.* Perrysburg, Ohio, Neal Publications, 1986, with permission.

Central tendency. Supervisor places most factors and most people in the middle of the rating scale

Recent behavior bias. Some event that happened recently outweighs other things and the supervisor shows a positive or negative trend in ratings

Personal bias. Supervisor shows either favoritism or negativism based on personal factors that should not have a bearing on performance (i.e., gender, age, race, ethnicity, sexual orientation, disabilities)

These practices are unfair, legally risky, and professionally inappropriate. They are also difficult to prove. Supervisors and managers should have an open line of communication with employees to be able to detect these practices in their areas. All employees should have opportunities to reply to the performance appraisals in writing within a given time period, and the appraisals should be reviewed by a senior administrative person. The senior person should also be available for employees to report their complaints to. Exit interviews or questionnaires should be done on all employees who resign or leave. This provides information for trending and potential problem areas.

The University of Texas M.D. Anderson Cancer Center has a survey form that is given to patients to inquire about the quality of the phlebotomists' services. Most hospitals have an employee who visits patients to ensure that the hospital services are acceptable. The phlebotomy manager may receive information in this manner. General areas of concern or recurring problems may serve as topics of in-service education, continuous quality improvement activities, or staff meetings.

In-service programs offer phlebotomy employees information on the latest advances in health care that affect their work or enhance their interest in their work. Generally, the employees are asked for topics of interest to them in preparation of the in-service programs. The manager can enhance interest by obtaining interesting guest speakers to present these topics. An evaluation of the in-service programs helps the manager improve the programs. Frequently, there is a coordinator of in-service education for the laboratory or the hospital who can assist in this activity. Suggestions for in-services include the following topics:

- Pediatric phlebotomy—review techniques
- Drawing from CVC lines
- Guest relations
- Listening skills
- Nonverbal communication
- Dressing to enhance professionalism
- Fire and biohazard safety
- IC procedures
- Review of workload

Staff meetings are usually held weekly in order to afford communication among employees, the manager, and the director. The employees should have an opportunity to bring problems or new ideas to the attention of the management. This also provides a time for management to share information about anticipated changes, new rules and regulations, and special events in the laboratory and hospital. Communication with the phlebotomy employees is the manager's most important function.

Becoming a Health Care Change Agent

New governmental regulations with the resultant cost containment pressures are creating new opportunities and new types of problems in the health care industry. Managing a phlebotomy team in this new health care environment requires that the team leader become a change agent. He or she needs to constantly consider new techniques that will increase phlebotomists' productivity levels without jeopardizing quality or safety. The supervisor must make it possible for phlebotomists to work more efficiently and to establish an environment that makes these employees want to work more effectively. To provide higher productivity, the leader of the phlebotomy team may wish to incorporate the following changes:

1. Plan goals that lead to high performance and continuous quality improvement
2. Improve scheduling through time studies that correlate workload and time of day, shift, weekend, and holidays
3. Establish better inventory control by studying dates of shipment and use of phlebotomy supplies and equipment
4. Improve the communication system by training employees in the proper use of the telephone, intercom system, and computer codes
5. Provide recognition and rewards (i.e., assignments with more authority or responsibility, commendatory memoranda, merit raises)

PLANNING A FORMAL PHLEBOTOMY EDUCATION PROGRAM

Medical technologists have recognized in recent years that the quality of their laboratory test results, those which provide information for diagnosis and treatment of patients, is directly affected by the quality of the collected blood sample. Many medical technologists expressing this concern to their respective administrations have met with approval and support in developing a formal training program for phlebotomists in the individual institution or as a service to the area's medical community.

Steps for Achieving Support from Management

Several steps should be followed to facilitate the development of a phlebotomy program. The first step is to develop a statement of need and the identification of goals. A few suggested methods for acquiring verification of a suspected need are

1. Circulate a questionnaire pertinent to specimen collection to laboratory department personnel and nursing staff for a hospital situation. A university department interested in developing a training program can circulate a similar questionnaire to hospitals or other clinical facilities in the surrounding area.
2. Produce minutes from interdepartmental meetings or by representatives concerned with specimen collection problem solving, suggesting formal phlebotomy education.
3. Review documented incidents or problems directly related to the current level of phlebotomy education.
4. Calculate vacancy and turnover rates for full-time and part-time phlebotomists. Calculate training time for new employees.

After the statement of need has been adequately supported with documentation, identification of the goals is in order. The goals should be fashioned to fulfill the statement of need while ultimately assuring quality laboratory blood specimen collection and thereby quality health care to the patient.

The second step to achieve support is to review the verification of need and submit a preliminary proposal for a formal educational program to the administration. If the response is favorable, continue with the development of the proposal.

The third step is the identification of educational resources. In a hospital-based program, the educational or in-service department personnel may be requested to advise and assist in writing objectives, providing classrooms, and suggesting a format for a course syllabus. It would be advisable to have input and thereby commitment from personnel in the other hospital departments who would be working with the phlebotomy students (e.g., Pharmacy and Nursing). In a university-based program, the medical technology faculty are accustomed to writing objectives, outlines, and formats. The majority of the work in this situation would involve juggling classroom time schedules and achieving affiliation agreements with clinical facilities for phlebotomy student clinical rotations.

The fourth step requires a literature review of standards and guidelines for phlebotomy instruction as well as a review of other types of phlebotomy education programs. Both the National Accrediting Agency for Clinical Laboratory Sciences (NAACLS) and the National Committee for Clinical Laboratory Standards (*NCCLS*) provide guidelines for proposing and conducting a phlebotomy training program as well as criteria for interviewing and selecting candidates.[10-12]

The fifth step begins the development of a course syllabus. A syllabus should contain the following information:

1. Prerequisites/requirements (minimum acceptable)
2. Intended audience (intrainstitution or public offer)
3. Class schedule (dates course is offered as well as agenda of a single course offering)
4. Purpose of course components (classroom, student lab, clinical site)
5. Course objectives
6. Instructor/faculty/institution/affiliation information
7. Course fee (if public offering)
8. Course description, content outline, and student policies
9. Credits/units/certificates
10. Contact for further information or application

The NCCLS also recommends having "didactic instruction" and "empirical training." The empirical portion would relate to observing then practicing the procedures.

The sixth and final step in proposing a formal phlebotomy educational program involves finances. At this point, hours of instruction and staffing costs must be calculated. Costs of purchasing equipment and supplies needed in a fiscal year per student take on new importance. Income resulting from tuition fees must be included in the financial evaluation. A realistic viewpoint is necessary to decide what facets of the educational program will fit budgetary allowances and still provide quality phlebotomists.

Providing the Basic Education and Training Program

The phlebotomy student must understand the objectives to be met and the expectations of the instructors at the beginning of the course. These objectives should be identified both verbally and in writing. The NCCLS standards for objectives of a training program require that upon completion of training the student should be able to:

1. Explain the physical layout of a blood drawing area and the hospital floors
2. Identify equipment used in collection of blood and describe its use
3. Identify the various documentation forms associated with blood collection
4. Identify collection sites normally used in blood collection
5. Perform collection techniques on a simulated arm (Figure 12–3)
6. Perform all steps of the venipuncture procedure with emphasis on patient identification accuracy.

Student Policies

Student policies may be written to express the objectives, goals, and expectations of the student. In this way, policy reinforces the path to meeting the objective and attaining the goals. Policies should cover:

1. Personal qualifications
2. Dress code
3. Time and attendance requirements, holidays, break times
4. Replacement of supplies and documents
5. Examinations and references for examination questions
6. Student liability
7. Health care of the student during the training session
8. Rules to follow at the clinical site

A special area in the policies should spell out grounds for failure. Time and attendance requirements should explain a mechanism for excused and unexcused absences and consequences. Makeup time and examination procedures should be covered carefully. Interjecting time and attendance policies provides a process for screening out the irresponsible phlebotomist who would not exercise responsibility in a patient care situation.

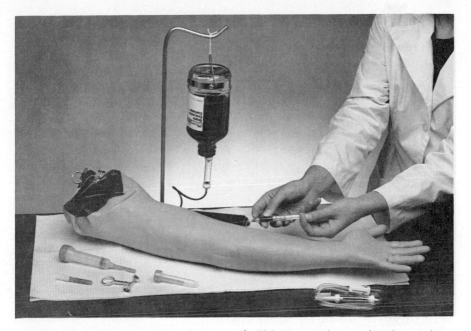

Figure 12 3. Nasco injectable training arm. A phlebotomy student needs to learn collection techniques using proper training equipment prior to patient collection. *(Courtesy of Nasco, Inc., Fort Atkinson, Wis.).*

Teaching Facilities

If the phlebotomy education process takes place in only one institution, arrangements need to be made for classroom space, for didactic instruction, and for access to patients for clinical instruction. Consideration should be given to whether or not students will collect blood on outpatients, inpatients, or both. Phlebotomy educational situations that include more than one facility may require an affiliation agreement, the input and support of supervisory personnel, and consideration of a variety of time schedules in the teaching agenda.

Equipment and Instructional Materials

Equipment and instructional materials important to a phlebotomy education experience include all the items that are listed for a venipuncture procedure or a skin puncture procedure (see Chapter 3). Additional items that would be desirable for proper training are:

- Phlebotomy training arms or devices (e.g., Nasco adult and pediatric training arms with Caucasian and African-American skin colors; Elektro Assemblies, Inc. Veni-Dot Phlebotomy Training Device)
- Collection trays
- Anatomic models

- Anatomic and circulatory charts
- Projectors—slide, VCR, overhead
- Chalkboards, tablets and markers, or both
- Teaching manuals and references

All of the equipment, supplies, and instructional materials must be planned and ordered well in advance of the time needed for instruction and must be stored when not in use.

Communication and Advertising

It is important to have a continuous flow of communication between the coordinator and the other instructors and affiliations. The nursing staff of the clinical facility should be informed in advance to render them cooperative with a program developed to improve patient care. Advertising the phlebotomy education program is a necessary activity if the program is to be marketed to clinical facilities or the public or both. This requires planning and publishing brochures detailing the course syllabus, as well as contacting the media and planning elements of exposure to the audience.

Selecting the Students

Selecting the students for each class requires specific selection criteria and a team of representatives involved in the selection. The criteria for most phlebotomy training programs require a high school diploma or General Education Development (GED) test certificate. The personal characteristics that are covered in the student policies may also be employed in the selection criteria.

A personal interview with the candidate for selection is important to a successful phlebotomy program. A candidate for a phlebotomy training program when interviewed should be poised, alert, pleasant, mature, enthusiastic, and sincere. Questioning the candidate should bring to surface characteristics of initiative, ability to speak well, cooperative attitude, and attention to detail. Because professional appearance is important for an occupational phlebotomist, a personal interview provides an opportunity to screen applicants in the areas of appearance and hygiene. An interview with a candidate also allows an opportunity for questioning the candidate and evaluating the responses. An acceptable candidate demonstrates good communication skills and self-confidence. Prior clinical experience and favorable references should be the first areas investigated. The desire to learn the skill of phlebotomy as a possible stepping stone into other medical careers is commonly expressed by candidates. Locomotion and agility must be considered because a phlebotomist walks and stands an excessive amount of time in most working situations. Strength (ability to lift up to 60 pounds) is often necessary for lifting equipment, supplies, and some patients. Reading, spelling, color-blindness, and mathematics entrance exams may be desirable because documentation, basic calculations, and differentiating tube colors in collection are essential capabilities for the practicing phlebotomist. A typical position summary or job description for a phlebotomist is as follows: performs venipunctures, skin punctures (finger and heel), collects and handles blood, urine, and other body fluid specimens, consults with supervisor and related health care team members, and maintains supplies needed for blood collection. Keeping a summary such as this in mind, it is easy to see why the above criteria must be specific. Also, as in other health care careers, phlebotomy candidates must be willing to work different shifts, holidays, and weekends if necessary.

Phlebotomy Program Content

It is suggested that a phlebotomy training program consist of both didactic and clinical instruction. The phlebotomy student should receive didactic instruction encompassing the topics covered in all chapters of this text prior to patient contact in the clinical instruction.

In the clinical setting, the phlebotomy student will have an opportunity to develop confidence through experience. The student should be carefully supervised in the initial attempts to collect blood specimens from patients. These first patients should be carefully selected for their large veins and cooperative attitudes. The supervising professional should remain close enough during these first experiences to take over as needed. Instruction on this level should contain elements of positive reinforcement, confidence in ability, reassurance, and the ever-important respect for self-esteem. The phlebotomy student needs much encouragement in the initial exposure to the patient.

Areas of information pertinent to the particular clinical facility that should be emphasized to a phlebotomy student during clinical instruction are:

1. Tasks on a checklist listing expected rate and level of performance of the student
2. Laboratory and institutional policies
3. Job description for phlebotomist
4. Medicolegal aspects relative to the particular institution
5. Safety, fire, and disaster plans: the role of the student in the event of an incident
6. First aid
7. Infection control and reporting
8. Specimen Collection Manual or File and standard protocol
9. Procedures for documentation: requisitions, logs, and so forth
10. Professional conduct and appearance

Class Schedule.   The length of the course in hours needs to be determined as soon as the program content has been developed. The times, dates, and locations of the individual classes must be carefully worked through. Phlebotomy educational programs mentioned in the literature review range from 40 hours to 150 hours in duration. Most programs have divided the time in the class schedule into periods, half of which are didactic instruction and the other half, clinical instruction. Some programs offer full-day instruction, whereas others offer instruction for only 4 hours each day.

The daily agenda should spell out reading assignments as well as activities for each day. This agenda, as part of the syllabus, aids the student in preparing for class as well as simplifies the task of course revision. Instructors can fill in for each other as needed if the lecture and laboratory outlines are available and the agenda is specific.

The National Accrediting Agency for Clinical Laboratory Sciences (NAA-CLS) conducts phlebotomy program approval to ensure that the phlebotomy graduates possess stated career entry-level competencies. Included in this Program Approval process is a presentation of the specific learning activities (lecture and laboratory class schedule), instructional resources utilized, evaluation methods, and criteria for acceptable performance that relate to each competency. The National Phlebotomy Association (NPA) also has guidelines for educational programs.

Certificates/Credits/Units.   A graduation ceremony for presentation of phlebotomy course certificates is highly recommended. The ceremony instills pride in the graduate and allows an opportunity to invite interested representatives from existing and future clinical affiliates. The certificate should contain the following:

1. Name of the course and the institution(s) (should include clinical affiliate)
2. Seals from the institution(s)
3. Number of hours of instruction/credits/units. (There are mechanisms for achieving college credits or continuing education units for a phlebotomy course from either a university, professional organization, or other educational accrediting group. Course credit is based upon contact hours of instruction.)[13]
4. Full name of the graduate
5. Date of graduation
6. Appropriate signatures (e.g., administrator, dean, director, instructor)

A phlebotomist graduating from a certificate program will be able to take this certificate to a prospective employer. With the advent of formal phlebotomy education programs, a phlebotomist now has a need for credentials when seeking employment.

In addition, graduates of a formal phlebotomy educational program are eligible to take the phlebotomy examination administered by the National Certification Agency for Medical Laboratory Personnel (NCA) and become certified as CLPlb (NCA).

The American Society of Clinical Pathologists (ASCP) and the National Phlebotomy Association (NPA) also offer certification examinations. Examination reviews or textbooks should be available to prepare students for taking objective-type examinations.[13,14]

Teaching Methods. It is recommended that for each skill taught, there should be five basic phases to the teaching process used in a phlebotomy education program.

Phase	Competency Tested
1. Preparation	Oral quiz, homework questions, written quiz
2. Familiarization	After seeing instructor demonstrations, oral quiz, homework questions, and written quiz
3. Observation	Oral quiz, student teaching instructor approach
4. Manipulation	Role-playing and practical exams for student to demonstrate technical competence
5. Operation	Clinically supervised bedside instruction according to checklist of tasks to master techniques in clinical setting[15]

The student must progress from one phase to another only after demonstrating competency. This is described as competency-based education. In the case of inability to demonstrate competence within the framework of the course, the student may be given another chance to achieve and demonstrate competence. He or she should be aware of how the scores will be counted (e.g., averaged together). Should the student fail to demonstrate the required level of competency on a second chance, the student should not continue in the program. Only students who have been able to demonstrate competence within the guidelines of the program for a particular phase of instruction are eligible to progress to the next phase. All areas of information should be covered in a comprehensive final examination. Failure to demonstrate competency on the final examination should preclude graduation from the program.

Several methods of instruction are recommended for use in a phlebotomy education program. Included are lecture, group discussion, demonstration, role-playing, case studies, independent study, and self-examination. Instructional aids include slide–tape programs, videocassettes, transparencies, computer assisted instruction, and opaque projections, films, models, and various charts and drawings.

Evaluation Techniques

Evaluating the Student. Phlebotomy students must be able to demonstrate skills in all three behavioral domains: cognitive, affective, and psychomotor. In the cognitive domain, the student must demonstrate knowledge, theory, understanding, and problem-solving skills; all of which can be evaluated through written examination or practical demonstration. However, evaluation of this nature cannot impose the stress, tension, and multitude of other variables affecting the performance of a phlebotomist in a "real life" situation. This is why evaluation of the affective domain is important to phlebotomy education.[16] Behavior reflecting attitude, coping capabilities, and methods of adjustment and adaptation must be tested and evaluated. Only the phlebotomist who is capable of maintaining an optimum attitude and necessary composure can successfully perform phlebotomy skills and manipulations. Role-playing between students and instructors is a good predecessor to patient contact and a way to give preliminary feedback about the student's attitude. A phlebotomist who has role-playing experience as a student often finds it easier to go step by step through a procedure in the real life situation.

Much of the behavior demonstrated in the affective domain is dependent upon personality. The important attitudinal characteristics should be listed in the screening process of phlebotomy applicants, if possible. Evaluating these characteristics is a difficult task that may be accomplished by using behavioral objectives incorporated in the policies and procedures taught. In this way, infractions that break policy will demonstrate incompetency. For example:

> Upon completion of the phlebotomy training program, the student will be expected to perform venipuncture procedures in accordance with the NCCLS Standard Procedures for the Collection of Diagnostic Blood Specimens by Venipuncture while exhibiting good communication skills, personable attitude, ethical conduct, self-confidence, organization, and responsibility, as well as professional appearance and hygiene.

A policy written in a similar fashion to the above (shorter versions are certainly advisable) would incorporate both performance and behavioral objectives. Behavioral objectives may be written to require professional behavior and appearance of a phlebotomy student, which can then be used as an evaluation tool for the affective domain in phlebotomy education.

Phlebotomy technical skills are evaluated in the psychomotor domain. This area may be tested with observations and simulated practicum in the classroom and with performance checklists and direct observation in the clinical setting.

Simulated Practicum. In the classroom situation, the phlebotomist should step through the basic venipuncture and basic skin puncture procedures using a teaching arm. A practicum of this nature allows evaluation of technique. To evaluate successful collection of blood specimens, collection from fellow phlebotomy students tests psychomotor skills under a greater level of stress and tension. This exercise resembles patient collection; however, classroom exercises do not completely prepare the student for patient contact, and initial patient collection must be closely supervised until the phlebotomy student has achieved a level of confidence that aids successful collection. Self-confidence is vital for phlebotomist performance. There should be defined limits in the program concerning the time when this self-confidence should evolve.

In the clinical rotation, a tool frequently used to evaluate the psychomotor domain is a task list of procedures with specific levels of acceptable and unacceptable performance per task. The tasks and rating levels should correspond to the course and procedure objectives. Evaluation of the psychomotor domain during clinical rotation should take place at the end of the Operation Phase of instruction.

Student Evaluation of Program.   Phlebotomy students sometimes synthesize from the educational process new ideas and better ways to get a message across. They are also good at pinpointing trouble spots in the instruction of the program.

Often the good students are complimentary and constructive, while the poor students are disgruntled and critical. An instructor can find useful information from an evaluation of a program by the students. After the comprehensive final exam but before the final grades have been posted is a good time to request filling out an evaluation of the program. Student evaluations of a program can be used to improve it as well as justify it as a service to the institution and community.

Instructor Evaluation of the Program.   Input and evaluation of the program by its instructors are invited. Providing an evaluation tool that lists questions with ratings and a place for comments stimulates instructors to respond or take time to note an idea for improvement. Instructor evaluations are valuable to justify a program, especially if evaluations come from instructors in affiliated clinical institutions. It is important to involve instructors in evaluation and revision of the phlebotomy education program to ensure their continued commitment to its success.

Seeking Employment

Interviewing skills and resume writing may be covered in the program to prepare phlebotomy students to embark on a new career. Role-playing helps here too. It is frustrating to a phlebotomist graduating at the top of the class to be passed up for a position because he or she lacks interviewing skills or experience composing a resume.

CONTINUING EDUCATION

The phlebotomist graduating from a formal training program needs to realize the importance of remaining current in the field. Continuing education is directly related to continued competence, particularly in areas of rapidly changing technology. Keeping the occupational phlebotomist updated is critical to competency in phlebotomy practice, which changes and improves constantly since it is an area of the medical field.

Workshops that teach trouble-shooting in phlebotomy are valuable to practicing phlebotomists. Communication skills are so important that revitalizing patient approach skills, especially with different kinds of patients, is good preventive maintenance for a phlebotomist. Because the phlebotomist is the most visible member of the laboratory, not just to patients but to other health care team members, in-service involving improving interdepartmental relationships should include the phlebotomist.

Phlebotomy is a stressful position, as described in Chapter 8. Patient contact and pressing importance of proper specimen collection render stress management exercises helpful to phlebotomists. Such exercises may aid a phlebotomist in communicating more effectively and discharging phlebotomy duties in a pleasant manner.

KEY TERMS

College of American Pathologists (CAP)	direct and indirect costs	NCCLS
Workload Recording Method	fixed and variable costs	paid productivity staffing
certification examinations	leadership management errors	strategic planning worked productivity

STUDY QUESTIONS

1. List six factors to be considered in planning a phlebotomy unit.
2. List four goals of a typical phlebotomy unit.
3. List five factors that dictate staffing requirements.
4. The phlebotomy collection procedure manual is used for [choose correct answer(s)]:

   a. recording the approved procedures for the phlebotomy unit.
   b. readily accessible performance by phlebotomists.
   c. criteria for acceptable performance by phlebotomists.
   d. a handy pocket reference to be carried by the phlebotomist.

5. List 10 basic characteristics of leadership.
6. List four factors that affect the scheduling of collections.
7. List five items to be considered in the preparation of a budget.
8. Name three reasons for monitoring.

For the remaining questions, circle the single best answer.

9. The statement of need for a phlebotomy education program expresses concern for the

   a. number of blood samples requiring collection.
   b. the variety of specimen collection criteria.
   c. effect of blood collection on test results.
   d. amount of time taken to correct phlebotomy errors.

10. The ultimate goal of a phlebotomy education program is to increase

    a. the number of phlebotomists.
    b. the time a medical technologist is at the bench.
    c. quality health care to the patient.
    d. the standards for phlebotomists.

11. The NCCLS standards for a phlebotomy training program are found in the NCCLS Approved Standard for Standard Procedures for

    a. skin puncture.
    b. venipuncture.
    c. collection devices.
    d. phlebotomy training programs.

12. The content outline for the didactic portion of the course should vary from the clinical rotation in order to emphasize

    a. clinical laboratory and institutional policies.
    b. interdepartmental relationships.
    c. equipment and supplies to use.
    d. application of acquired knowledge.

13. An example of proper training equipment for teaching venipuncture technique is a(an)

    a. model of the circulatory system.
    b. injectable arm.
    c. venipuncture demonstration film.
    d. ample supply of syringes and Vacutainer systems.

14. Instructional materials can be used to

    a. enhance understanding prior to application.
    b. replace clinical application.
    c. explain the process after application.
    d. determine the ability to apply knowledge.

15. Methods of instruction used may be

    a. lecture and group discussion.
    b. demonstration and role-playing.
    c. case studies and independent study.
    d. all of the above.

16. The recommended phase training theory uses five phases:

(1) familiarization   (4) manipulation
(2) preparation   (5) observation
(3) operation

These phases must progress in which order?

a. (2), (5), (4), (3), (1)   **c.** (2), (4), (3), (5), (1)
b. (2), (4), (5), (3), (1)   **d.** (2), (1), (5), (4), (3)

REFERENCES

1. Karni KR, Viskochil KR, Amos PA (ed): *Clinical Laboratory Management*. Boston, Little, Brown, 1982.
2. Lorimor KK, Collins FL: Monitoring quality control in the clinical laboratory, in Becan-McBride K (ed): *Textbook of Clinical Laboratory Supervision*. New York, Appleton-Century-Crofts, 1982, pp 146–244.
3. McGregor D: *The Human Side of Enterprise*. New York, McGraw-Hill, 1960.
4. Blake R. Mouton J: *The Managerial Grid*. Houston, Gulf, 1964.
5. Likert R: *New Patterns of Management*. New York, McGraw-Hill, 1961.
6. Murphy MB: Personnel relationships, in Becan-McBride (ed): *Textbook of Clinical Laboratory Supervision*. New York, Appleton-Century-Crofts, 1982, pp 107–113.
7. Duplantis D: Budgetary considerations, in Becan-McBride K (ed): *Textbook of Clinical Laboratory Supervision*. New York, Appleton-Century-Crofts, 1982, p 238.
8. College of American Pathologists (CAP): Workload Recording Method and Personnel Management Manual, 1992 Edition. Northfield, Ill., CAP, 1991.
9. Day CM: Counciling and performance appraisal: A planning perspective. *Am J Med Tech* 49:6, 415–419, June 1983.
10. National Committee for Clinical Laboratory Standards, NCCLS Approved Standard: *ASH-3 Standard Procedures for the Collection of Diagnostic Blood Specimens by Venipuncture*. 3rd ed, H4-A3, 11(11), July 1991.
11. College of American Pathologists: So You're Going to Collect a Blood Specimen. College of American Pathologists, Northfield, Ill., 1989.
12. National Accrediting Agency for Clinical Laboratory Sciences (NAACLS): Phlebotomy Program Approval Guide. Chicago, Ill., NAACLS, Nov. 1989.
13. The National Phlebotomy Association (NPA): Continuing Education Programs. NPA, 7610 Georgia Avenue, N.W. Suite 2, Washington, D.C. 20012, 1980.
14. Becan-McBride K, Garza D: Phlebotomy Examination Review. Norwalk, Conn., Appleton & Lange, 1989.
15. Golden TH: A college course for phlebotomists. *MLO* 1981.
16. Grimaldi PQ: Phase training: A systematic approach to lab instruction. *MLO* 1981.

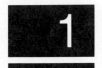

Basic Requests in English, Spanish, French, German, Russian, and Japanese

The following translations are designed to present the phlebotomist with a *very basic* means of communicating with patients who speak Spanish, French, German, Russian, or Japanese. Before speaking with patients, it is recommended that the phlebotomist practice using these phrases with someone who knows the correct pronunciation. Otherwise the patient may be even more confused. Another alternative is to have the key phrases printed on cards that the phlebotomist may point to or use as a reference when communicating with the patient.

The Russian and Japanese translations are written phonetically so that the words are written as they sound in English. The authors felt that this would be more useful to English-speaking phlebotomists than using Russian or Japanese characters. The German includes exclamation points (!) after imperatives, in accordance with German grammar.

English	**Spanish**
One	uno
Two	dos
Three	tres
Four	cuatro
Five	cinco
Six	seis
Seven	siete
Eight	ocho
Nine	nueve
Ten	diez
Twenty	veinte

Thirty	trenta
Forty	cuarenta
Fifty	cinquenta
Sixty	sesenta
Seventy	setenta
Eighty	ochenta
Ninety	noventa
One hundred	cien
Hello	Hola
Good day	Buenos dias
Good morning	Buenos dias
Good afternoon	Buenas tardes
Good evening	Buenas noches
Mother	Madre/Mama
Father	Padre/Papa
Sister	Hermana
Brother	Hermano
Son	Hijo
Daughter	Hija
Husband	Esposo, Marido
Wife	Esposa
Infant/Baby	Niño, niña
Grandfather	Abuelo
Grandmother	Abuela
Friend	Amigo/Amiga
Mister	Señor
Mrs.	Señora
Miss	Señorita
Doctor	Doctor
Nurse	Enfermera
My name is . . .	Me llamo . . .
I work in the laboratory	Trabejo en el laboratorio.
I speak . . .	Hablo . . .
We are going to analyze	Vamos analizar
. . . your blood	. . . su sangre
. . . your urine	. . . su orina
. . . your sputum	. . . su esputo
Do you understand?	Entiende Usted(ud.)?
I do not understand.	No entiendo.
Please (pls.)	Por favor (p.f.)
Thank you	Gracias
You are welcome.	De nada.
Speak slower, pls.	Hable mas despacio, p.f.
Repeat, pls.	Haga me el/favor de repetir.

Relax	Relajese
What is your name?	Como se llama?
What is your address?	su domicilio?
What is your birthdate?	En que fecha nacio?
How old are you?	Cuantos años tiene ud.?
Have you been here before?	Ha estado ud. aqui antes?
Who is your doctor?	Quien es su doctor?
Your doctor wrote the order.	El doctor/la doctora escribio la orden.
Here is the bathroom.	Aqui esta el baño.
Here is the call light.	Aqui esta la luz de emergencia.
You may not eat/drink anything except water.	No debe de comer/beber nada solamente agua.
You may not smoke.	No puede fumar.
Have you had breakfast?	Ya tomo el desayuno?
We need a blood/urine/stool sample.	Necesitamos una muestra de su sangre/orina/del excremento.
Please	Haga me el favor de (*or* Por favor . . .)
. . . make a fist	. . . cerrar el puño
. . . bend your arm	. . . doblar el brazo
. . . roll up your sleeve	. . . levantarse la manga
. . . open your hand	. . . abrir la mano
. . . sit down here	. . . sientese aqui
. . . change your position	. . . cambiarse de posicion
. . . turn over	. . . voltearse
. . . change to the left	. . . cambiarse a la izquierda
. . . change to the right	. . . cambiarse a la derecha
I need to	Necesito
. . . take a blood sample	. . . sacar sangre
. . . stick/prick your finger	. . . picarle su dedo
It will hurt a little.	Le va a doler un poquito.
The needle will stay in your arm while I am collecting the blood sample.	La aguja se quedara en su brazo durante el tiempo necesario para obtener la muestra.
I am finished.	Ya termine.
Press this gauze on your arm or finger until I can make sure that the bleeding has stopped.	Comprese esta banda en su brazo o su dedo asta que pare la sangre.
Are you lightheaded? *or* Do you feel like you are going to faint?	Esta usted mareado? *or* Se siente como si se va a desmayar?
You must lie down.	Necesita acostarse.
Collect the midstream portion of the urine in the container or bottle.	Coleccione la porcion del medio de la orina en el vaso.

English	French
One	un, une
Two	deux
Three	trois
Four	quatre
Five	cinq
Six	six
Seven	sept
Eight	huit
Nine	neuf
Ten	dix
Twenty	vingt
Thirty	trente
Forty	quarante
Fifty	cinquante
Sixty	soixante
Seventy	soixante-dix
Eighty	quatre-vingt
Ninety	quatre-vingt-dix
One hundred	cent
Hello	Allo
Good day/Good morning	Bonjour
Good afternoon	Bonsoir
Good evening	Bonsoir
Mother	Mére
Father	Pére
Sister	Soeur
Brother	Frére
Son	Fils
Daughter	Fille
Husband	Mari
Wife	Femme/Epouse
Infant/Baby	Enfant/Bébé
Grandfather	Grand-pére
Grandmother	Grand-mére
Friend	Ami/Amie
Mister	Monsieur
Mrs.	Madame
Miss	Madamoiselle
Doctor	Docteur
Nurse	Infirmière
My name is . . .	Je m'appelle . . .
I work in the laboratory.	Je travaille au laboratoire.

I speak . . .	Je parle . . .
We are going to analyze	Nous allons analiser
. . . your blood	. . . votre sang
. . . your urine	. . . votre urine
. . . your sputum	. . . votre gachat
Do you understand?	Comprenez-vous?
I do not understand.	Je ne comprend pas.
Please (pls.)	Si'l vous plait (s.v.p.)
Thank you	Merci
You are welcome.	De rien
Speak slower, pls.	Parlez plus lentment, s.v.p.
Repeat, pls.	Repetez, s.v.p.
Relax	Relaxez-vous
What is your name?	Comment vous-appelez vous?
What is your address?	Quelle est votre adresse?
What is your birthdate?	Quel est que votre anniversaire?
How old are you?	Quel âge avez-vous?
Have you been here before?	Êtes-vous veni ici avant?
Who is your doctor?	Qui est votre docteur?
Your doctor wrote the order.	Le docteur/la doctoresse à écrit l'ordre.
Here is the bathroom.	Voilà la salle de bain.
Here is the call light.	Ça c'est la lumiere d'appel en cas d'urgence.
You may not eat/drink anything except water.	Il ne faut rien manger/boire excepté de l'eau.
You may not smoke.	Il ne faut pas fumer.
Have you had breakfast?	Avez-vous pris le petit dejeuner?
We need a blood/urine/stool sample.	Nous avons besoin d'un echantillon de sang/urine/selle.
Please	
. . . make a fist	Faites un poing, s.v.p.
. . . bend your arm	Pliez votre bras, s.v.p.
. . . roll up your sleeve	Roulez votre manche, s.v.p.
. . . open your hand	Ouvrex votre main, s.v.p.
. . . sit down here	Asseyez-vous ici, s.v.p.
. . . change your position	Changez votre position, s.v.p.
. . . turn over	Tournez-vous, s.v.p.
. . . change to the left	Tournez à gauche, s.v.p.
. . . change to the right	Tournez à droit, s.v.p.
I need to	Il faut que
. . . take a blood sample	. . . je prenne du sang
. . . stick/prick your finger	. . . je pique votre doigt pour prendre du sang.

It will hurt a little.

The needle will stay in your arm while I am collecting the blood sample.

I am finished. I have finished.

Press this gauze on your arm or finger until I can make sure that the bleeding has stopped.

Are you lightheaded? *or* Do you feel like you are going to faint?

You must lie down.

Collect the midstream portion of the urine in the container or bottle.

Ça va faire un peu mal.

L'aiguille restera dans votre bras pendant que je fais un prise de sang.

Je suis fini. J'ai fini.

Appayez ce gaze su votre bras ou doigt jusqu'a ce que je suis sûre que vous ne saignez pas.

Avez vous la tête léger? *or* Sentez vous que vous allez vous evanouir?

Couchez-vous s.v.p.

Recueillez la "portion du milieu"? quand vous urinez dans le récipient (la bouteille).

English	German
One	eins
Two	zwei
Three	drei
Four	vier
Five	fünf
Six	sechs
Seven	sieben
Eight	acht
Nine	neun
Ten	zehn
Twenty	zwanzig
Thirty	dreißig
Forty	vierzig
Fifty	fünfzig
Sixty	sechzig
Seventy	siebzig
Eighty	achtzig
Ninety	neunzig
One hundred	einhundert
Hello	Guten Tag! Hallo! (informal)
Good day	Guten Tag!
Good morning	Guten Morgen!
Good afternoon	Guten Nachmittag!
Good evening	Guten Abend!
Mother	die Mutter

Father	der Vater
Sister	die Schwester
Brother	der Bruder
Son	der Sohn
Daughter	die Tochter
Husband	der Mann
Wife	die Frau
Infant/Baby	das Kind
Grandfather	der Großvater
Grandmother	die Großmutter
Friend	der Freund (male) die Freundin (female)
Mister	(der) Herr
Mrs.	(die) Frau
Miss	(das) Fräulein (used primarily for those less than 16 yrs. old)
Doctor	der Arzt
Nurse	die Krankenschwester or die Schwester
	der Krankenpfleger (male nurse)
My name is . . .	Ich heiße . . .
I work in the laboratory.	Ich arbeite im Laboratorium
I speak . . .	Ich spreche . . .
We are going to analyze	Wir werden _____ analysieren.
. . . your blood	das Blut
. . . your urine	den Urin
. . . your sputum	den Auswurf
Do you understand?	Verstehen Sie?
I do not understand.	Ich verstehe nicht.
Please (pls.)	Bitte schön
Thank you	Danke schön
You are welcome.	Bitte.
Speak slower, pls.	Sprechen Sie langsamer, bitte!
Repeat, pls.	Wiederholen Sie, bitte!
Relax	Entspannen Sie sich!
What is your name?	Wie heißen Sie?
What is your address?	Was ist Ihre Adresse?
What is your birthdate?	Wann ist Ihr Geburtstag?
How old are you?	Wie alt sind Sie?
Have you been here before?	Sind Sie schon einmal hier gewesen?
Who is your doctor?	Wer ist Ihr Arzt?
Your doctor wrote the order.	Ihr Arzt hat es Ihnen verordnet.
Here is the bathroom.	Hier ist die Toilette ("W.C.").

Here is the call light.	Sie können mit diesem Licht rufen.
You may not eat/drink anything except water.	Sie dürfen nichts, außer Wasser, essen oder trinken.
You may not smoke.	Sie dürfen nicht rauchen!
Have you had breakfast?	Haben Sie Frühstück gegessen?
We need a blood/urine/stool sample.	Wir brauchen eine _____
	Blutprobe
	Urinprobe
	Stuhl probe
Please	Bitte . . .
. . . make a fist	machen Sie eine Faust!
. . . bend your arm	biegen Sie sich den Arm!
. . . roll up your sleeve	krempeln Sie den Ärmel hoch!
. . . open your hand	Öffnen Sie die Hand!
. . . sit down here	setzen Sie sich hier!
. . . change your position	stellen Sie sich anders!
. . . turn over	drehen Sie sich um!
. . . change to the left	zum links
. . . change to the right	zum rechts
I need to	
. . . take a blood sample	Ich muß eine Blutprobe nehmen.
. . . stick/prick your finger	Ich muß Ihnen in den Fingern stechen.
It will hurt a little.	Es wird ein bißchen schmerzen.
The needle will stay in your arm while I am collecting the blood sample.	Die Nadel bleibt in dem Arm während ich die Blutprobe nehme.
I am finished.	Ich bin jetzt fertig.
Press this gauze on your arm or finger until I can make sure that the bleeding has stopped.	Drücken Sie diese Gaze auf den Arm (der Finger), bis ich sicher wissen kann, daß es nicht mehr blut!
Are you lightheaded? *or* Do you feel like you are going to faint?	Fühlen Sie sich schwindlig? *or* Werden Sie ohnmächtig?
You must lie down.	Sie müssen sich hinlegen!
Collect the midstream portion of the urine in the container or bottle.	Lassen Sie das mittlerer Teil des Urins in die Flasche fließen!

English	Russian
One	adeen
Two	dva
Three	tree
Four	chyeteeri
Five	pyat
Six	shaist
Seven	syem
Eight	vosyem
Nine	dyevyat
Ten	desyat
Twenty	dvadtsut
Thirty	treetsut
Forty	sorok
Fifty	pyatdesyat
Sixty	shestdesyat
Seventy	syemdesyat
Eighty	vosyemdesyat
Ninety	devyenosto
One hundred	stoc
Hello	zdrastvooytyeh
Good day/Good afternoon	dobree dyen
Good morning	dobraya ootra
Good evening	dobree vyechyer
Mother	mat(ye)
Father	atyets
Sister	sestra
Brother	brat
Son	syn
Daughter	doch
Husband	moojh
Wife	jyena
Infant/Baby	mladenets/beybee
Grandfather	dyedooshka
Grandmother	babooshka
Friend	droog/padroog
Mister	gospodeen
Mrs./Miss	gospoyha
Doctor	doktor
Nurse	myetsyestra
My name is . . .	Mynya zavoot . . .
I work in the laboratory.	Ya rabotayoo v laboratoreah.
I speak . . .	Ya gavaryoo . . .

We are going to analyze
   . . . your blood
   . . . your urine
   . . . your sputum
Do you understand?
I do not understand.
Please (pls.)
Thank you
You are welcome.
Speak slower, pls.

Repeat, pls.
Relax
What is your name?
What is your address?
What is your birthdate?
How old are you?
Have you been here before?
Who is your doctor?
Your doctor wrote the order.
Here is the bathroom.
Here is the call light.
You may not eat/drink anything except water.
You may not smoke.
Have you had breakfast?
We need a blood/urine/stool sample.
Please
   . . . make a fist
   . . . bend your arm
   . . . roll up your sleeve
   . . . open your hand
   . . . sit down here
   . . . change your position
   . . . turn over
   . . . change to the left
   . . . change to the right
I need to
   . . . take a blood sample
   . . . stick/prick your finger
It will hurt a little.
The needle will stay in your arm while I am collecting the blood sample.

My boodyem analeezeeravat
   . . . vasha krov
   . . . vasha macha
   . . . vasha slyuna
Ve paneemaetye?
Ya nye paneemayoo.
Pozhalusta
Spaseeba
Nye za shto.
Gavareetye pomyedlyeneye pazhalusta.
Pavtaryeetye pazhalusta.
Rasslaptyes.
Kak vas zavoot?
Kakoi vash adriss?
Kagda vy radilis?
Skolka vam lyet?
Ve bylee zdyes ranshye?
Kto vash doktor?
Vash doktor vypisal retsept.
Vot tualet.
Vot vyzav myetsyestry.
Vam nyelzya nichevo yest eelee peetz kromi vady.
Vam nyelzya kooreetz.
Ve oozhye zavtrakali?
Nam nuzhna vzyat krof/machu/kala.
Pazhalusta
   . . . sazhmitye ruku f koolak.
   . . . sagnitye ruku v laktye.
   . . . zasuchitye rukaf.
   . . . razazhmitye ruku.
   . . . syadtye syuda.
   . . . izmenitye pozu.
   . . . pyeryevyernites.
   . . . pavyernityes na lyevo.
   . . . pavyernityes na pravo.
Mnye noozhna
   . . . vzyat analeez krovee.
   . . . prakalot vash paletz.
Boodyet nyemnoga bolna.
Eegla boodyet v rookye paka ya nye vazmu analeez krovee.

I am finished.

Press this gauze on your arm or finger until I can make sure that the bleeding has stopped.

Are you lightheaded? *or* Do you feel like you are going to faint?

You must lie down.

Collect the midstream portion of the urine in the container or bottle.

Ya koncheel(a) (f.)

Dyerzhitye etat tampon paka krof nye astanovitsa.

U vas kruzhista galava? *or* Vam plokha?

Ve dalzhnee lyetch.

Sabyeritye f steklyanny sasut machu f syeryedinye machei spuskania.

English	Japanese
One	Ichi
Two	Ni
Three	San
Four	Shi, Yon
Five	Go
Six	Roku
Seven	Shichi, Nana
Eight	Hachi
Nine	Ku, Kyu
Ten	Ju
Twenty	Niju
Thirty	Sanju
Forty	Yonju
Fifty	Goju
Sixty	Rokuju
Seventy	Shichiju, Nanaju
Eighty	Hachiju
Ninety	Kuju
One hundred	Hyaku
Hello	Kon-nichiwa, Moshimoshi
Good day	Kon-nichiwa
Good morning	Ohayo
Good afternoon	Kon-nichiwa
Good evening	Konbanwa
Mother	Haha
Father	Chichi
Sister	Shimai
Brother	Kyodai
Son	Musuko
Daughter	Musume
Husband	Otto

Wife	Tsuma
Infant/Baby	Kodomo/Akanbo
Grandfather	Oji-isan, Sofu
Grandmother	Oba-asan, Sobo
Friend	Tomodachi
Mister	. . . San
Mrs.	. . . San
Miss	. . . San
Doctor	Isha (. . . Sensei)
Nurse	Kangohu
My name is . . .	Watashino namaewa . . . desu.
I work in the laboratory.	Watashiwa kensashitsude hataraiteimasu
I speak . . .	Watashiwa . . . o shaberimasu.
We are going to analyze	Warewarewa anatano ketsueki, nyo, tan o shirabemasu
. . . your blood	
. . . your urine	
. . . your sputum	
Do you understand?	Anatawa wakarimasuka?
I do not understand.	Watashiwa wakarimasen
Please (pls.)	Dozo
Thank you	Arigato
You are welcome.	Doitashimashite
Speak slower, pls.	Dozo yukkuri hanashite kudasai
Repeat, pls.	Dozo kurikaeshite kudasai
Relax	Yuruyakani shitekudasai
What is your name?	Anatano namae wa nan desuka?
What is your address?	Anatano jusho wa doko desuka?
What is your birthdate?	Anatano tanjobi wa itsudesuka?
How old are you?	Anatano toshi wa ikutsudesuka?
Have you been here before?	Anatawa kokoe koraretakotoga arimasuka?
Who is your doctor?	Anatano ishawa daredesuka?
Your doctor wrote the order.	Anatanoishaga shigio kaita.
Here is the bathroom.	Kokoga benjodesu.
Here is the call light.	Korega yobirindesu.
You may not eat/drink anything except water.	Anatawa mizuigai tabetari nondarishitewa ikemasen
You may not smoke.	Anatawa tobako a suttewa ikemasen
Have you had breakfast?	Anatawa choshokuo tabemashitaka?
We need a blood/urine/stool sample.	Warewarewa ketsueki/nyo/ben o shitsuyotoshimasu.

Please

Dozo

... make a fist — Teonigittekudasai

... bend your arm — Udeo magetekudasai

... roll up your sleeve — Udeo makkutekudasai

... open your hand — Teo aketekudasai

... sit down here — Kokoe suwattekudasai

... change your position — Ichio kaetekudasai

... turn over — Negaerio uttekudasai

... change to the left — Hidarie kawattekudasai

... change to the right — Migie kawattekudasai

I need to — Watashiwa

... take a blood sample — Ketsuekio toru

... stick/prick your finger — Anatano ubiotsuku

Shitsuyoga-arimasu

It will hurt a little. — Korewa sukashi itamimasu

The needle will stay in your arm while I am collecting the blood sample. — Konohariwa watashiga ketsuekio totteiruaida anatanoudeni tomatteimasu.

I am finished. — Watashiwa owarimashita.

Press this gauze on your arm or finger until I can make sure that the bleeding has stopped. — Watashiga shiketsushitakoto-o tashikamerukotoga dekirumade kono gazeo anatanoudeka ubini oshitekudasa;

Are you lightheaded? *or* Do you feel like you are going to faint? — Anatawa memaigashimasuka? *or* Soretomu kizetsushisodesuka?

You must lie down. — Anatawa yokuninatte kudasai

Collect the midstream portion of the urine in the container or bottle. — Nyono nakahodonobubun o yokika bin-ni atsumetekudasai

2 Units of Measurement and Symbols

Å	angstrom
α	alpha
≅	approximately
amp	ampere (units of electric current)
°C	degrees Centigrade or Celsius (unit of temperature; convert to Fahrenheit by multiplying by 1.8 and adding 32)
c	centi- (10^{-2})
cc	cubic centimeter (same as mL, $^1/_{1000}$ L)
cd	candela (units of luminous intensity)
cm	centimeter
cu mm or mm³	cubic millimeter
d	deci- (10^{-1})
da	deca- (10^1)
dL	deciliter ($^1/_{10}$ of a liter)
°F	degrees Fahrenheit (unit of temperature; convert to Centigrade by subtracting 32 and multiplying by 0.555)
g or gm	gram ($^1/_{1000}$ of a kilogram, unit of mass)
hpf	high-power field on microscope
G%	grams in 100 mL
h	hecto- (10^2)
IU	international unit
k	kilo = (10^3)
°K	degrees Kelvin (thermodynamic temperature; convert to centigrade by subtracting 273.15)
kg	kilogram (1000 g, or 2.2 lb)
L	liter (1000 mL or 1000 cc, unit of volume)
lpf	low-power field on microscope
m	meter (unit of length)

'lli- (10^{-3})	
-(10^{-6}); micron	
gram ($^1/_{1000}$ mg)	
licurie	
milliequivalent	
milligram ($^1/_{1000}$ g)	
milligrams in 100 mL (same as dL)	
minutes	
milliinternational unit ($^1/_{1000}$ IU)	
milliliter ($^1/_{1000}$ L, same as cc)	
mm	millimeter ($^1/_{10}$ cm)
cu mm or mm³	cubic millimeter
mm Hg	millimeters of mercury
mmole	millimole
mol, M	mole (units of substance)
mOsm	milliosmol
N	normality
n	nano- (10^{-9})
ng	nanogram ($^1/_{1000}$ mg)
p	pico- (10^{-12})
pg	picogram ($^1/_{1000}$ ng)
QNS	quantity not sufficient
sec	second (unit of time)
SI	international system
sp g	specific gravity
U	international enzyme unit
μ	micro
μg (mcg)	microgram ($^1/_{1000}$ mg)
wt	weight
w/v	weight/volume
μCi	microcurie ($^1/_{1000}$ mCi)
WNL	within normal limits
WNR	within normal range
≤	less than or equal to
≥	greater than or equal to
+ or (+)	positive
− or (−)	negative
Σ	sum

3 Metric Conversion Chart

Length	1 inch (in.) = 2.54 centimeters (cm)
	1 foot (ft) = 30.48 centimeters (cm)
	39.37 inches (in.) = 1 meter (m)
	1 mile (mi) = 1.61 kilometers (km)
Mass	1 ounce (oz) = 28.35 grams (g)
	1 pound (lb) = 453.6 grams (g)
	2.205 pounds (lb) = 1 kilogram (kg)
Volume	1 fluid ounce (fl oz) = 29.57 milliliters (mL)
	1.057 quarts (qt) = 1 liter (liter or L)
	1 gallon (gal) = 3.78 liters (liter or L)

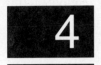

Formulas and Calculations

Area	square meter (sq m or m^2)
Clearance	liter/second (L/s)
Concentration and conversions	
Mass	kilogram/liter (kg/L)
Substrate	mole/liter (mol/L)

%$^{w/v}$ to M or vice versa:

$$M = \frac{\%^{w/v} \times 10}{\text{molecular wt (mol wt)}}$$

%$^{w/v}$ to N or vice versa:

$$N = \frac{\%^{w/v} \times 10}{\text{eq wt}}$$

mg/dL to mEq/L or vice versa:

$$mEq/L = \frac{mg/dL \times 10}{\text{eq wt}}$$

M to N:

$$N = M \times \text{valence}$$

N to M:

$$M = \frac{N}{\text{valence}}$$

Density	kilogram/liter kg/L
Dilutions	Final concentration = Original concentration × dilution 1 × dilution 2, and so forth
Electrical potential	volt $V = kg\ m^2/s^3A$
Energy	joule $J = kg\ m^2/s^2$
Force	Newton $N = kg\ m^2/s^2$

hertz   Hz = 1 cycle/sec.

Mean corpuscular volume (MCV) = average volume of red cells; expressed in cubic microns (μ^3) or femtoliters (fL)

$$MCV = \frac{Hct \times 10}{RBC\ count\ (in\ millions)}$$

Hct = hematocrit value

Mean corpuscular hemoglobin (MCH) = average weight of hemoglobin in RBC; expressed in picograms (pg)

$$MCH = \frac{hgb\ (g) \times 10}{RBC\ count\ (in\ millions)}$$

hgb = hemoglobin value

Mean corpuscular hemoglobin concentration = hemoglobin concentration of average RBC

$$MCHC = \frac{hgb\ (g)}{Hct} \times 100\%$$

Red blood cell distribution width (RDW) = numerical expression of variation of RBC size, dispersion of red cell volumes about the mean.

$$RDW = \frac{SD\ (standard\ deviation)\ of\ RBC\ size}{MCV}$$

Pressure	Pascal (Pa) = (kg/m)s^2
Quality control math	Variance (s^2):

$$s^2 = \frac{(x - \bar{x})^2}{n - 1}$$

Standard deviation(s):

$$s = \sqrt{s^2}$$

% Coefficient of variation:

$$\% \ CV = \frac{s}{\bar{x}} \times 100$$

Relative centrifugal force (rcf)	Measures force of centrifugation acting on blood components and allowing

them to separate. Can be used to calibrate centrifuges.

$$rcf = 1.118 \times 10^{-5} \times r \times n^2$$

r   = rotating radius (centimeters)

n   = speed of rotation (revolutions per minute)

Solutions

Percent (%)

To find amount of solute needed to make a given volume of solution:

$$g \text{ (or mL) of solute to be diluted up to desired volume} = \frac{\% \times \text{desired volume}}{100}$$

To find % solution when amount of solute and total volume of solution are known:

$$\% = \frac{g \text{ (or mL) solute} \times 100)}{\text{volume}}$$

Molarity (M)

$$g/L = \text{mol weight} \times M$$

$$M = \frac{g/L}{\text{mol wt}}$$

$$\text{mmole}/L = \frac{mg/L}{\text{mol wt}}$$

Osmolarity (Osm/L):

$$\text{Osm}/L = M \times \text{particles/molecule after ionization}$$

$$\text{mOsm}/L = \text{mmole}/L \times \text{particles/molecule after ionization}$$

$$\text{Osm}/L = \frac{\Delta \text{ temperature}}{1.86}$$

$$\text{mOsm}/L = \frac{\Delta \text{ temperature}}{0.00186}$$

Normality (N)

$$\text{eq wt} \times N = g/L$$

$$N = \frac{g/L}{eq\ wt}$$

Specific gravity (sp g):

$$sp\ g = \frac{wt\ of\ solid\ or\ liquid}{wt\ of\ equal\ volume\ of\ H_2O\ at\ 4°C}$$

Temperature

Celsius or Centigrade:

$$(°C = K - 273.15;\ °C = °F - 32 \times 0.555)$$

Kelvin:

$$°K = °C + 273.15\ or\ 5/9\ °F + 255.35$$

Fahrenheit:

$$°F = (°C \times 1.8) + 32$$

Volume

deciliter (dL) = $^1/_{10}$ of a liter
10 dL = 1 L

centiliter (cL) = $^1/_{100}$ of a liter
100 cL = 10 dL = 1 L

milliliter (mL) = $^1/_{1000}$ of a liter
1000 mL = 100 cL = 10 dL = 1 L

5 Abbreviations and Medical Terminology

a	without (e.g., aphasia, inability to speak)
α	alpha
ab-	deviating (e.g., abnormal)
Ab	antibody
ABG	arterial blood gases
ABO	blood types
ABR	absolute bed rest
a.c.	ante cibum, L., before meals
AC	alternating current
ACD	acid citrate dextrose, anticoagulant
A-CHO	Group A, carbohydrate
ACTH	adrenocorticotrophic hormone
ACU	acupuncture
ad-	toward (e.g., adduction)
aden/o-	gland (e.g., adenopathy)
ADH	antidiuretic hormone
ADH	arginine dihydrolase
ad lib	at pleasure; as described
ADP	adenosine 5-diphosphate
aer/o	air (e.g., aerobic)
AFB	acid-fast bacillus
AFP	alpha-fetoprotein
Ag	silver
Ag-Ab	antigen—antibody reaction
A/G	albumin/globulin ratio
Agg	agglutination
AGL	acute granulocytic leukemia
AH	antihyaluronidase

AHG	antihemophilia globulin
AIDS	acquired immune deficiency syndrome
AIHA	autoimmune hemolytic anemia
AK	above the knee
Al	aluminum
-al	pertaining to (suffix; e.g., hormonal)
ALA	delta-aminolevulinic acid
ALL	acute lymphocytic leukemia
ALT	alanine amino transferase (term for SGPT)
alges-	overly sensitive to pain (e.g., algesia)
-algia	pain (suffix; e.g., neuralgia)
alveol/o-	alveolus
AM	morning
AML	acute myeloblastic leukemia
an-	without (e.g., anemia)
ANA	antinuclear antibodies
angi/o-	vessel
ante-	before (e.g., anterior)
anti-	against (e.g., antisepsis)
Approx	approximately
APPT	activated partial thromboplastin time (PTT)
ARA	arakinose (sugar)
ARD	antibiotic removal device
arthro-	pertaining to joint(s) (e.g., arthritis)
-ary	pertaining to (suffix; e.g., coronary)
As	arsenic
ASAP	as soon as possible
ASK	antistreptokinase
ASO	antistreptolysin O titer
AST	asparate amino transferase (term for SGOT)
ATCC	American type culture collection
atel/o-	imperfect, incomplete (e.g., atelectasis)
ATP	adenosine triphosphate
Au	gold
aur-	ear
auto-	self
Auto-trans	autologous transfusion
AV	Atrioventricular, arteriovenous
B	boron
BAP	blood agar plate
Ba	barium
baso-	basophils

β	beta
BBT	basal body temperature
B cell	lymphocyte derived in bone marrow
BC	blood culture
BCP	biochemical profile; birth control pills
BFP	biologically false-positive
BHI	brain heart infusion agar
Bi	bismuth
bi-	two (e.g., bifurcate)
b.i.d.	bis in die; twice daily
bio-	life (e.g., biology)
BM	bowel movement
BMR	basal metabolic rate
bp	boiling point
B/P	blood pressure
Br	bromide
brady-	slow (e.g., bradycardia)
bronch-	windpipe (e.g., bronchitis)
BS	blood sugar
BSA	body surface area
BSP	bromsulphalein dye for liver function
BUN	blood urea nitrogen

C	carbon, compliance, clearance, coulomb
c̄	with
C_3 C_4	complement factors
C&S	culture and sensitivity
Ca	calcium, cancer
CAB	coronary artery bypass
capnia	carbon dioxide (e.g., capnophilic)
carcin/o-	cancer (e.g., adenocarcinoma)
caudal	near tail
cardio-	heart (e.g., cardiopulmonary)
CAT	computerized axial tomography scan
CBC	complete blood count
CCU	coronary care unit
CDC	Centers for Disease Control
CEA	carcinoembryonic antigen
-cele	herniation (suffix; e.g., meningiomyelocele)
-centesis	surgical puncture (suffix; e.g., amniocentesis)
cephalo-	head (e.g., cephalic)
cerebro-	cerebrum, brain (e.g., cerebrospinal fluid)
CEU	continuing education units

CF	complement fixation
CHOC	chocolate agar
CH_3OH	methanol
$(C_2H_5)OH$	ethanol
$C_6H_{12}O$	glucose
CIE	counter immunoelectrophoresis
CIT	citrate (sodium)
CK	creatine kinase
Cl	chloride
CLIA	Clinical Laboratory Improvement Act
CML	chronic myelogenous leukemia
Co	cobalt
co-	together, with (e.g., coagulation)
-coccus	berry-shaped bacteria (suffix; e.g., streptococcus)
CO	carbon monoxide, carboxyhemoglobin
CO_2	carbon dioxide (Pco_2 = partial pressure of CO_2)
$CO(NH_2)_2$	urea
contra-	against (e.g., contraceptive)
COPD	chronic obstructive pulmonary disease
CNS	central nervous system
CPD	citrate phosphate dextrose, anticoagulant
CPK	creatine phosphokinase
CPR	cardiopulmonary resuscitation
CPT-4	Common Procedural Terminology, 4th edition
CQI	continuous quality improvement
Cr	chromium
cranial	near head
-crin/o	secrete (suffix; e.g., endocrine)
Crit	hematocrit
CRP	C-reactive protein
crypt/o	hidden
CSF	cerebrospinal fluid
Cu	copper
cutaneo	skin
CV	curriculum vitae, biographical data
CV	coefficient of variation
CVC	central venous catheter
CVP	central venous pressure
cyan/o-	blueness (e.g., cyanotic)
cyst/o-	fluid sac, bladder (e.g., encystment)
cyt/o-	cells (e.g., cytopathology)
δ	delta
D&C	dilatation and curettage

DC	direct current
D/C	discontinue
derm/o-	skin (e.g., dermatophyte)
dia-	through (e.g., diaphragm)
DIC	disseminated intravascular coagulation
Diff	differential (white blood cells)
Dis	disease
Distal	away from body trunk
DNA	deoxyribonucleic acid
DNase	deoxyribonuclease
DOA	dead on arrival
dorsal	back
DPT	diphtheria, pertussis, tetanus vaccine
DRG	diagnosis-related group
-dyno/o	pain (e.g., carotodynia)
dys-	painful, difficult (e.g., dysmenorrhea)
EBV	Epstein-Barr virus
ECG, EKG	electrocardiogram
ECHO	echocardiogram (based on sound)
-ectasia	dilatation (suffix; e.g., bronchiectasis)
ect/o-	outside (e.g., ectoparasite)
ectomy	excision by surgery (suffix; e.g., appendectomy)
EDTA	ethylenediaminetetraacetate
EEG	electroencephalogram
EIA	enzyme immunoassay
ELISA	enzyme-linked immunosorbent assay
EM	electron microscopy
EMB	eosin methylene blue agar
em-	in (e.g., empyema)
-emia	blood (suffix; e.g., leukemia)
end/o-	inner (e.g., endotracheal tube)
ENT	ear, nose, throat
entero/o	small intestine (e.g., enteritis)
cos	eosinophils
epi-	over, near, upon (e.g., epidemic)
epitheli-	epithelium; protective covering
ER	emergency room
erythro-	red (e.g., erythrocyte)
ESR	erythrocyte sedimentation rate
etio-	cause (of disease)
EtOH	ethanol
ex/o-	out from
extra-	outside, beyond (e.g., extrasensory)

F	fluorine
FA	fluorescent antibody test
FBS	fasting blood sugar
FDA	Food and Drug Administration
Fe	iron
FEP	free erythrocyte porphyrins
fibro	fibrous tissue
FLK	funny-looking kid
FSH	follicle-stimulating hormone
FSP	fibrin split products
FTA	fluorescent treponemal antibody
FUO	fever of unknown origin

γ	gamma
g	centrifugal force
gastr/o-	stomach (e.g., gastroenteritis)
GC	gonococcus (gonorrhea)
-gen	agent that causes something (suffix; e.g., pathogen)
-genesis	origin, cause (suffix; e.g., pathogenesis)
-genic	producing, causing (suffix; e.g., pathogenic)
geri-	old age (e.g., geriatrics)
gest-	bear, carry (e.g., gestation)
GFR	glomerular filtration rate
GFT	graft (e.g., skin)
GH	growth hormone
GI	gastrointestinal
GLU	glucose
glyco-	sweet, sugar (e.g., glycolysis)
G6PD	glucose-6-phosphatase dehydrogenase
-gram	record, x-ray (suffix; e.g., radiogram)
-graph	instrument used to record (suffix; e.g., radiograph)
GTT	glucose tolerance test
gtts	drops
GVH	graft-versus-host reaction
gynec/o-	woman (e.g., gynecology)

H	hydrogen
HAA	hepatitis-associated antigen (Australian antigen)
HAT	heterophile antibody titer
HAV	hepatitis A virus
H_3BO_3	boric acid
H_2O_2	hydrogen peroxide

H_2S	hydrogen sulfide
H_2SO_4	sulfuric acid
Hb (Hgb)	hemoglobin
HBD	hydroxybutyric dehydrogenase
HB_SAg	hepatitis B surface antigen
HBV	hepatitis B virus
HCG	human chorionic gonadotropin
HCO_3	bicarbonate
HCl	hydrochloric acid
Hct	hematocrit
HDL	high-density lipoprotein
HDN	hemolytic disease of the newborn
He	helium
H&E	hematoxylin and eosin stain
hema-	blood (e.g., hematology)
hemi-	half (e.g., hemisphere)
hepato-	liver (e.g., hepatocyte)
hetero-	other (e.g., heterosexual)
Hg	mercury
5HIAA	5-hydroxyindoleacetic acid
HIV	human immunodeficiency virus
hidro-	sweat (e.g., hidrodenitis)
HNO_3	nitric acid
H_2O	water
hpf	high power field
hr	hours
h.s.	at bedtime
H_2SO_4	sulfuric acid
HTLV	human T-cell lymphotropic virus
hydro-	watery (e.g., hydrocephalic)
hyper-	above, more than normal (e.g., hyperplasia)
hypo-	under, less than normal (c.g., hyponatremia)

I	iodine
-ia	condition (suffix; e.g., leukemia)
-iasis	formation or presence of (suffix; e.g., psoriasis)
IBC	iron-binding capacity
ICSH	interstitial cell-stimulating hormone (LH in females)
ICSH	International Committee for Standardization in Hematology
ICU	intensive care unit
Ident	identification (ID)
IFA	immunofluorescence antibody test
Ig	immunoglobulin (e.g., IgA, IgM)

I.M.	infectious mononucleosis
IM	intramuscular
inferior	away from head
inter-	between (e.g., interdependent)
intra-	within (e.g., intrauterine)
I&O	intake and output
-ist	one who (suffix; e.g., microbiologist)
-itis	inflammation (suffix; e.g., conjunctivitis)
IV	intravenous
IU	international unit
IUD	intrauterine device

κ	kappa
K	potassium
Kary/o-	nucleus (e.g., karyotype)
kerat/o-	hard tissue (e.g., keratin)
17-KGS	17-ketogenic steroids
KOH	potassium hydroxide

LAL	limulus amoebocyte lysate test
later-	side, away from body midline (e.g., lateral)
lb	pounds
λ	lambda
LDH, LD	lactic dehydrogenase
LDL	low-density lipoprotein
LE prep	lupus erythematous test
-lei/o	smooth (suffix; e.g., nuclei)
leuk-	white (e.g., leukocytosis)
LFT	liver function tests
LH	luteinizing hormone (ICSH in males)
Li	lithium
lipo-	fatty (e.g., lipoproteins)
lith-	stone, calculus (e.g., lithiasis)
lob/o-	part that hangs down (e.g., lobe of lungs, ear, liver, brain)
LP	lumbar puncture
lpf	low powerfield
lymph-	lymph (e.g., lymphocyte)
-lysis	breaking down (suffix; e.g., hemolysis)
Lytes	electrolytes (Na, Cl, K, bicarbonate)

MAC	MacConkey agar
macro-	large (e.g., macrocyte)

mal-	bad, abnormal (e.g., malaria)
malac/o	softening (e.g., malacoma)
mast/o-	breast (e.g., mastectomy)
MBC	minimal bactericidal concentration
MCH	mean corpuscular hemoglobin (RBC indices)
MCHC	mean corpuscular hemoglobin concentration (RBC indices)
MCV	mean corpuscular volume (RBC indices)
medial	toward body midline
megal/o-	enlarged (e.g., megaloblastic)
mening/o-	membrane (e.g., meningitis)
meta-	after, beyond, change (e.g., metaphase)
metr-	uterus (e.g., endometrium)
metr/o-	measure (e.g., metric)
Mg	magnesium
MHA	microhemagglutination test
MI	myocardial infarction
MIC	minimal inhibitory concentration
MIF	migration inhibition factor
micro-	small (e.g., microcytic)
MMR	measles, mumps, rubella vaccine
mo	months
mono	monocytes
muco	relative to mucus (e.g., mucosal lining)
multi-	many
myc/o-	fungal (e.g., mycosis)
myelo-	marrow (e.g., myeloblastic)
myo-	muscle (e.g., myocardium)

N	nitrogen
N	normal
NA	not applicable
Na	sodium
NaCl	sodium chloride (salt)
$NaHCO_3$	sodium bicarbonate
NaOH	sodium hydroxide
naso	pertaining to the nose (e.g., nasopharyngeal)
nat-	birth (e.g., natal)
NBS	National Bureau of Standards
NC	normal color
Neg	negative
ne/o-	new (e.g., neoplasm)
necro-	death (e.g., necrotic)
nephr-	kidney
neuro-	nerve

NG	nasogastric
NH_3	ammonia
Ni	nickel
NL	normal, normal limits
NMR	nuclear magnetic resonance
no	number
noct/i-	night (e.g., nocturnal sweats)
noso-	disease (e.g., nosocomial)
NPN	nonprotein nitrogen
NPO	nothing per os (by mouth)
NR	nonreactive
NRBC	nucleated red blood cell

O_2	oxygen (Po_2 = partial pressure of oxygen)
OB	obstetrics
17-OH	17-hydroxysteroids
-oid	like, resembling (suffix; e.g., lymphoid tissue)
-ologist	one who studies (suffix; e.g., microbiologist)
-ology	the study of (suffix; e.g., microbiology)
-oma	tumor-related (suffix; e.g., lymphoma)
onco-	tumor-related (e.g., oncology)
onycho-	nail (e.g., onychomycosis)
O&P	ova and parasites
ophthalm/o-	eye (e.g., ophthalmology)
-opsy	to view (suffix; e.g., biopsy)
OR	operating room
organ/o-	organ (e.g., organelles)
-orrhagia	hemorrhage (suffix)
-orrhea	excessive discharge (suffix; e.g., dismenorrhea)
orth/o-	straight (e.g., orthodontic)
os	mouth
OSHA	Occupational Safety and Health Administration
-osis	condition, usually abnormal (suffix; e.g., dermatosis)
oste/o-	bone (e.g., osteomyelitis)
-ostomy	surgical forming of an opening (suffix; e.g., colostomy)
OTC	over-the-counter (drugs)
-otomy	surgical forming of an opening (suffix; e.g., tracheotomy)
-oxia	oxygen (suffix; e.g., hypoxia)

P	phosphorus
PA	pernicious anemia
pachy-	thickening (e.g., pachyderma)

pan-	all; complete (e.g., pandemic)
para-	beside, around, near (e.g., paracystitis)
paralysis	loss of movement
path/o-	disease (e.g., pathology)
path/o-	to bear; to carry (e.g., pathogen)
Pb	lead
PBI	protein-bound iodine (outdated)
p.c.	after meals
PCV	packed cell volume (hematocrit)
PCP	*Pneumocystis carnii* pneumonia
pedi/a-	child (e.g., pediatrics)
ped/o-	foot (e.g., pedicle)
-penia	decrease in (suffix; e.g., leukopenia)
peri-	around (e.g., periorbital)
pexy	surgical fixation
pH	hydrogen ion concentration
-phagia	eating, swallowing (suffix; e.g., onychophagia)
phonia	sound, voice
PID	pelvic inflammatory disease
PKU	phenylketonuria
-plas/o	formation (suffix; e.g., neoplasty)
-plasm	growth, formation (suffix; e.g., cytoplasm)
-plast/o	surgical repair, reconstruction (suffix; e.g., mammoplasty)
Pl.ct.	platelet count
pleuro-	pertaining to the pleura (e.g., pleurisy)
Plts.	platelets
PM	evening
PMNs	polymorphonuclear cells (type of WBC)
pneumo-	lungs, air (e.g., pneumonia)
pod/o-	foot (e.g., podiatry)
poly-	too many (e.g., polyploid)
Pos	positive
post-	behind; after (e.g., posterior)
PP or PC	postprandial (or after meals)
PPLO	pleuropneumonia-like organism (characteristics between virus and bacteria)
pre-	before; in front of (e.g., prenatal)
PRN	as needed
pro-	in front of (e.g., proenzyme)
proct-	rectum, anus (e.g., proctoscope)
proximal	near body trunk
PRP	platelet rich plasma
pseudo-	false (e.g., pseudopregnancy)
PSI	pounds per square inch

PSP	phenosulfonphthalein (dye for renal excretion test)
psych/o-	soul; mind (e.g., psychology)
PT	prothrombin time
PTH	parathyroid hormone or parathormone
-ptosis	prolapse; sagging (suffix; e.g., ophthalmoptosis)
PTT	partial thromboplastin time (see also APTT)
PVA	polyvinylalcohol
py/o-	pus (e.g., pyogenic)
pyr/o-	fire; fever (e.g., pyrophobia)

QA	quality assurance
QC	quality control
q.d.	quaque die, every day
q.h.	quaque hora, every hour
q.2h.	every 2 hours
q.i.d.	quarter in die, four times daily
QNS	quantity not sufficient
q.o.d.	every other day
quad	quadruple, four

R	reactive
RA	rheumatoid arthritis
Radi-	ray (e.g., radiotherapy)
RAI	radioactive iodine
RAST	radioallergosorbent test
RBC	red blood cell
rcf	relative centrifugal force
RDW	red cell distribution width
re-	back; again (e.g., remission)
ren/o-	kidney (e.g., renal)
Retic	reticulocyte count
retr/o-	behind; in back of (e.g., retroperitoneal)
RF	rheumatoid factor (also called RA factor)
Rh	rhesus; Rh factor in blood
rhin/o-	pertaining to the nose (e.g., rhinoplasty)
rhabd/o-	rod shaped, striated
RIA	radioimmunoassay
RNA	ribonucleic acid
R/O	rule out
rpm	revolutions per minute
RPR	rapid plasma reagin (test for syphilis)
RR	recovery room

RT	room temperature
Rx	medication
S	sulfur
Σ	sigma, sum of
s̄	without
S&A	sugar and acetone
sagittal	lengthwise
sarc/o-	flesh, connective tissue
scler/o-	hard (e.g., sclerosis)
-scop/o	to examine; look at (suffix; e.g., proctoscopy)
seb/o-	oily
sed/rate	sedimentation rate
segs	segmented neutrophils of WBC
semi	half (e.g., semisynthetic)
sep-	decay (e.g., septic)
SG	specific gravity
SGOT	serum glutamicoxaloacetic transaminase (newer name is AST)
SGPT	serum glutamicpyruvic transaminase (newer name is ALT)
SI	system of international units
Si	silicon
SIDS	sudden infant death syndrome
sine	without
SMA	sequential multiple analyzer (SMA-6 does 6 tests; SMA-12, 12 tests)
SOB	shortness of breath
son/o-	sound (e.g., sonogram)
SOP	standard operating procedure
spasm	contraction; twitching
sp. gr.	specific gravity
spir/o-	breathing (e.g., respiration)
SS	social security
Staphyl/o-	grapelike clusters (e.g., staphylococcus)
-stasis	stopping; controlling (suffix; e.g., hemostasis)
Stat	immediately, now
STD	sexually transmitted diseases
sten/o-	narrow (e.g., stenosis)
strept/o-	twisted chains (e.g., streptococcus)
STS	serologic or standard test for syphilis
sub-	below; under (e.g., suborbital)
super-	above; more than normal (e.g., superior)
supra-	above; more than normal (e.g., suprapubic)

Surg	surgery
system/o-	system

T_3	triiodothyronine
T_4	thyroxine
tact-	touch (e.g., tactile)
tach/y-	rapid; fast (e.g., tachycardia)
TAT	tattoo
TB	tuberculosis
TBG	thyroid-binding globulin
TBI	total body irradiation
T&C	type and cross-match
TC	to contain
T cell	lymphocyte derived from thymus
TD	to deliver
thromb/o-	clot (e.g., thrombosis)
TIBC	total iron-binding capacity
t.i.d.	ter in die, three times daily
-tome	instrument for cutting (suffix; e.g., microtome)
tox-	poison (e.g., toxicology)
TP	total protein
TPI	*Treponema pallidum* immobilization
TPR	temperature, pulse, respiratory
TQM	total quality management
trache/o-	pertaining to the trachea (e.g., tracheostomy)
trans-	across (e.g., transtracheal)
TRH	thyroid-releasing hormone
tri-	three (e.g., trisomy)
trich-	hair
-tripsy	surgical crushing (e.g., lithotripsy)
troph/o-	nourishment; development (e.g., trophology)
T&S	type and screen
TS meter	refractometer
TSH	thyroid-stimulating hormone (thyrotropin)
TSP	total serum proteins
TSS	toxic shock syndrome
TT	thrombin time

UA	urinalysis
UC	urine culture
uni-	one; single (e.g., unilocular)
UrAc	uric acid

URI	upper respiratory infection
ur/o-	urine (e.g., urology)
UTI	urinary tract infection
UV	ultraviolet

vas/o-	vessel (e.g., vasoconstriction)
VD	venereal disease
VDRL	Venereal Disease Research Laboratory (test for syphilis)
ven/o-	vein (e.g., venipuncture)
ventral	front
viscer-	viscera, internal organs
VLDL	very low-density lipoprotein
VMA	vanillylmandelic acid

WBC	white blood cell; white blood count
WNL	within normal limits
WNR	within normal range

X match	cross-match (of blood)
X	female chromosome

Y	male chromosome
yr	years

Zn	zinc
ZN	Ziehl–Neelsen stain

Appendix References

Abbott Laboratories: *Common Medical Terminology and Abbreviations.* North Chicago, Ill., 1982.

Colorado Association for Continuing Medical Laboratory Education: *Introduction to Phlebotomy,* Denver, Colo., 1988.

Corbett JV: *Laboratory Tests and Diagnostic Procedures with Nursing Diagnoses,* 3rd ed. Norwalk, Conn., Appleton & Lange, 1992.

Henry JB: *Todd-Sanford-Davidsohn Clinical Diagnosis and Management by Laboratory Methods,* 19th ed. Philadelphia, W.B. Saunders, 1990.

LaFleur MW, Starr WK: *Exploring Medical Language—A Student Directed Approach,* 2nd ed. St. Louis, C.V. Mosby, 1989.

NCCLS: *Approved Guidelines: Use of Devices for Collection of Skin Puncture Blood Specimens.* Villanova, Penn., National Committee for Clinical Laboratory Standards, 5(9); July 1985.

NCCLS: *Approved Standard: Procedures for the Collection of Diagnostic Blood Specimens by Venipuncture,* 3rd ed. Villanova, Penn., National Committee for Clinical Laboratory Standards, 11(10):H3—A3; July, 1991.

Answers to Study Questions

CHAPTER 1

1. a   4. a
2. b   5. b
3. c

CHAPTER 2

1. a, b   4. b, d
2. d   5. c
3. a, d

CHAPTER 3

1. a, b, c   5. b
2. d   6. a
3. b   7. b
4. c   8. c

CHAPTER 4

1. a, b   6. a
2. b, c   7. d
3. a, b, c   8. a, c, d
4. b, c   9. b, d
5. d   10. a, b, c, d

CHAPTER 5

1. The thumb has a pulse that may be confused with the patient's own pulse.
2. Once the site is decided upon, the area should be cleaned well with Betadine and allowed to dry.
3. The Duke method is difficult to standardize and does not allow ample surface area to repeat the test, if needed. If bleeding is excessive, it is difficult to control at this site. It also causes undue apprehension in some patients.
4. After locating a vein, the phlebotomist should release the tourniquet and scrub the entire area well with soap for about 2 min. A sterile alcohol pad is used to remove the soap from the puncture site moving out in increasing

circles. The alcohol is allowed to dry and Betadine is applied in the same manner and allowed to dry.

5. Skin tests are a simple, relatively inexpensive way to determine if a patient has ever had contact with particular antigens and has produced antibodies to that antigen.

6. The patient should be instructed to eat normal, well-balanced meals for 3 days prior to the test. Twelve hours before the test is to start, the patient should be fasting completely except for water. Water intake is encouraged throughout the test. No other beverage is allowed. Cigarette smoking and gum chewing should be discouraged until the completion of the test.

7. Because both tolerance tests rely on the injection of the stimulants into a vein, the phlebotomist may only assist the physician or other qualified personnel in the test and draw the required blood specimens as directed.

8. In the diagnosis of cystic fibrosis.

9. a. Weight—donors should weigh at least 110 lb.
   b. Temperature—oral temperature may not exceed 37.5°C.
   c. Pulse—should be strong, regular beats; 50 to 100 beats/min.
   d. Blood pressure—the systolic blood pressure should be between 90 and 180 mm Hg and the diastolic blood pressure should be between 50 and 100 mm Hg.
   e. Skin lesions—both arms should be examined for signs of drug addiction.
   f. General appearance—if the donor looks ill, excessively nervous, or under the influence of alcohol or drugs, he should be deferred.
   g. Hematocrit or hemoglobin—the hematocrit must be no less than 38 percent for females and no less than 41 percent for males. The hemoglobin value may be no less than 12.5 g/dL for female donors and no less than 13.5 g/dL for male donors.

10. About 405 to 495 mL.

11. Therapeutic phlebotomy is used in the treatment of some myeloproliferative diseases such as polycythemia or other conditions in which the removal of blood benefits the patient.

12. Timed specimens, fasting specimens, stat specimens.

13. First, he or she must be completely familiar with all of the equipment and well versed in all blood collecting procedures. Second, the phlebotomist must be able to follow directions quickly and correctly.

CHAPTER 6

1. d
2. b, c, d
3. b, c
4. a, b, c, d, e
5. b
6. b, c, d

CHAPTER 7

1. Manuals, procedures (technical, administrative, safety, quality control), continuing education, staff meetings, performance evaluations, memoranda, and bulletin boards.
2. Be consistent in format and headings; allow enough space for patient descriptions, printouts, imprints, or handwriting; have adequate number of copies; make it clear and concise; be convenient to handle, store, sort, and attach to a patient's chart.
3. Hand delivered, hospital transportation department, pneumatic tube system.
4. Medical records, staff on inpatient floors, laboratory, hospital business office.
5. Test requisitioning.
6. On-line computer input of test request information by the requesting authority is the most error-free method because computer systems have the capability of performing automatic checks on the input.
7. Correct and proper identification of the patient should be made prior to obtaining the specimen.

CHAPTER 8

1. a. Greet the patient.
   b. Identify yourself.
   c. Ask the patient's name.
   d. Ask the patient's address. Required by some hospitals.
   e. Check the laboratory request slip with the patient's ID number on his wristband.
   f. Label the tube of blood before leaving the patient's bedside.
2. a. Have the patient apply pressure to the venipuncture site.
   b. After labeling the tube(s), check the condition of the site and general condition of the patient.
   c. Observe the patient after she stands up to make sure there are no adverse signs (fainting, bleeding).
   d. Thank the patient.
3. a. Language barriers   c. Tone of voice
   b. Hearing disabilities   d. Age
4. a. Eye contact   d. Posture
   b. Eye level   e. Comfort zone
   c. Grooming

5. a. Rolling eyes; boredom
    b. Squirming; nervous, anxious
    c. Sighs; boredom, reluctance
    d. Crossed arms; defensive
    e. Smoking; distracting

6. a. Get ready
    b. Concentrate
    c. Listen
    d. Be objective
    e. Feedback
    f. sense nonverbal signs
    h. Look for true meaning
    i. "Tell me more"
    j. Paraphrase

7. The patient has the right to
    a. Considerate and respectful care
    b. Know who is performing a procedure and what the procedure is
    c. Refuse treatment
    d. Privacy of person, treatment
    e. Privacy of method and condition of payment
    f. Reasonable service
    g. Continuity of care
    h. Know what rules are important to his or her care (instructions for preparation of patient for laboratory testing normally given by phlebotomist)
    i. An environment free of conflict

8. Maslow's hierarchy of needs is: physiological, safety, love, esteem, and self-actualization

CHAPTER 9

1. The JCAHO's 10 step process includes the following:
    Assign responsibility, delineate the scope of care, identify key aspects of care, construct indicators, define thresholds of evaluation, collect and organize data, evaluate data, develop a corrective action plan, assess actions and document improvement, and communicate relevant information.

2. Five characteristics of TQM for a phlebotomy service are:

    1. The organized total quality management approach must permeate areas of the laboratory and specimen collection section, both horizontally and vertically.
    2. The objective of TQM must be continuous improvement instead of meeting fixed, predetermined standards.
    3. Groups, teams, or quality circles must include multidisciplinary individuals; preferably experts from the major groups that contribute to the process being studied.
    4. The groups or teams must be accountable to customers.
    5. There must be commitment to customer satisfaction.

3. Ten "customers" served by members of the phlebotomy team are: Internal inpatients, outpatients, blood donors, clinical laboratory scientists, clinical

laboratory technicians, pathologists, nurses, administrators, human resources personnel and students.

4. Poor patient outcomes that have been described as the "5 D's" are: death, disease, disability, discomfort, and dissatisfaction.

5. Please refer to Figure 9–1 for the flow chart format. Insert steps from Fig. 4–13.

6. Five possible monitors for specimen collection include: response time, patient waiting time, number of hematomas, number of patients who faint.

7. Eight sources of information for quality assessments include: medical records, incident reports, accident reports, written complaints, patient questionnaires, customer focus groups, quality circles, and committee reports.

CHAPTER 10

1. a, b   4. b, c, d
2. b, c, d   5. a, b, d
3. b, c, d

CHAPTER 11

1. The four factors that are considered in negligence cases are:

   1. Duty: what duties or responsibilities the hospital or health care worker had toward the patient; it also includes all the individuals who had a duty toward the patient.
   2. Breach of duty: whether or not the duty was breached and if it was avoidable.
   3. Proximate Causation: whether or not the breach of duty actually contributed to or caused injury; it also concerns all parties involved in contributing to the alleged injury.
   4. Damages: whether or not the plaintiff was actually injured and when these injuries were discovered.

2. Informed consent: If the patient requires treatment that is of potential risk, the physician must explain risks and alternatives prior to asking the patient to sign an Informed Consent form. The form is required for surgical, experimental, or other invasive procedures.

   Invasion of privacy: The physical intrusion upon a person; the publishing of confidential information, though true, but of such objectionable or personal nature as to be offensive.

   Liable refers: Under legal obligation, as far as damages are concerned.

   Malpractice: Improper or unskillful care of a patient by a member of the health care team or any professional misconduct, unreasonable lack of skill, or fidelity in professional or judiciary duties.

3. The basic purposes of the medical records are the following: Allows for continuity of patient's care plan; provides document of the patient's illness and treatment; documents communication between the physician and the health care team; provides a legal document which can be used by patients, hospital or health care workers to protect their legal interests.

4. A generic model of Risk Management might involve: Risk identification and analysis, risk treatment, education, risk transfer or postponement, and risk evaluation.

CHAPTER 12

1. a. source and number of patients
   b. age and sex of patients
   c. socioeconomic or ethnic background of patients
   d. proportion of ambulatory patients to bed patients
   e. the location of the phlebotomy unit
   f. availability of a computer

2. a. draw or collect specimens as required by physicians
   b. provide a liaison service between the physicians and the laboratory
   c. deliver specimens to appropriate section and communicate results promptly
   d. under direction of physician or nurse to aid in delivery of patient care as required

3. a. volume of specimens
   b. permanent assignment or daily flexible assignments
   c. number of times that collections will be made
   d. other duties in addition to specimen collection
   e. the special nature of the patient population

4. a, c

5. a. understanding
   b. respect for others
   c. knowledge of situation
   d. adaptability
   e. enthusiasm
   f. objectivity
   g. communication skills
   h. confidence in oneself and one's subordinates
   i. proper use of authority
   j. providing recognition

6. a. number of critical care areas
   b. time of delivery of food service
   c. time of first surgery scheduled
   d. emergency or trauma center patients

7. a. volume of specimens and other work anticipated
   b. human hours required and level of skills needed
   c. materials and outside services
   d. equipment
   e. revenue and rate setting
8. a. to evaluate progress of unit
   b. to evaluate personnel performance
   c. to identify adjustments that need to be made
   d. to fulfill responsibility for equipment and supplies
9. c   13. b
10. c   14. a
11. b   15. d
12. d   16. b

Index

Page numbers followed by t and f indicate tables and figures, respectively.